INFANTS BORN AT RISK

Physiological, Perceptual, and Cognitive Processes

INFANTS BORN AT RISK
Physiological, Perceptual, and Cognitive Processes

Edited by

TIFFANY FIELD, Ph.D.
Associate Professor
Departments of Pediatrics and Psychology
Mailman Center for Child Development
University of Miami Medical School
Miami, Florida

ANITA SOSTEK, Ph.D.
Associate Professor
Departments of Pediatrics and Obstetrics/Gynecology
Georgetown University School of Medicine
Washington, D.C.

(G&S)

GRUNE & STRATTON
A Subsidiary of Harcourt Brace Jovanovich, Publishers
New York   London
Paris   San Diego   San Francisco   São Paulo
Sydney   Tokyo   Toronto

Library of Congress Cataloging in Publication Data
Main entry under title:

Infants born at risk.

Bibliography
Includes index
1. Infants (Premature)—Psychology.   2. Infants
(Premature)—Physiology.   3. Infants (Newborn)—
Psychology.   4. Infant psychology.   5. Developmental
psychology.   I. Field, Tiffany.   II. Sostek, Anita.
BF720.P7I53   1983   618.92′8   83-1606
ISBN 0-8089-1563-0

Grune & Stratton, Inc.
111 Fifth Avenue
New York, New York 10003

Distributed in the United Kingdom by
Academic Press Inc. (London) Ltd.
24/28 Oval Road, London NW 1

Library of Congress Catalog Number 83-1606
International Standard Book Number 0-8089-1563-0
Printed in the United States of America

Contents

v

Preface

Four years ago we published a volume entitled *Infants Born at Risk: Behavior and Development*. That collection of research papers has been well received by an ever increasing number of researchers studying infants born at risk. In the intervening years researchers have explored further the physiological, perceptual, and cognitive processes that underlie the behavior and development of infants born at risk; this volume represents a more intensive analysis of those processes.* Among the conditions studied are anoxia, low birth weight, prematurity, respiratory distress syndrome, bronchopulmonary dysplasia, and Down's syndrome. Inasmuch as these authors have concentrated their efforts on the investigation of neonates, infants, and young children, this focus provides a natural organization of the chapters into three sections: the neonatal period, the infancy stage, and the follow-up assessments during childhood.

The section on the neonatal period includes data presentations for a number of different functions considered critical to neonatal well-being. In Chapter 1 Stephen W. Porges describes preliminary research using heart rate patterns in the neonate as a potential diagnostic assessment to investigate mild forms of central nervous system dysfunction that may be responsible for a wide range of developmental disabilities, such as mental retardation and learning disabilities. After a discussion on the limitations of the early assessment instruments, he provides a rationale for the estimation of vagal tone. He then shows how spectral analysis can be used to determine the vagal component of the heart rate pattern that can reflect central nervous system dysfunction. In this way Porges suggests that the evaluation of heart rate patterns in the neonate may provide a diagnostic window to the developing brain.

---

*We have arbitrarily defined "infants born at risk" as those who suffered perinatal medical complications that might contribute to later developmental delays or deficits.

In a similar use of spectral analysis, Philip Sandford Zeskind illustrates how neonatal crying can be related to other biobehavioral systems of the neonate and how it, too, can be used as a diagnostic procedure. Short of providing a record of cry sounds, Zeskind's illustrations of cry patterns from a number of different risk groups provide convincing data that this very natural behavior of the newborn can be used as a valuable diagnostic tool.

In the subsequent chapter, Susan A. Rose reviews a number of studies conducted by her colleagues and herself directed toward understanding the sensory and perceptual capabilities of the preterm infant. In several of those studies the responses of preterm infants to tactile and visual stimulation during different states have been compared to that of full-term infants. This research has focused primarily on (1) the sensitivity and responsivity of preterm and term infants to different intensities of stimulation, (2) the interrelation between behavior and the concomitant psychophysiological indices of responsivity, (3) autonomic lability and activation, and (4) the role of the sleep state in modulating responsivity. Similarly, Judith M. Gardner and Bernard Z. Karmel (Chapter 4) focused their studies on the responses of preterm infants to stimulation in the visual and auditory modalities as compared with those of the term infant. These researchers provided these stimuli at varying sleep–wakefulness states and note that stimulus-frequency preferences interact with the arousal level. They suggest that the infants who have a limited capacity to modulate their states of arousal, such as preterm infants, will be at some risk for poor developmental outcome.

Reactivity patterns of preterm infants to auditory stimulation are also the focus of a study by Elizabeth E. Krafchuk, Edward Z. Tronick, and Rachel K. Clifton in Chapter 5. Their study suggests that the reactivity of preterm infants to auditory stimulation is a function of the degree of risk at birth, the type of response system (behavioral activity versus heart rate), and the type of stimulus. Their data characterize the preterm infant, especially the more stressed infant, as hypo- and hyperreactive. The preterm infant appears to have both an elevated sensory threshold and a lowered defensive-reaction threshold that may function protectively and make the preterm infant less reactive, except to stimuli that are strong enough to pass the defensive threshold. In addition the preterm infant has greater difficulty habituating, which makes the infant appear more reactive once responding is initiated, and finally, the preterm infant's reaction patterns seem to be global and diffuse. The authors suggest that, in combination, these functional qualities produce an infant who is less available to stimulation but more reactive once a response is initiated.

The following chapter by Gene Cranston Anderson, Arlene K. Burroughs, and Carol Porter Measel reports data from a series of studies suggesting that providing nonnutritive sucking opportunities for preterm infants is not only a safe but also an effective treatment. The paradigm of giving nonnutritive nipples to very small preterm infants has yielded data suggesting that these preterm infants may require fewer tube feedings, show greater weight gain, and be discharged from the intensive care unit after fewer treatment days than preterm infants not given this opportunity. Confirmatory data from other laboratories suggest that this may be a cost-effective form of treatment for preterm neonates.

Finally, in this first section on the neonatal period, Barry M. Lester, Cynthia T. Garcia Coll, and Carol Sepkoski provide data on a very interesting study of the neonatal outcomes of teenage pregnancies in the Puerto Rican and American black cultures, one of the first to compare teenage pregnancy cross-culturally. Their results show that the outcome for neonates born to Puerto Rican teenage mothers was superior to that of infants born to mainland teenage mothers (principally black mothers) of equivalent socioeconomic status. One of the interpretations offered for this difference was that the Puerto Rican mothers were more often married and thus possibly received more support or experienced less stressful pregnancies. Differences in the infants' development might be expected to persist beyond the neonatal period not only because of the different support systems of those cultures but also because of their different attitudes toward child rearing. The findings of this study suggest that infants of teenage mothers may differ from infants of older mothers, particularly in the organization of state behavior, but these effects are subtle and the effects of maternal age on neonatal behavior are increased in the presence of prenatal and perinatal risk factors.

Together these chapters suggest, therefore, that some of the more critical physiological processes, including heart rate patterns, crying behavior, sucking patterns, state organization or arousal levels, and thresholds to stimulation, are affected by prenatal and perinatal risk factors that tend to limit the infant's performance in various neonatal stimulation contexts.

In the section on infancy the focus is less on physiological and perceptual processes and more on cognitive processes, as befits the increasing cognitive abilities of the developing infant. In Chapter 8 Wendy S. Masi and Keith G. Scott discuss their investigation of the preterm and full-term infants' ability to discriminate their mothers' face from strangers' faces. Although both the preterm and full-term infants were observed to make this discrimination at 1 and 2 months of age and, in fact, showed a preference for their mothers' face, the preterm infants required more testing time than the full-term infants, they were fussier, and it took longer for them to orient to the faces. The authors attribute the preterm infants' lesser attentiveness to their more limited information-processing abilities.

In the next chapter Albert J. Caron, Rose F. Caron, and Penny Glass introduce a new measure of cognitive functioning that may be effective in predicting cognitive outcomes for infants at risk. This measure taps the infant's ability to detect and abstract a particular aspect of environmental information, namely, its configural or relational characteristics. The authors assume that the ability to interrelate elements of experience is an essential ingredient of intellect, and thus the infant's competence in processing relational information may provide an early index of future functioning. The authors briefly review their data on comparisons between preterm and full-term infants; both groups had essentially processed aspects of the habituation stimuli, but the preterm infants focused primarily on the elements of the stimuli while the full-term infants focused on the relations between elements, suggesting a greater degree of sophistication in this cognitive process by term infants. Encouraged by these results, Caron et al. tested the sensitivity of these tasks even more stringently in order to determine whether the performance on relational tasks might reveal subtle effects associated with perinatal events within groups of full-term infants. Infants who failed to meet the criteria usually associated with normal full-term infants, such as 40 weeks gestation and Apgars of 8/9 or better, were categorized as nonoptimal, and, like the preterm infants of their earlier studies, these nonoptimal infants did not perform as well as the optimal infants on the same relational tasks. Additional comparisons of infants who had Apgars of 6 or less and postterm infants yielded similarly poor performance, suggesting that this type of task may reflect more subtle perinatal complications. Although there is a question as to whether these differences merely represent transient effects or have long-term consequences, the data offered by Caron et al. suggest that, at least in normal term infants, there are some moderate correlations between performance on these relational tasks during early infancy and performance on IQ tasks during childhood.

Another cognitive-functioning task that is thought to differentiate normal from at-risk infants is that of visual-recognition memory. In the chapter by Lynn Twarog Singer, Dennis Drotar, Josph F. Fagan III, Linda Devost, and Robin Lake, data are presented on visual-recognition-memory-task performance and Bayley scale scores of normal, organic failure to thrive, and nonorganic failure to thrive infants. The results of their studies suggest that both groups of failure to thrive infants perform significantly more poorly than normal control infants on the Bayley scale but only the organic failure to thrive infants perform more poorly on the visual-recognition-memory test. The authors suggest that the heavy reliance on the Bayley test for sensorimotor and productive-language functioning may result in lower scores in very young children and may be misleading as an estimate of intellectual potential. Perceptual–cognitive measures, such as the visual-recognition task, may be less influenced by sensorimotor factors and more representative of the types of information-processing tasks characteristic of cognitive functioning. On the basis of the visual-recognition task, the organic failure to thrive infants are considered at greater risk for intellectual delay than nonorganic failure to thrive infants.

In the subsequent chapter (Chapter 11), Edward Goldson presents data on comparisons between infants who experience severe bronchopulmonary disease (BPD) and those who experience mild BPD or lung disease during the neonatal period. Children with more severe lung disease performed more poorly on developmental testing, particularly on the Bayley scale, than did the healthier children. In addition, the sicker children had a higher incidence of pathological findings on the neuromotor assessment than did the healthier children. Although the children with no disease or only mild lung disease were performing better on these assessments, all of these children had suspicious neuromotor findings, suggesting that none of these lower birth-weight infants are completely normal at 2 years of age. These data are disconcerting inasmuch as recent literature suggests that children with suspicious neuromotor assessments may have learning difficulties requiring special education at school age.

Down's syndrome infants are the focus of the next chapter written by Peter M. Vietze, Mary McCarthy, Susan McQuiston, Robert MacTurk, and Leon J. Yarrow. These investigators studied infants with Down's syndrome at 6 and 12 months of age using procedures designed to investigate exploratory behavior in challenging situations. The youngest children showed extensive visual exploration while the older children appeared to spend more time in manual exploration. Measures of exploratory behavior that index mastery were correlated with Bayley scale scores. Visual attention, however, was not related to mental development at any age. The fact that the time spent in nontask-related behavior is negatively correlated with mental development suggested to the authors that exploratory behavior may facilitate mental development. The authors conclude that the major difference in the performance of Down's syndrome and normal infants is in the amount of time they spend in more instrumental behavior, such as manual exploration or what the authors call "mastery behavior." They suggest that Down's syndrome infants, with their characteristic hypotonia, may take longer to make contact with objects placed before them—or that the caretakers of these infants do not wait long enough for the infants to make contact—and the infants thus have limited experience with handling objects.

In the last section, on follow-up, three of the longest follow-up studies of infants born at risk are reported. All three studies assessed preterm infants with varying degrees of risk status and used similar measures during the 5-year follow-up periods.

In the first chapter of this section, Marian D. Sigman focuses primarily on individual variability in attentiveness to visual stimulation. Her thesis is that preterm neonates who are neurologically more intact should be better able to initiate and maintain their attention to visual stimuli. Visual fixations of the infants were measured using a checkerboard for a stimulus. Then at 5 years, the children were given the Stanford-Binet scale. The neonatal visual-attention measure was one of the major predictors of the outcome at 5 years. The author suggests that, since this measure contributed more to the outcome than socioeconomic status did, the visual-attention measure operates independently of this demographic factor.

In a 5-year follow-up of even smaller and more premature infants, Linda S. Siegel reports that these preterm infants are at subsequent risk for learning disabilities, and that the infant test scores as well as a medical risk index can be used as predictors of these disabilities. Early in development, perceptual–motor functions, such as eye–hand coordination on manipulation items of the Bayley mental and motor scales, are the best predictors of subsequent outcome, whether it is language or perceptual–motor performance. The cognitive items of the Bayley become predictive at about 8 months, but it is not until 12 months that the language items become predictive. Environmental and demographic variables contributed more to the prediction of language functioning and delay, while prenatal and reproductive variables contributed more to the prediction of perceptual–motor function.

Finally, in Chapter 15 by Tiffany Field, Jean Dempsey, and H. H. Shuman, 5-year-old children who had experienced preterm delivery and respiratory distress syndrome, as well as infants who had experienced post-term delivery and postmaturity syndrome, were compared to a normal term group. Data are reported for the annual assessments made up to 5 years as well as regression analyses in which variables from the earlier assessment periods are entered to determine the predictive validity of early assessment measures. Those variables that most frequently entered the regression analyses were the 8-month Bayley motor scale score, the 2-year Bayley mental scale score, the 4-month mother–infant interaction rating, and the years of maternal education. That the 8-month Bayley motor and the 2-year Bayley mental scale scores were predictive of 5-year cognitive performance is inconsistent with several longitudinal studies that failed to show any relation between infant developmental assessments and later IQ scores. This inconsistency might be explained by the greater correspondence between Bayley and McCarthy scale items than between Bayley and the traditionally used Stanford-Binet scale items.

In summary, the contributors of this volume have taken us a step further in understanding the developmental delays of high-risk infants by examining some of the physiological, perceptual, and cognitive processes of early development. Converging evidence suggests that these infants may be less organized physiologically and may have more difficulty modulating arousal and sustaining alertness. Their thresholds to stimulation may be higher and their less developed attentional processes and information-processing skills may limit performance on early developmental assessments. At school age these children appear to perform within the normal range on IQ tests, but their delays in language production and behavior problems, such as limited attention span, may place them at risk for learning disabilities. Further research will be needed to understand the relations between these early physiological, perceptual, and cognitive processes and the later development of infants born at risk.

Contributors

Gene Cranston Anderson, R.N., Ph.D., F.A.A.N. _____

Professor and Research Coordinator
College of Nursing
The J. Hillis Miller Health Center
University of Florida
Gainesville, Florida

Arlene K. Burroughs, R.N., M.Ed. _____

Assistant Professor
College of Nursing
University of Illinois
Medical Center
Chicago, Illinois

Albert J. Caron, Ph.D. _____

Research Professor in Psychology
Co-Director, Infant Research Laboratory
The George Washington University
Silver Spring, Maryland

Rose F. Caron, Ph.D. _____

Research Professor in Psychology
Director, Infant Research Laboratory
The George Washington University
Silver Spring, Maryland

Rachel K. Clifton, Ph.D.

Professor, Department of Psychology
University of Massachusetts
Amherst, Massachusetts

Cynthia T. Garcia Coll, Ph.D.

Assistant Professor of Pediatrics
Department of Pediatrics
Brown University
Providence, Rhode Island

Jean Dempsey, M.A.

Research Associate
Neonatology Department
Baystate Medical Center
Springfield, Massachusetts

Linda Devost, B.S.

Research Associate
Infant Growth Project
University Hospitals
Cleveland, Ohio

Dennis Drotar, Ph.D.

Associate Professor
Departments of Pediatrics and Psychiatry
Case-Western Reserve University Medical School
Rainbow Babies and Children's Hospital
Cleveland, Ohio

Joseph F. Fagan III, Ph.D.

Professor, Department of Psychology
Case-Western Reserve University
Cleveland, Ohio

Tiffany Field, Ph.D.

Associate Professor
Departments of Pediatrics and Psychology
Mailman Center for Child Development
University of Miami Medical School
Miami, Florida

Judith M. Gardner, Ph.D.

Research Associate
Department of Psychiatry
Albert Einstein College of Medicine
Bronx, New York

Penny Glass, M.A.

Research Associate
The George Washington University
Silver Spring, Maryland

Edward Goldson, M.D.

Director, Newborn Follow-up Program
The Children's Hospital and
Assistant Professor of Pediatrics
University of Colorado School of Medicine
Denver, Colorado

Bernard Z. Karmel, Ph.D.

Associate Professor
Department of Psychology
University of Connecticut
Storrs, Connecticut, and
Visiting Associate Professor
Department of Pediatrics
Mt. Sinai Medical Center
New York, New York

Elizabeth E. Krafchuk, M.S.

Research Associate
Department of Psychology
University of Massachusetts
Amherst, Massachusetts

Robin Lake, Ph.D.

Research Associate
Standard Oil Company
Corporate Research Center
Cleveland, Ohio

Barry M. Lester, Ph.D.

Assistant Professor of Pediatrics
Harvard Medical School and
Director, Developmental Research
Child Development Unit
Children's Hospital Medical Center
Boston, Massachusetts

Robert MacTurk, Ph.D.

Research Associate
Child and Family Research Branch
National Institute of Child Health
and Human Development
National Institutes of Health
Bethesda, Maryland

Wendy S. Masi, Ph.D.

Assistant Director
The Family Center of Nova University
Ft. Lauderdale, Florida

Mary McCarthy, Ph.D.

Research Associate
Child and Family Research Branch
National Institute of Child Health
and Human Development
National Institutes of Health
Bethesda, Maryland

Susan McQuiston, Ph.D.

Research Associate
University of Illinois
Chicago, Illinois

Carol Porter Measel, R.N., M.S.N.

Assistant Professor
Wayne State University
Detroit, Michigan

Stephen W. Porges, Ph.D.

Professor, Department of Psychology
University of Illinois at Urbana-Champaign
Champaign, Illinois

Susan A. Rose, Ph.D.

Associate Professor of Psychiatry (Psychology)
Albert Einstein College of Medicine
Bronx, New York

Keith G. Scott, Ph.D.

Professor, Departments of Pediatrics and Psychology
University of Miami
Mailman Center for Child Development
Miami, Florida

Carol Sepkoski, M.A.

Research Associate
Children's Hospital Medical Center
Boston, Massachusetts, and
University of Florida
Gainesville, Florida

H. H. Shuman, M.D.

Associate Director
Neonatology Department
Baystate Medical Center
Springfield, Massachusetts

Linda S. Siegel, Ph.D.

Professor, Department of Psychiatry
Faculty of Health Sciences
McMaster University
Hamilton, Ontario, Canada

Marian D. Sigman, Ph.D.

Associate Professor
Department of Psychiatry
UCLA School of Medicine
Center for Health Sciences
Los Angeles, California

Lynn Twarog Singer, Ph.D.

Assistant Professor
Department of Pediatric Psychology
Case-Western Reserve University Medical School
Rainbow Babies and Children's Hospital
Cleveland, Ohio

Edward Z. Tronick, Ph.D.

Professor, Psychology Department
University of Massachusetts
Amherst, Massachusetts

Peter M. Vietze, Ph.D.

Health Scientist Administrator
Mental Retardation and Developmental
Disabilities Branch
National Institute of Child Health
and Human Development
National Institutes of Health
Bethesda, Maryland

Leon J. Yarrow, Ph.D. (deceased)

Branch Chief
Child and Family Research Branch
National Institute of Child Health
and Human Development
National Institutes of Health
Bethesda, Maryland

Philip Sandford Zeskind, Ph.D.

Assistant Professor of Psychology
Department of Psychology
Virginia Polytechnic Institute and State University
Blacksburg, Virginia

I   THE NEONATAL PERIOD

Heart Rate Patterns in Neonates:
A Potential Diagnostic Window to the Brain

Stephen W. Porges

The identification of physiological variables that are predictive of behavioral sequelae is a basic objective in the study of infants born at risk. Whether this objective may be reached is debatable and depends on three theoretical issues: (1) the relationship between neural function and observable behavior, (2) the reversibility of nervous system abnormalities, and (3) the continuity between early nervous system organization and subsequent behavioral development.

A monotonic relationship is often assumed between physiological activity and behavior. The empirical evidence in support of this assumption has been weak owing to the limitations of instruments available to assess the nervous system in infants. Although behavorial scientists often rely on medical assessment to categorize "at risk" infants, medical assessment lacks the specificity necessary to rank infants along meaningful dimensions of nervous system organization. Thus research that does not support tight

The preparation of this chapter was supported in part by Research Scientist Development Award K02-MH-0054 from the National Institute of Mental Health and grant HD15968 from the National Institutes of Health. The newborn data were collected at Cook County Hospital in Chicago in collaboration with Drs. Srinivasan and Pildes of the Department of Neonatology. I wish to thank Michael N. Cheung, who aided in the collection of the data, the analyses, and the development of the computer software necessary to analyze the data. The spectral analysis methodology described in this manuscript is a product of a long and productive collaboration with Dr. Robert E. Bohrer of the Department of Mathematics at the University of Illinois.

monotonic relationships between diagnostic indices and behavior does not preclude the possibility that there are parallels.

In the absence of sensitive biomedical measurement techniques, it is assumed that mild forms (i.e., unmeasurable) of central nervous system dysfunction are responsible for a wide range of developmental disabilities, including forms of mental retardation and learning disabilities. Medical assessments have focused on the question of viability and not on evaluating individual differences in central nervous system status that may be related to gradations in intellectual and behavioral performance. There is thus a large void between the *needs* of the behavioral scientist and the current status of assessment procedures. This chapter will describe preliminary research using heart rate patterns in the neonate as a potential diagnostic assessment to investigate this clinical and research problem.

ASSESSMENT: LIMITATIONS AND CONSEQUENCES

Limitations of Available Early Assessment Instruments

At present there are no definitive neurological tests for identifying infants at risk (Parmelee & Michaelis, 1971). The existing neurological and medical assessment instruments function well only in extreme cases. Prediction is most reliable at the low end of the continuum (Honzik, 1976). In cases of obvious or severe central nervous system damage, however, additional screening may not be necessary. Gallagher and Bradley (1972) reviewed the literature on early identification measures and child development scales and concluded that the available instruments were far from infallible in detecting potentially handicapping conditions. The most commonly used clinical evaluations of the newborn, the Apgar (1966) and the neurological (Prechtl & Beintema, 1964; Parmelee & Michaelis, 1971), are successful in identifying gross central nervous system abnormalities but are not as effective in detecting milder forms of neural dysfunction.

A more recent and promising instrument is the Brazelton Neonatal Behavioral Assessment Scale (Brazelton, 1973). This scale is a broad-based newborn behavioral and neurological examination that attempts to capture the complexity of behavioral responses to social stimuli as a function of behavioral state. At this time the scale is limited to full-term infants, although a modification suitable for premature infants has been developed (Als, Lester, & Brazelton, 1979). Unfortunately, like all infant assessment tests, predictive validity to later infant or childhood behavior has not been demonstrated. Present research by other investigators is addressing this problem.

A major problem in assessment is posed by the infant without apparent anomaly who has been exposed to stressful circumstances (e.g., anoxia, prolonged labor) often in combination with prematurity. Parmelee, Kopp, and Sigman (1976) pointed out that although some of these infants may develop normally, others may have developmental difficulties at a later age when the behavioral repertoire becomes more complex. The challenge is to identify the infants who need continued monitoring and who may at some future time benefit from clinical intervention.

Consequences of Risk: Intellectual and Behavioral Deficits _____

There are specific populations that appear to be "at risk" for intellectual and behavioral dysfunctions. Infants weighing less than 1.5 kg at birth appear to define a particularly high risk group for poor intellectual development (Caputo, Goldstein, & Taub, 1979; Drillien, 1964; Weiner, Rider, Oppel, & Harper, 1968; Wright, Blough, Chamberline, Ernest, Halstead, Meier, Moore, Naunton, & Newell, 1972). These children have a higher probability of manifesting disabilities such as low IQs, behavior disorders often associated with hyperactivity, poor attention span, and difficulties in school adjustment. Many complications of pregnancy and parturition such as asphyxia, hypoglycemia, as well as other conditions potentially injurious to the central nervous system, such as respiratory distress syndrome, are among the problems of premature infants. Often these problems are subtle and result in an apparent reduction in the developmental potential. For example, Field, Dempsey, and Shuman (1979) reported that although the IQs of 4-year-old respiratory distress survivors were within the normal range, their scores were at the low end of the distribution and they exhibited deficits in hearing and language production. Moreover, they exhibited significantly more symptoms associated with hyperactivity, short attention span, distractability, and inattentiveness when compared to appropriate controls.

Drillien (1964) reported that by school age 75 percent of infants weighing 3 pounds or less had some congenital defect or were mentally retarded. Lubchenco, Delivoria-Papadopoulos, and Searles (1972) found that 66 percent of infants weighing less than 1.5 kg had visual or central nervous system handicaps. Wright et al. (1972) found that 34 percent of infants weighing less than 1.5 kg at birth had IQs less than 80. The reduced mortality rate of low birth weight infants may exacerbate these problems. Less than 50 years ago infants born weighing less than 1500 g were classified as "previable." During the past 20 years, the survival rate in the 1–1.5 kg weight group has increased from less than 50 percent to over 70 percent (Ross & Leavitt, 1976). Given this change in the number of survivors, there is a need for reliable assessment to enable appropriate placement in intervention programs.

Consequences of Delay in Accurate Assessment

There is an unfortunate delay in the identification of infants who need remediation, because the infant assessment procedures have been generally unreliable until the child is several years of age (McCall, Hogarty, & Hurlburt, 1972). This delay is disturbing to all interested in ameliorating the infants' disabilities. Aldrich (see de la Cruz, 1976) investigated a variety of factors related to mental retardation, including the age at which children were first suspected and confirmed as mentally retarded. The average age for suspected retardation ranged from 7.8 months for the profoundly retarded to 34.5 months for the mildly retarded. The average elapsed time between suspicion and confirmation of mental retardation ranged from 6.2 months for the profoundly retarded for 12.0 months for the mildly retarded.

Assessment of Psychophysiological Function

It is obvious that a component of behavior is determined by the nervous system and that central nervous system damage results in a qualitative change in behavior. This is readily observed in infants who have suffered from severe insults during labor and delivery. However, the relationship between individual differences in the nervous system and behavior is not so readily demonstrated in the vast population of infants who have been considered normal or mildly stressed. A goal of applied developmental psychophysiological research is the identification of psychological disorders at the earliest possible age. By measuring physiological responses as indices of cognitive processes, psychophysiological tests may be able to evaluate infants prior to the emergence of verbal or complex motor behaviors. These early measures may potentially contribute to the development of valid methods for assigning neonates to categories at risk for cognitive and behavioral development.

There is a substantial literature demonstrating and examining psychological processes such as habituation and classical conditioning in the neonate with physiological dependent variables (e.g., Clifton & Nelson, 1976; Fitzgerald & Brackbill, 1976; Porges, 1974; Stamps & Porges, 1975). Many of these studies have selected the heart rate response as an index of cognitive activity. It is important to note that although the heart may beat in the absence of central nervous system influences, the heart rate response to experimental manipulations (responses with latencies shorter than those of metabolic or endocrine influences) may *only* be mediated by the central nervous system.

There are studies demonstrating that the heart rate response during conditioning and attention-demanding tasks differentiates groups of normal individuals from groups of severely brain-damaged individuals (Karrer, 1976; Krupski, 1975). Overall, the findings have been consistent enough to encourage the application of psychophysiological paradigms as methods for identifying certain classes of nervous system dysfunction in the neonate.

In spite of its promising potential, psychophysiological assessment would suffer from three major limitations: (1) it has a high attrition rate, since many subjects are unable to maintain a constant behavioral state (e.g., sleep, crying) throughout the testing session; (2) at present, based upon the literature, it would only discriminate the severely dysfunctioning infant from the total population; and (3) validity may be questioned because physiological responses may be a function of a deficit in a specific sensory or visceromotor system and not monotonically related to centrally mediated cognitive processes.

A New Alternative: The Continuity Model

If it were possible to assess the status of the neural control of the heart (i.e., the influence of the central nervous system on the heart), it might be possible to obtain information similar to that derived from psychophysiological paradigms. Since central nervous system influences on the heart are encoded within the pattern of heart rate, it might be possible to use heart rate patterns as an indexing variable for underlying nervous system dysfunction (i.e., a diagnostic window to the brain). For example, brain death produces a constant heart rate without beat-to-beat variability (Kero, Antila, Ylitalo, & Valimaki, 1978). Moreover, pediatricians and obstetricians have frequently used the beat-to-beat variability measure as a clinical index of the general status of the nervous system (Lowensohn, Weiss, & Hon, 1977; Nelson, 1976). Although heart rate variability appears promising, one must be cautious in its interpretation, since it reflects both neural and extraneural influences.

For the past 15 years my research has focused on the hypothesis that individual differences in the heart rate pattern would provide important information regarding the central nervous system and would therefore be predictive of autonomic and behavioral response patterns (i.e., organized psychophysiological responses). During the past decade the research program has shifted from evaluating a global measure of heart rate variability (containing both neural and extraneural influences) to more precise measures of neural influence on the heart by partitioning the variability of heart rate through the use of spectral analysis.

The relationship between central nervous system dysfunction, causal in many forms of behavior disorders, and autonomic nervous system activity may be theoretically conceptualized as a *continuity model* (see Porges & Smith, 1980). This approach assumes important continuities between the central and autonomic nervous systems. The approach emphasizes the patterning of autonomic activity such as heart rate and respiration and assumes that information regarding brain dysfunction may be derived from analysis of autonomic patterns.

The continuity model assumes that the centrally mediated autonomic control system is a complex homoeostatic system consisting of peripheral and central afferent–efferent feedback mechanisms. The model makes no inference regarding afferent feedback on perceptual sensitivity, the underlying basis of Lacey's (1967) intake–rejection hypothesis. Moreover, the model acknowledges that small shifts in autonomic activity, mediated by the central nervous system, may be insignificant in terms of the effector organ's contribution to biological survival (e.g., Obrist, Webb, Sutterer, & Howard, 1970). Physiological survival may be a function of the rate at which the heart beats, while the patterning of heart rate (e.g., respiratory sinus arrhythmia) may represent varying neural influences and thus reflect central nervous system status.

Although seldom explicitly stated, the prevalence of heart rate as a variable in psychophysiological research is a function of an *assumed* relationship between the central nervous system and the heart. The impact of this assumption has been to shift the role of heart rate monitoring from that of a global index of arousal or emotion to a sensitive index of cognitive processing. This assumption underlies the burgeoning field of cognitive psychophysiology. Ironically, psychophysiological research evaluating neural influences on the heart is scant.

The identification of a physiological substrate that parallels individual differences in attention has been one of the primary research objectives of psychophysiology. The general approach has been within the context of the mechanistic world view (see Reese & Overton, 1970; Overton & Reese, 1973) associated with the traditional behavioristic stimulus–response model. In the context of this model, physiological responses parallel the task demands necessitating attention. Experimental procedures have often taken the form of manipulating task difficulties and identifying physiological responses that are hypothesized to parallel the increasing task demands (e.g., Walter & Porges, 1976). This approach has resulted in the identification of relatively consistent physiological response patterns.

The heart rate response pattern in neonates has been investigated (Porges, Arnold, & Forbes, 1973; Porges, 1974; Porges, Stamps, & Walter, 1974; Stamps & Porges, 1975). The research consistently identified directional heart rate responses to changes in stimulation. Moreover, a relationship between spontaneous heart rate variability and reactivity to visual and auditory stimuli was identified. These findings are consistent with the pediatric literature that had identified a relationship between neonatal well-being and heart rate variability; newborns with high heart rate variability were autonomically responsive to the external environment.

In research with adults, spontaneous heart rate variability was cor-

vagal tone that is characterized by increases in heart period and in the amplitude of rhythmic oscillations in heart period associated with respiration. We have conducted research with pharmacological manipulations that are known to increase (phenylephrine) and decrease (atropine) vagal tone (Yongue, McCabe, Porges, Rivera, Kelley, & Ackles, 1982): $\hat{V}$ was suppressed by atropine, increased following the time course of phenylephrine, and was unaffected by saline.

It has been assumed that the vagal control of the heart follows a developmental trend. Based upon previous research (e.g., Ashida, 1972; Adolph, 1967), it has been hypothesized that the vagal control of the heart of the rat does not fully mature until approximately 14–21 days postpartum. If $\hat{V}$ is a sensitive measure of vagal tone to the heart, measurement of heart rate patterns in the rat pup during the first few weeks postpartum should provide an experimental preparation with which to evaluate the development of vagal tone to the heart. Larson and Porges (1982) described the ontogeny of $\hat{V}$ in rats from birth through 24 days postpartum. The developmental trend of $\hat{V}$ is characterized by monotonic increases in $\hat{V}$ during the first 18 days postpartum, a period in which the development of vagal control of the heart is assumed to occur.

CENTRAL NERVOUS SYSTEM DYSFUNCTION AND HEART RATE PATTERNS IN THE NEONATE

The application of spectral analysis enables the evaluation of a component of the heart rate pattern that is directly influenced by the brain. Conceptually, this approach treats components of the heart rate pattern (e.g., $\hat{V}$) as *indexing variables* of underlying neurological function (see the continuity model). Thus, in a sense, heart rate that is easily monitored may provide critical information regarding the central nervous system.

In Figure 1-1 the heart period patterns and associated spectra are presented for two neonates. (Heart period is the reciprocal of heart rate.) One neonate was normal and the other was diagnosed as brain death following severe birth asphyxia. The spectral analysis decomposes the heart period patterns into constituent periodicities. Note that the spectrum of the normal neonate's heart period pattern exhibits a peak within the normal frequency band of respiration (i.e., 0.3–1.5 Hz, or approximately 30–90 breaths per minute) whereas the asphyxiated neonate's spectrum is flat. The $\hat{V}$ statistic is calculated by summing the spectral density estimates within the frequency band associated with breathing. Although the heart rate is much faster (i.e., shorter heart periods) for the asphyxiated neonate, there are numerous examples of brain death neonates having normal heart rates. These two neonates provide the boundary examples for the interpretation of $\hat{V}$.

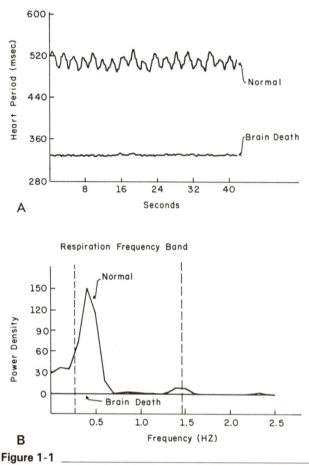

A

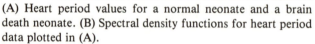

B

Figure 1-1

(A) Heart period values for a normal neonate and a brain death neonate. (B) Spectral density functions for heart period data plotted in (A).

In a preliminary study, $\hat{V}$ was evaluated in a group of clinically normal neonates and a group of neonates characterized by a variety of clinical pathologies, including severe brain damage. Heart period variability and mean heart period were also calculated. Figure 1-2A represents the natural logarithm of heart period variability for the normal and pathological neonates; Figure 1-2B represents the natural logarithm of $\hat{V}$ for the same infants. The letters on the scale represent the diagnosis or insult associated with the individual infants. There is an apparent monotonic relationship between $\hat{V}$ and the severity of clinical dysfunction. The one hydrocephalic infant who appears to be misclassified by $\hat{V}$ was subsequently evaluated by

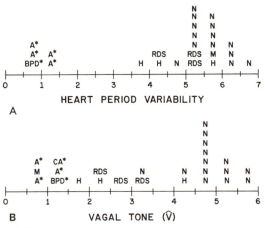

Figure 1-2

(A) The natural logarithm of heart period variability for normal and pathological infants. (B) The natural logarithm of $\hat{V}$ for the same infants. The letters on the scales represent the diagnosis or insult associated the individual infants (A, asphyxia; BDP, bronchiopulmonary dysplasia; CA, cardiac arrest; H, hydrocephalus; M, microcephalus; N, normal; RDS, respiratory distress syndrome). Infants who subsequently died are denoted by an asterisk. (Reprinted with permission from Porges, S. W., McCabe, P. M., & Yongue, B. G. Respiratory–heart-rate interactions: Psychophysiological implications for pathophysiology and behavior. In J. Cacioppo & R. Petty (Eds.), *Perspectives in cardiovascular psychophysiology*. New York: Guilford Press, 1982.)

the pediatrician to be functioning within the bounds of normal intellectual and social development. When the same infants were ranked in terms of heart period variability, there was a clear distinction between those who died and all other neonates. Heart period variability clearly distinguished between infants diagnosed as brain death, with their characteristic absence of neural influence on the heart, and all other infants. Heart period variability did not distinguish among the various neural tube defects, respiratory distress syndrome, and normal neonates. Heart period level did not reliably discriminate among the various pathologies, although there was a tendency for the severely brain damaged neonates to have shorter heart periods (i.e., faster heart rate). Classification by heart period variability partitioned the neonates into two global categories, whereas $\hat{V}$ classified the infants along a continuum of apparent severity of neuropathology. Thus, although heart period variability is sensitive to gross dysfunction, in this preliminary study $\hat{V}$ seems to be more sensitive to individual differences in central nervous system dysfunction.

There is evidence in the literature supporting the hypothesis that vagal tone is monotonically related to gestational age. Schifferli and Caldeyro-Barcia (1973) reported that fetal heart rate increased when atropine was administered to the pregnant mothers. Moreover, the magnitude of the change in heart rate was correlated with gestational age, with the more mature fetuses exhibiting greater increases in heart rate in response to atropine. Similarly, one would expect that premature newborns without major identifiable complications would also exhibit a relationship between an estimate of vagal tone and gestational age. To evaluate this possibility of an early developmental trend in the neural control of the heart, a preliminary study (Porges, Srinivasan, Cheung, Shanker, Pildes, & Bohrer, 1980) was conducted. To assess the relationship between $\hat{V}$ and gestational age, data were collected from term and preterm infants who were free from clinical complications. Figure 1-3 illustrates the relationship between $\hat{V}$ and gestational age. The correlation between gestational age and $\hat{V}$ was .82. This correlation is similar to the correlation of .74 between weeks of pregnancy and increase in fetal heart rate in response to atropine reported by Schifferli and Caldeyro-Barcia (1973).

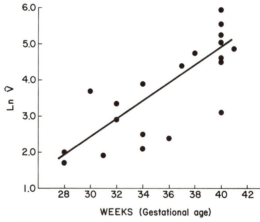

Figure 1-3 _____

Natural logarithm of $\hat{V}$ in preterm and term infants. (Reprinted with permission from Porges, S. W., McCabe, P. M., & Yongue, B. G. Respiratory–heart-rate interactions: Psychophysiological implications for pathophysiology and behavior. In J. Cacioppo & R. Petty (Eds.), *Perspectives in cardiovascular psychophysiology*. New York: Guilford Press, 1982.)

CONCLUSION

The evaluation of heart rate variability provides a simple example of the difference between medical assessment and the "individual difference" approach. Heart rate variability functions well in evaluating viability, but functions less adequately when a monotonic individual difference dimension is sought. In contrast, the continuity model with an objective to partition neural influences in the heart period pattern generates a potentially more useful method for characterizing individual differences. Research is currently being conducted to relate individual differences in $\hat{V}$ to evoked heart rate responses in the newborn, as well as to more traditional assessment procedures and cognition in the older infant.

In the ontogeny of behavioral sequelae, dysfunction could occur on a variety of levels. To elaborate on this point and to relate the preceding sections on heart period pattern to behavioral anomalies, a hierarchial model of "neurobehavioral" organization has been developed. The model has four major levels, each level being based upon the preceding level of organization and reflecting the condition of the central nervous system.

Level I represents the organization of a specific physiological system. For example, heart rate in the normal healthy neonate is rhythmically organized. If the neonate is severely stressed, the rhythmic components of the heart rate pattern start to deteriorate. The heart rate pattern may still exhibit variability; however, the pattern would be more like "white noise." If the insult to the neonate continues, as in the case of the prolonged hypoxia characteristic of severe fetal distress, the heart rate pattern will no longer exhibit variability. There is thus a continuum from no variability to "white noise" variability to rhythmic "organized" variability. Paralleling this continuum is a continuum of the general status of the central nervous system.

Level II represents the coordination of physiological systems. Within the body the nervous system attempts to coordinate via complex homeostatic feedback mechanisms the interplay of numerous physiological systems. It is conceivable that on a univariable level each system reflects organizational qualities that appear to be appropriate but which in terms of coordinated function may be disorganized. This level of disorganization may result in more subtle deficiencies and is more difficult to assess. Coordination reflects dynamic interactions between systems and most strategies for assessing physiological activity are both univariate and static. An example of level II organization would be the coordination between respiration and heart rate. As discussed earlier, respiration "gates" heart rate. This results in increases in heart rate during inhalation and decreases in heart rate during exhalation. This gating operation is conducted through a complex neural network in the brainstem. Interestingly, there are individual differences in the degree of predictability of the heart rate pattern from the respiration (although both patterns may exhibit similar rhythmicities). Simply stated, there may be unpredictable variability in the time delay between the respiratory input to the brainstem and the vagal output to the heart. Moreover, this individual difference seems to be related to behavior. For example, the variability of the time delay is significantly decreased in hyperactive children when methylphenidate is administered (Porges et al., 1981). Also, in adult subjects (see Porges & Coles, 1982) only the individuals with predictable coupling exhibit anticipatory heart rate decelerations during a reaction time task. The predictability of the temporal coupling is determined via cross-spectral analysis, and the statistic that assesses the coupling is called coherence (Porges, Bohrer, Cheung, Drasgow, McCabe, & Keren, 1980).

Level III reflects the organization of the overt behavior of an individual. Overt behavior is obviously dependent upon multivariable physiological organization. A deficiency in the organizational characteristics of the nervous system as reflected in underlying physiological activity would be manifested in dysfunctional overt behavior. It is also possible to have appropriate functioning on levels I and II and defective functioning on level III. This could be a function of inappropriately learned behavior or the interaction between other psychological processes and the overt behavior.

Level IV reflects the pinnacle of organization, the coordination of the social dyad. It is this level that is functionally responsible for processes such as affectional bonding and socialization.

It is important to note that a dysfunction on a lower level is manifested as dysfunction on each higher level, whereas, a dysfunction on a higher level is not necessarily accompanied by dysfunction on a lower level. In the former case the "hierarchial rule" holds, in which more complex processes necessitate appropriately functioning underlying processes. In the latter case, this implies that the locus of the dysfunction is associated with the mechanisms reflecting the organization of the specific "level." The mechanisms on levels III and IV need not be neurophysiological but may be psychological.

This discussion of levels of neurobehavioral organization forces us to evaluate the methods available to answer our research questions. Many of us are interested in level III and level IV questions. We assume either a monotonic relationship between some global construct of nervous system status and behavior or an independence between behavior and neurophysiological mechanisms. Neurobehavioral systems are dynamic and interactive. Unfortunately, methods for evaluating dynamic and interactive systems generally have not been applied in the study of behavior and neurophysiology. The use of spectral analysis to study univariable organization (e.g., rhythmic heart rate patterns) and the use of cross-spectral analysis to study multivariable coordination (e.g., coupling between heart rate and respiration) may provide an important response to this problem. Thus, the evaluation of heart rate patterns, which at first appears to be greatly removed from many of the research problems that behavioral scientists study, may provide the building blocks for more complex behaviors and function as a diagnostic window to the brain.

REFERENCES

Adolph, E. F. Ranges of heart rate and their regulation at various ages (rat). *American Journal of Physiology*, 1967, *212*, 595–602.

Als, H., Lester, M. B., & Brazelton, T. B. Dynamics of the behavioral organization of the premature infant: A theoretical perspective. In T. Field, S. Goldberg, A. Sostek, & H. H. Shuman (Eds.), *The high risk newborn*. New York: Spectrum, 1979.

Apgar, V. A. The newborn (Apgar) scoring system. *Pediatric Clinics of North America*, 1966, *13*, 645.

Ashida, S. Developmental changes in the basal and evoked heart rate in neonatal rats. *Journal of Comparative and Physiological Psychology*, 1972, *78*, 368–374.

Brazelton, T. B. *Neonatal behavioral assessment scale*. Clinics in Developmental Medicine, No. 50. Philadelphia: Lippincott, 1973.

Caputo, D. V., Goldstein, K. M., & Taub, H. B. The development of prematurely born children through middle childhood. In T. Field (Ed.), *Infants born at risk*. New York: SP Medical and Scientific Books, 1979.

Chess, G. F., Tam, M. K., & Calaresu, R. F. Influences of cardiac neural inputs on rhythmic variation of heart period in the cat. *American Journal of Physiology*, 1975, *228*, 775–780.

Clifton, R. K., & Nelson, M. N. Developmental study of habituation in infants: The importance of paradigm, response system and state. In T. J. Tighe & R. N. Leaton (Eds.), *Habituation: Perspectives from child development, animal behavior, and neurophysiology*. Hillsdale, N.J.: Lawrence Erlbaum Associates, 1976.

de la Cruz, F. F. Pediatric care and training: A paradox? In J. D. Tjossem (Ed.), *Intervention strategies for high risk infants and young children*. Baltimore: University Park Press, 1976.

Drillien, D. M. *The growth and development of the prematurely born infant*. Baltimore: Williams and Wilkins, 1964.

Field, T. M., Dempsey, J. R., & Shuman, H. H. Developmental assessments of infants surviving the respiratory distress syndrome. In T. Field (Ed.), *Infants born at risk*. New York: SP Medical and Scientific Books, 1979.

Fitzgerald, H. E., & Brackbill, Y. Classical conditioning in infancy: Development and constraints. *Psychological Bulletin*, 1976, *83*, 353–376.

Gallagher, J. J., & Bradley, R. H. Early identification of developmental difficulties. In I. J. Gordon (Ed.), *Early childhood education*. Chicago: University of Chicago Press, 1972.

Honzik, M. P. Value and limitations of infant tests: An overview. In M. Lewis (Ed.), *Origins of intelligence: Infancy and early childhood*. New York: Plenum, 1976.

Karrer, R. (Ed.) *Developmental psychophysiology of mental retardation: Concepts and studies*. Springfield, Ill.: Charles C. Thomas, 1976.

Katona, P. G., & Jih, F. Respiratory sinus arrhythmia: Non-invasive measure of parasympathetic cardiac control. *Journal of Applied Physiology*, 1975, *39*, 801-805.

Kero, P., Antila, K., Ylitalo, V., & Valimaki, I. Decreased heart rate variation in decerebration syndrome: Quantitative clinical criterion of brain death? *Pediatrics*, 1978, *62*, 307-311.

Krupski, A. Heart rate changes during a fixed reaction time task in normal and retarded adult males. *Psychophysiology*, 1975, *12*, 262-267.

Lacey, J. I. Somatic reponse patterning and stress: Some revisions of activation theory. In M. H. Appley & R. Trumbell (Eds.), *Psychological stress: Issues in research*. New York: Appleton-Century-Crofts, 1967.

Larson, S. K., & Porges, S. W. The ontogeny of heart period patterning in the rat. *Developmental Psychobiology*, 1982, *15*, 519-528.

Lopes, O. U., & Palmer, J. F. Proposed respiratory "gating" mechanism for cardiac slowing. *Nature*, 1976, *264*, 454-456.

Lowensohn, R. I., Weiss, M., & Hon, E. H. Heart-rate variability in brain damaged adults. *Lancet*, March 19, 1977, 626-628.

Lubchenco, L. O., Delivoria-Papadopoulos, M., & Searles, D. Long-term follow-up studies of prematurely born infants. *Journal of Pediatrics*, 1972, *80*, 509-512.

McCabe, P. M., Porges, S. W., & Yongue, B. G. Spectral analysis of heart rate during depressor nerve stimulation: The validation of a non-invasive estimate of vagal tone. *Society for Neurosciences Abstracts*, 1979, *5*, 156.

McCall, R. B., Hogarty, P. S., & Hurlburt, N. Transition in infant sensory-motor development in the prediction of childhood IQ. *American Psychologist*, 1972, *27*, 728-748.

Nelson, N. M. Respiration and circulation before birth. In C. A. Smith and N. M. Nelson (Eds.), *The physiology of the newborn infant*. Springfield, Ill.: Charles C. Thomas, 1976.

Obrist, P. A., Webb, R. A., Sutterer, J. R., & Howard, J. L. Cardiac deceleration and reaction time: An evaluation of two hypotheses. *Psychophysiology*, 1970, *6*, 695-706.

Overton, W. F., & Reese, H. W. Models of development: Methodological implications. In J. R. Nesselroade and H. W. Reese (Eds.), *Life-span developmental psychology: Methodological issues*. New York: Academic Press, 1973.

Parmelee, A. H., Kopp, C. B., & Sigman, M. Selection of developmental assessment techniques for infants at risk. *Merrill-Palmer Quarterly*, 1976, *22*, 177-199.

Parmelee, A. H., & Michaelis, R. Neurological examination of the newborn. In J. Hellmuth (Ed.), *The exceptional infant* (Vol. 2). New York: Brunner/Mazel, 1971.

Porges, S. W. Heart rate variability and deceleration as indexes of reaction time. *Journal of Experimental Psychology*, 1972, *92*, 103-110.

Porges, S. W. Heart rate variability: An autotomic correlate of reaction time performance. *Bulletin of the Psychonomic Society*, 1973, *1*, 270-272.

Porges, S. W. Heart rate indices of newborn attentional responsivity. *Merrill-Palmer Quarterly*, 1974, *20*, 231–254.

Porges, S. W., Arnold, W. R., & Forbes, E. J. Heart rate variability: An index of attentional responsivity in human newborns. *Developmental Psychology*, 1973, *8*, 85–92.

Porges, S. W., Bohrer, R. E., Cheung, M. N., Drasgow, F., McCabe, P. M., & Karen, G. New time-series statistic for detecting rhythmic co-occurrence in the frequency domain: The weighted coherence and its application to psychophysiological research. *Psychological Bulletin*, 1980, *88*, 580–587.

Porges, S. W., Bohrer, R. E., Keren, G., Cheung, M. N., Franks, G. J., & Drasgow, F. Cardiac–respiratory coupling and hyperkinetic children: A physiological manifestation of the influence of methylphenidate. *Psychophysiology*, 1981, *18*, 42–48.

Porges, S. W., & Coles, M. G. H. Individual differences in respiratory–heart period coupling and heart period responses during two attention demanding tasks. *Physiological Psychology*, 1982, *10*, 215–220.

Porges, S. W., & Humphrey, M. M. Cardiac and respiratory responses during visual search in nonretarded children and retarded adolescents. *American Journal of Mental Deficiency*, 1977, *82*, 162–169.

Porges, S. W., McCabe, P. M., & Yongue, B. G. Respiratory–heart-rate interactions: Psychophysiological implications for pathophysiology and behavior. In J. Cacioppo & R. Petty (Eds.), *Perspectives in cardiovascular psychophysiology*. New York: Guilford Press, 1982.

Porges, S. W., & Smith, K. M. Defining hyperactivity: Psychophysiological and behavioral strategies. In C. K. Whalen & B. Henker (Ed.), *Hyperactive children: The social ecology of identification and treatment*. New York: Academic Press, 1980.

Porges, S. W., Srinivasan, G., Cheung, M. N., Shanker, H., Pildes, R., & Bohrer, R.E. Spectral analysis of neonatal heart rate and respiratory patterns. Paper presented at the International Conference on Infant Studies, New Haven, April 1980.

Porges, S. W., Stamps, L. E., & Walter, G. F. Heart rate variability and newborn heart rate responses to illumination changes. *Developmental Psychology*, 1974, *10*, 507–513.

Prechtl, H., & Beintema, D. *The neurological examination of the full term newborn infant*. Clinics in Developmental Medicine, No. 12. London: Heinemann, 1964.

Reese, H. W., & Overton, W. F. Models of development and theories of development. In L. R. Goulet and P. B. Baltes (Eds.), *Life-span developmental psychology: Theory and research*. New York: Academic Press, 1970.

Ross, L. E., & Leavitt, L. A. Process research: Its use in prevention and intervention with high risk children. In T. D. Tjossem (Ed.), *Intervention strategies for high risk infants and young children*. Baltimore: University Park Press, 1976.

Sayers, B. M. Analysis of heart rate variability. *Ergonomics*, 1973, *16*, 17–32.

Schifferli, P. Y., & Caldeyro-Barcia, R. Effects of atropine and beta-adrenergic drugs on the heart rate of the human fetus. In L. Boreus (Ed.), *Fetal pharmacology*. New York: Raven Press, 1973.

Stamps, L. E., & Porges, S. W. Heart rate conditioning in newborn infants: Relationships among conditionability, heart rate variability, and sex. *Developmental Psychology*, 1975, *11*, 424–431.

Walter, G. F., & Porges, S. W. Heart rate and respiratory responses as a function of task difficulty: The use of discriminant analysis in the selection of psychologically sensitive physiological responses. *Psychophysiology*, 1976, *13*, 563–571.

Weiner, G., Rider, R. V., Oppel, W. C., & Harper, P. A. Correlates of low-birth weight. *Pediatric Research*, 1968, *2*, 110–118.

Wright, F. H., Blough, R. F., Chamberline, A., Ernest, T., Halstead, W. C., Meier, P., Moore, R. Y., Naunton, R. F., & Newell, F. W. A controlled follow-up study of small prematures born from 1952 through 1956. *American Journal of Disabled Children*, 1972, *124*, 506–522.

Yongue, B. G., McCabe, P. M., Porges, S. W., Rivera, M., Kelly, S. L., & Ackles, P. K. The effects of pharmacological manipulations that influence vagal control of the heart on heart period, heart-period variability and respiration in rats. *Psychophysiology*, 1982, *19*, 426–432.

2

Production and Spectral Analysis of Neonatal Crying and Its Relation to Other Biobehavioral Systems in the Infant at Risk

Philip Sandford Zeskind

Finding meaning in the variations of infant cry sounds has long been of interest to those who study behavioral development. Early studies used devices such as musical notation (Gardiner, 1938), photographs, line drawings (Darwin, 1965), and wax cylinders (Flatau & Gutzman, 1906) to record variations in vocal expression as they characteristically related to different biological states or levels of arousal. In more recent years, sound spectrographic analyses have been used to describe the relation between various changes in the infant's biological system, such as hunger or pain, and corresponding characteristic variations in rhythmical (Wolff, 1967) and harmonic features of infant crying (Wasz-Hockert, Lind, Vuorenkoski, Partanen, & Valanne, 1968). For example, in response to a presumably painful stimulus, initial portions of the cry show longer pauses and expirations of sound (Wolff, 1967) and more sudden shifts to higher pitch (Wasz-Hockert et al., 1968) than cries in response to presumably less arousing conditions. Some evidence suggests that as infant arousal subsides, the rhythmical (Wolff, 1967) and harmonic (Blinick, Tavolga, & Antopol, 1971) characteristics of the pain cry may become more similar over time to the cries in response to less arousing conditions.

This chapter is based, in part, on a dissertation submitted in partial fulfillment of the requirements for the Ph.D. degree at the University of North Carolina at Chapel Hill. The research was supported by the Biomedical Research Fellowship awarded to the author from the University of North Carolina at Chapel Hill.

While there may be some characteristic variations in cry sounds associated with different eliciting conditions, different infants may produce different cry sounds in response to similar eliciting conditions. For example, Truby and Lind (1965) classified infant cries in response to a skin pinch as (1) phonated, characterized by a smooth, regular harmonic structure (400–500 Hz), (2) dysphonated, characterized by turbulence and noise at higher pitch, or (3) hyperphonated, characterized by an abrupt, upward shift in pitch (up to 2000 Hz). The hyperphonated cry was described as a most vociferous response to discomfort which results from motor constriction in the vocal apparatus. While the motoric activity of the infant's laryngeal and respiratory mechanisms produce the hyperphonated sound (Golub, 1981), individual differences in nervous system control of the peripheral vocal mechanisms may determine whether this high-pitched sound will occur. For example, variations in the characteristics of crying may reflect the capacity of the infant's nervous system to be activated and then to inhibit that activation (Parmelee, 1962). As Parmelee (1962) suggested, a "good" cry can be described by the amount of stimulation required to produce a sustained cry, the duration of crying, and the tonal quality of the cry. Variations in the threshold, duration, and pitch of crying may thus tell us something about the manner in which the nervous system of an individual infant responds to a particular eliciting condition.

Characteristic variations in these cry features may then be useful in the identification and assessment of the infant who is at risk due to events which may affect nervous system functioning. For example, a higher threshold for cry elicitation, a shorter duration of crying, and an unusually high-pitched cry sound have differentiated low risk infants from infants in the normal newborn nursery who showed obstetric (Zeskind & Lester, 1978) and anthropometric (Zeskind & Lester, 1981) indices of high risk. Although similar responsivity (Karelitz & Fisichelli, 1962) and harmonic (Wasz-Hockert et al., 1968) characteristics of crying have been used to support the clinical diagnosis of brain damage, among relatively healthy infants these cry variations have been hypothesized to reflect the capacity of the nervous system to mediate the biobehavioral activities of the infant (for a review, see Lester & Zeskind, 1979, 1982; Zeskind, in press-a); that is, rather than necessarily indicating structural central nervous system pathology, the differential cry features may be related to the functional organization of the nervous system as it responds to internal and external sources of stimulation.

The autonomic nervous system, with its sympathetic and parasympathetic components, may be implicated in this biobehavioral response system. Activation of the sympathetic nervous system is associated with heightened arousal and excitation; conversely, activation of the parasympathetic nervous system is associated with the inhibition of arousal. The fluctuating balance between these two autonomic nervous system components is manifested in a wide range of biobehavioral activities such as heart rate, respiratory changes, and state fluctuations. Following the conceptualization of infant crying as a complex motor response comprised of a cry *act* and a cry *sound* (Truby & Lind, 1965), one model of variations in these cry features suggest that the production (*act*) and spectral (*sound*) characteristics, respectively, are related to these activities of the sympathetic and parasympathetic nervous systems (Lester & Zeskind, 1982). According to this model, the *excitatory* action of the sympathetic nervous system is hypothesized to influence the threshold and duration of infant crying, while the *inhibitory* action of the parasympathetic nervous system and its effect on the tone of the vagus nerve is hypothesized to affect the tension of the laryngeal muscles and thus the fundamental frequency of the cry sound. Frequent shifts in pitch, such as between phonated ("normal") and hyperphonated (high-pitched) cry sounds, may be a reflection of poor modulation of the cry signal caused by an imbalance between the opposing excitatory and inhibitory elements of the autonomic nervous system. Although infants may demonstrate high thresholds for crying (production) and produce high-pitched cry sounds, these production and spectral features are posited to tap into different biobehavioral systems. Depending on the nature of the nonoptimal prenatal and/or perinatal events which increase the risk status of the infant, it is possible that infants may differ in one response class and not another. Because there are reliable individual differences in the cry features *within* groups of infants with nonoptimal prenatal experiences (Zeskind & Lester, 1981), the variations in cry features may be sensitive to individual differences in the infant's biobehavioral functioning within a group of infants categorically described as at increased risk.

Performance on the Neonatal Behavioral Assessment Scale (NBAS) (Brazelton, 1973) may be one way by which we can index biobehavioral functioning in the infant. For example, studies of infants who show anthropometric signs of increased risk such as a low ponderal index (which indicates that an infant is of low birth weight relative to its birth length) perform poorly on the NBAS when compared to infants with an average ponderal index (Als, Tronick, Adamson, & Brazelton, 197.; Lester, 1979; Zeskind, 1981). Preliminary studies of these infants at risk show relations between individual differences in NBAS performance and neonatal pain cry variations. Among a group of infants who ranged from average weight for length to underweight for length, multiple regression analysis showed that the combination of a poor performance on the NBAS (all four a priori dimensions), a low ponderal index, and a short gestation was associated with infant cries of short duration, high average fundamental frequency, and high maximum frequency and fewer numbers of harmonics in the cry sound (Lester & Zeskind, 1978).

The NBAS was analyzed in terms of the four a priori dimensions of social interactive processes, motoric process, state modulation, and physiological response to stress (Als et al., 1976). Performance on the motoric dimension of the NBAS was the greatest predictor of the number of harmonics in the cry. In an analysis of a subsample of these infants, the average fundamental frequency of the cry was reliably related to all four NBAS dimensions (Lester, 1979). These preliminary findings have indicated that combined behavioral and physical growth measures may account for a substantial portion of the variation in neonatal pain cry sounds. Examining the relation between neonatal cry features and newborn behavior among infants of differential fetal growth may thus help us to understand how particular cry variations are associated with different aspects of biobehavioral functioning.

The purposes of this study were to examine further the cry features of infants with nonoptimal patterns of fetal growth and the relation of individual differences in these cry features to performance on the NBAS.

1. Recent studies of neonatal cry features (Zeskind & Lester, 1981) and NBAS scores (Zeskind, 1981) indicate that overweight- and underweight-for-length infants show similar behaviors which differentiate them from average weight-for-length infants. Whereas previous research relating cry sounds to behavior (Lester, 1979, Lester & Zeskind, 1978) investigated only average weight- and underweight-for-length newborn, this study will include overweight-for-length newborn and thus examine infants along a more complete weight–length continuum.

2. Whereas previous research has used the four a priori dimensions of the NBAS (Als et al., 1976) for assessments of biobehavioral functioning (e.g., Lester & Zeskind, 1978; Zeskind, 1981), this study will use a system which separates the NBAS scale items into seven conceptual clusters and allows for a more fine-grained analysis of behavior (Lester, Als, & Brazelton, 1982).

3. Previous cry research of infants with nonoptimal fetal growth has studied the average fundamental frequency of the first pain cry expiration. While this has been useful because of its standardization and diagnostic value, the average fundamental frequency, by definition, averages the variability in pitch and may thus homogenize a heterogeneous sound. Furthermore, studying only the first cry expiration limits our understanding of how the cry may change as infant arousal subsides. So, in addition to cry threshold and duration, this study will examine both the highest and lowest dominant frequencies (not the average) found in both the initial and final segments of the pain cry. A randomly selected segment of a cry occurring during administration of the NBAS will also be studied. Whereas only the highest dominant frequency of this cry segment was previously reported (Zeskind, 1981) for the infants in this study, the lowest dominant frequency of that NBAS cry sound will also be examined here.

4. In order to provide a descriptive categorization of the pain and NBAS cry segments, the three cry segments will be classified by the pattern of variability in the sound. The study of these infants' cry features and behaviors will enable us to examine how different components of the cry differentiate the infant groups and how these components are related among themselves and to the seven clusters of neonatal behavior.

METHOD

Subjects

Subjects were selected from a sample of 109 2-day-old infants who were born at a university-affiliated teaching hospital and resided in the normal newborn nursery. From this larger sample, only those infants who were full-term (range 38–42 weeks gestation), showed no gross abnormal clinical signs on routine newborn examinations, and were not circumcised were included for study. The ponderal index (PI), a birth-weight–birth-length ratio, was calculated for each infant. Birth weight was obtained from the hospital records. Birth length was derived from the consensus of two examiners who elicited a tonic neck reflex and measured the crown–heel length. The PI ratios were used to classify infants as belonging to a low-PI (PI $\leq$ 2.28), average-PI (PI = 2.29–2.81), or high-PI group (PI $\geq$ 2.82). The low- and high-PI criteria respectively, represent the 10th and 90th percentiles of the neonatal weight-for-length scale (see Miller & Hassanein, 1971).

A total of 13 average-PI and 13 high-PI infants were randomly chosen for comparison with the 13 low-PI infants found in this sample. The results of chi-square analyses suggested that among the three PI groups distributions of race [$\chi^2(2) < 0.21, p = .90$], sex, [$\chi^2(2) = 0.82, p < .66$], and presence of maternal obstetric medication [$\chi^2(2) = 2.17, p < .34$] did not reliably differ from those expected by chance. Analyses of variance showed that the low-, average-, and high-PI infant groups also did not reliably differ in Apgar scores at both 1 min [$F(2,36) = 0.39, p < .68$] and 5 min [$F(2,36) = 0.06, p < .94$] or in the number of nonoptimal obstetric conditions listed in the medical records [$F(2,36) = 0.45, p < .64$].

Procedure

Informed consent was obtained and midway between scheduled feedings the infant was taken to a quiet room in the nursery. With the infant in a supine position in a bassinet, a cry was elicited by snapping the infant's foot with a standard rubber band stretched 15 cm along the edge of a ruler. If a cry of at least 10 sec was not elicited, the infant's foot was again snapped, to a maximum of five snaps. The duration of crying activity was measured by a research assistant using a stopwatch. Unlike the 30-sec limit for the length of crying used in previous reports, infants were allowed to cry up to 60 sec before being quieted, because a 30-sec time limit may produce a "ceiling effect" on the individual differences in crying length (Zeskind & Lester, 1981). This procedure and the ensuing cry was recorded on magnetic tape (Sony model TC-150) with a Sony Electret condenser microphone held 20 cm midline from the infant's mouth by the research assistant. The investigator and research assistant were unaware of the infant's PI classification throughout the data collection and analyses.

Midway between scheduled feedings and 8 hours after the recording session of the pain cry, infants were administered the NBAS by a trained examiner who was blind to the infant's PI classification. For this study, the NBAS scores were broken down into seven behavioral clusters, which are shown in Table 2-1 along with the behavioral items included in each cluster.

Table 2-1
Seven Brazelton Neonatal Behavioral Assessment Scale Dimensional Clusters

Items*	Clusters
	Habituation
Light (1)	Raw score of each
Rattle (2)	
Bell (3)	
Pinprick (4)	
	Orientation
Inanimate visual (5)	Raw score of each
Inanimate auditory (6)	
Animate visual (7)	
Animate auditory (8)	
Visual auditory (9)	
Alertness (10)	
	Motor
Tonus (11)	Recode: 9/1 = 1; 8/2 = 2; 7/3 = 3; 4 = 4; 5 = 5; 6 = 6
Maturity (12)	Raw score
Pull to sit (13)	Raw score
Defense (15)	Raw score
Activity (20)	Recode: 9/1 = 1; 8/2 = 2; 7/3 = 3; 4/6 = 4; 5 = 5

	Range of State
Peak of excitement (17)	Recode: 9/1 = 1; 8/2 = 2; 4/3 = 3; 7/5 = 4; 6 = 5
Rapidity of buildup (18)	Recode: 9/1 = 1; 8/2 = 2; 7/3 = 3; 4 = 4; 5 = 5; 6 = 6
Irritability (19)	Recode: 9/1 = 1; 8 = 2; 7 = 3; 6 = 4; 5 = 5; 2,3,4 = 6
Lability of state (24)	Recode: 1,7,8,9 = 1; 5,6 = 2; 4 = 3; 3 = 4; 2 = 5

	Regulation of State
Cuddliness (14)	Raw score of each
Consolability (16)	
Self-quieting (25)	
Hand to mouth (26)	

	Autonomic Stability
Tremors (21)	Recode: invert 9 = 1; (1 = 9); 8 = 2 (2 = 8); etc.
Startles (22)	Recode: if 1, drop; otherwise invert 2–9 on 8-point scale
Skin (23)	Recode: 9,1 = 1; 8 = 2; 7 = 3; 6 = 4; 5 = 5; 3,4 = 6; 2 = 7

Reflexes

An abnormal score is defined as 0, 1, or 3 for all reflexes except clonus, nystagmus, tonic neck reflex, where 0, 1, and 2 are normal and 3 is abnormal. The reflex score is the total number of abnormal reflex scores.

Reprinted with permission from Lester, B. M., Als, H., & Brazelton, T. B. Regional obstetric anesthesia and newborn behavior: A reanalysis toward synergistic affects. *Child Development*, 1982, *53*, 687–692. © The Society for Research in Child Development, Inc.
*Numbers in parentheses represent NBAS item number.

Each NBAS behavioral item, according to this system is redefined to a linear scale with a score of 9 denoting an optimal performance. The behavioral items included in each cluster are summed and averaged for each infant's cluster score, except for the reflex cluster, which included the sum total of the deviant reflexes found. During the administration of the NBAS, the first crying state of the infant was tape-recorded. The state of crying was determined by the NBAS examiner, but the 15-sec criterion for a complete state change did not apply to this cry sound. Two infants in each of the three PI groups did not cry during the examination.

Cry Analysis

Spectral features of the beginning and ending segments of the pain cry sound and a randomly chosen segment of the NBAS cry were determined from spectrograms produced by a Voice Print model 700 sound spectrograph using a narrow band filter and a linear expansion production of the spectrogram for enhanced accuracy of measurement. Measurements were made in the absence of knowing the PI classification of the infant.

Eight cry features were selected for analysis, of which six were selected from the pain cry: (1) the threshold, the number of rubber band snaps required to elicit a 10-sec cry; (2) the activity, the total amount of time in seconds the infant cried in response to the final rubber band snap; (3) the initial peak frequency, the highest dominant frequency in the initial 2.4 sec of the pain cry phonation; (4) the final peak frequency, the highest dominant frequency in the final 2.4 sec of the pain cry phonation; (5) the initial lowest frequency, the lowest dominant frequency in the initial 2.4 sec of the pain cry phonation; and (6) the final lowest frequency, the lowest dominant frequency in the final 2.4 sec of the pain cry phonation. Whereas only the NBAS peak frequency (the highest dominant frequency in the randomly selected 2.4-sec segment of crying during the NBAS examination), the seventh feature, was presented in a previous report (Zeskind, 1981), the NBAS lowest frequency (the lowest dominant frequency in the same randomly selected segment of crying during the NBAS examination) was the eighth feature analyzed in this study. The selection of these eight cry features allowed for the study of (1) the *production* features of the pain cry; (2) the *spectral* features of not only the initial pain cry segment, but also the end segment of that pain crying bout and a cry segment that occurred during a period of handling the infant; and (3) the high- and low-pitch variabilities within a cry segment.

In addition to the quantitative measurement of the frequencies of the cry sounds, a classification of the harmonic structure of the cry sound represented on the spectrogram was made from the unenhanced spectrograms. Consensus with a research assistant was necessary to classify each spectrogram as evidence of either hyperphonation, partial hyperphonation, or phonation. As with the other cry analyses, this classification of cry patterns was conducted with the investigator and assistant blind to the infant's identity or PI status.

RESULTS

Group Comparisons

Two multivariate analyses of variance were conducted to compare the six pain cry features of the three infant groups. The first multivariate analysis included the cry threshold, activity, and the highest dominant frequencies of both the initial and final pain cry segments. A significant linear combination of the four variables was indicated [$F(8,66) = 5.11, p < .001$]. The univariate tests and subsequent Neuman-Keuls analyses (p's $< .005$) showed that low- and high-PI infants had a higher threshold for cry response, a shorter duration of crying activity, and a higher peak dominant frequency in both the initial and final segments of the pain cry than the average-PI infants. No reliable differences were found between the low- and high-PI groups on these four cry features.

The second multivariate analysis, incorporating the lowest dominant frequencies of the initial and final pain cry segments, did not show a significant effect for PI group membership [$F(4, 70) = 1.15, p < .34$]. The lack of a significant effect indicates that there was no reliable difference between any of the groups on the lowest dominant frequencies in the initial and final pain cry segments. To test whether the lowest frequency of the NBAS cries differentiated the three PI groups, an analysis of variance was conducted and yielded a nonsignificant result. Thus, like the spectral features of the pain cry, the highest pitch of the cry occurring during the NBAS differentiated the low- and high-PI infants from the average-PI infants (Zeskind, 1981), but the lowest pitch of that cry did not. Table 2-2 shows the means, standard deviations, and results of the appropriate univariate tests for these eight cry variables.

Box (1953) tests for homogeneity of variance were conducted to compare the within-groups variabilities of all eight cry features among the three PI groups. For the cry threshold, activity, and the highest dominant frequencies of the three cry segments, the variances of the low- and high-PI infant groups were reliably different from those of the average-PI group (all p's $< .001$). No reliable differences were found between the low- and high-PI groups on these cry features. Furthermore, no reliable differences were found in the variances of the lowest dominant frequencies of the three cry segments among any of the three PI groups. That is, the five cry features that differentiated the low- and high-PI infants from average-PI infants by tests of mean differences also differentiated the groups by tests of the individual differences within the groups. Because the finding of differences among the variances of the cry features may violate the assumption of homogeneity of variance in the univariate tests, the univariate tests were repeated after being adjusted for the heterogeneous variances. The results of these tests showed the same pattern of results as reported in Table 2-2.

Correlations Among Cry Features

Table 2-3 shows the Pearson product–moment correlations of the eight cry features. Overall, the correlations ranged from .03 to .75, with a median of .30. Cry threshold was inversely related to the duration of crying activity, but was not related to the spectral features of the cry sound. Crying activity

Table 2-2 _____

Means, Standard Deviations, and the Results of Univariate Tests
of Cry Features

Cry Feature	Low PI	Average PI	High PI	F	df	p
		Group				
Threshold (Number of snaps)						
X	2.0	1.1	2.4	4.79	2,36	<.01
SD	1.1	0.4	1.3			
Activity (sec)						
X	14.8	30.1	15.0	8.28	2,36	<.001
SD	5.5	17.1	6.5			
Initial peak frequency (Hz)						
X	1606.1	545.9	1602.7	9.45	2,36	<.001
SD	827.9	213.9	899.7			
Final peak frequency (Hz)						
X	1049.5	538.5	993.1	4.24	2,36	<.02
SD	677.2	85.9	506.1			
NBAS peak frequency (Hz)						
X	1140.2	524.4	990.5	4.78	2,30	<.01
SD	602.7	129.3	575.6			
Initial lowest frequency (Hz)						
X	556.7	388.2	465.1	NA		
SD	227.6	133.7	219.0			
Final lowest frequency (Hz)						
X	414.3	358.7	389.0	NA		
SD	120.2	71.3	131.9			
NBAS lowest frequency (Hz)						
X	395.6	385.5	380.4	0.12	2,30	<.88
SD	79.1	79.5	58.6			

showed small but significant correlations with the initial peak frequency
and NBAS peak frequency, but was unrelated to the other spectral cry
features.

An examination of the correlations among the peak dominant frequencies of the cry segments showed a range of .43–.75. The correlations
show that the peak dominant pitch of the initial pain cry segment was
reliably related to the peak dominant pitch at the conclusion of that pain
cry and that both measures of the pain cry were reliably related to the
highest pitch of the cry occurring during the NBAS examination. The
NBAS cry segment had a higher correlation with the final pain cry segment
than with the initial pain cry segment.

Table 2-3

Correlations Among Cry Features

	Activity	Initial Peak Frequency	Final Peak Frequency	NBAS Peak Frequency	Initial Low Frequency	Final Low Frequency	NBAS Low Frequency
Threshold	−.41†	.07	.08	.21	.06	.03	−.09
Activity		−.21*	−.18	−.30*	−.16	−.20	−.09
Initial peak frequency			.43†	.62†	.31†	.42†	.20
Final peak frequency				.75†	.38†	.38†	.34*
NBAS peak frequency					.45†	.55‡	.47†
Initial lowest frequency						.45†	.08
Final lowest frequency							.20

*$p < .05$.
†$p < .01$.
‡$p < .001$.

Analysis of Harmonic Structure

Spectrograms displaying examples of hyperphonated, partially hyperphonated, and phonated cry sound segments from the infants in this study are shown in Figure 2-1. The hyperphonated cry segment (Fig. 2-1A) would be characterized as a continuously high-pitched whistlelike sound in comparison to the "normal" lower-pitched sound of the phonated cry segment (Fig. 2-1C). The partially hyperphonated cry segment (Fig. 2-1B) would be characterized as a lower pitched "normal" cry sound broken by a sudden shift to the high-pitched whistlelike sound that quickly reverts to the "normal" pain cry sound.

To examine the relations among the PI group, cry segment, and cry pattern, the number of initial pain cry segments, final pain cry segments, and NBAS cry segments that were classified as one of the three cry patterns were determined for each of the three PI groups. Table 2-4 shows the frequencies and percentages of each cry pattern for the cry segments of the group of low- and high-PI infants and the group of average-PI infants.

Table 2-4 shows that the hyperphonated cry pattern was comprised of pain-elicited cry segments from low- and high-PI infants; no NBAS cry segments of the low- and high-PI infants or any cry segments of average-PI infants appeared in this category. The partially hyperphonated cry pattern was comprised of cry segments from low- and high-PI infants, but showed proportionately the same number of pain-elicited and NBAS cry segments. Seven average-PI infant cry segments were also classified into this category of cry patterns, six of which were from pain-elicited cries. The phonated cry pattern was predominated by the pain and NBAS cry segments of average-PI infants.

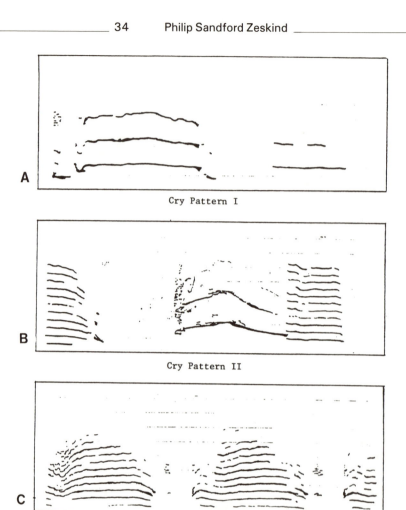

A
Cry Pattern I

B
Cry Pattern II

C
Cry Pattern III

Figure 2-1

Spectrograms displaying examples of hyperphonated (A), partially hyperphonated (B) and phonated (C) cry segments.

The association between differential fetal growth and the occurrence of infant cry hyperphonation was determined by pooling the number of cry segments classified as either hyperphonated or partially hyperphonated for a combined group of low- and high-PI infants and for the group of average-PI infants. Chi-square analyses showed that the distribution of phonated versus hyperphonated cries for the different PI groups departed from that which would be expected by chance in the cases of the initial pain cry segment [$\chi^2(1) = 19.5, p < .001$], the final pain cry segment [$\chi^2(1) = 6.3, p < .01$], and the NBAS cry segment [$\chi^2(1) = 8.8, p < .003$].

Table 2-4

Distribution of Cry Patterns for Low- and High-PI Infants and Average-PI Infants

	Group			
	Low- and High-PI Infants		Average-PI Infants	
Cry Segment	(*n*)	(%)	(*n*)	(%)
Initial Pain Cry Segment				
Hyperphonated	8	31	0	0
Partially hyperphonated	16	62	3	23
Phonated	2	7	10	77
Final Pain Cry Segment				
Hyperphonated	3	11	0	0
Partially hyperphonated	14	54	3	23
Phonated	9	35	10	77
NBAS Cry Segment				
Hyperphonated	0	0	0	0
Partially hyperphonated	14	64	1	9
Phonated	8	36	10	91

Relations Among Neonatal Cry Features and NBAS Behavioral Clusters

In order to examine the relations among the eight neonatal cry features and the seven NBAS behavioral clusters, the 39 infants were treated without regard to PI group membership. Table 2-5 shows the means and standard deviations of the 15 dependent measures of this sample of infants. A Person product–moment correlation matrix was derived from these variables and showed correlations ranging from .00 to .75. A principal–component factor analysis with varimax rotation and iterations was conducted. The first step of the factor analysis resulted in the extraction of five factors with eigenvalues greater than unity that accounted for 70.3 percent of the variance of the unreduced correlational matrix.

The results of the revised factor matrix and the denotation of the factor on which each variable was loaded the highest are shown in Table 2-6. A minimum criterion of .40 was used for significant factor loading. Factor I accounted for 45.3 percent of the variance of the revised matrix and showed the highest factor loadings of the motor behavioral cluster, all four spectral features of the pain cry, and the highest pitch of the NBAS cry. Factor II accounted for 23.1 percent of the variance and showed the highest factor loadings of the threshold and activity features of the pain cry and the orientation and autonomic stability behavioral clusters. Factors I and II shared contributions from the orientation and motor behavioral clusters. The motor cluster was also represented in factor III. Factor III accounted for

Table 2-5

Means and Standard Deviations of Cry Features and NBAS Clusters for Entire Sample

Neonatal Behavior	$\overline{X}$	SD
Habituation	5.8	1.4
Orientation	5.4	1.5
Motor	5.0	0.9
Range of states	3.2	1.0
Regulation of states	5.4	1.3
Autonomic stability	5.2	0.7
Reflexes	3.7	0.3
Initial lowest frequency	470.0	205.0
Initial peak frequency	1251.0	861.0
Final lowest frequency	387.0	110.0
Final peak frequency	860.0	530.0
NBAS lowest frequency	387.0	71.0
NBAS peak frequency	885.0	541.0
Threshold	1.8	1.1
Activity	20.0	12.9

Table 2-6

Revised Factor Matrix

Items	Factors				
	I	II	III	IV	V
Habituation	.273	.364	.273	−.069	−.040
Orientation	−.411*	.599†	.246	.235	−.202
Motor	−.484†	.434*	.421*	.236	−.135
Range of states	−.039	.010	−.005	.053	.671†
Regulation of states	.233	.166	.610†	−.012	−.037
Autonomic stability	.276	.502†	.116	−.123	−.336
Reflexes	−.041	−.203	−.848†	.248	−.067
Initial lowest frequency	.657†	.010	−.185	−.056	−.057
Initial highest frequency	.577†	−.109	−.130	.216	−.196
Final lowest frequency	.708†	−.005	.259	.160	−.092
Final highest frequency	.610†	−.146	−.156	.385	.195
NBAS lowest frequency	.121	.068	−.078	.675†	.059
NBAS highest frequency	.681†	−.145	−.189	.648	−.025
Threshold	.099	−.521†	−.072	−.032	−.039
Activity	−.193	.719†	.168	−.102	.445*

*Significant loading on factor.
†Highest loading of item.

13.3 percent of the variance and showed the highest factor loadings of the regulation of state and reflex behavioral clusters. Factor IV accounted for 10.4 percent of the variance and showed the highest factor loading of the lowest pitch of the NBAS cry and a significant contribution from the highest pitch of that cry segment. Lastly, factor V accounted for 7.9 percent of the variance of the revised factor matrix and showed the highest factor loading of the range of state behavioral cluster and a significant contribution from the activity feature of the cry.

DISCUSSION _____

The results of this study partially replicate and extend the findings of previous studies of infants who showed different patterns of fetal growth. As was found in another sample (Zeskind & Lester, 1981), low- and high-PI infants showed similar cry features which differentiated them from average-PI infants. The methods used in this study resulted in the differentiation of infant groups by both production features of infant crying such that low- and high-PI infants required more stimulation to elicit crying and had shorter periods of crying activity than average-PI infants. As was previously found in the average fundamental frequency of the initial pain cry expiration (Zeskind & Lester, 1981), the peak dominant frequency in both the initial and final segments of the pain cry distinguished the low- and high-PI infants from the average-PI infants. Although the high pitch was evident thoughout the pain cry sound and was found in a more naturally occurring cry (Zeskind, 1981), this study also shows that the cry was not uniformly high pitched and that there were components of the cry sounds of the low- and high-PI infants that did not differentiate them from average-PI infants. As can be seen in cry pattern II in Figure 2-1B, an infant may produce markedly different dominant frequencies in the same cry expiration; that is, the cry sound can suddenly shift to a high pitch from a lower pitched "normal" cry sound.

The qualitative categorization of the cry sounds indicates that this shift to a higher pitch may reflect differences in infant arousal which occur as a function of both the intensity of the eliciting condition and the manner in which the biological system of the infant responds. Of the cry segments of the low- and high-PI infants, 74 percent showed a hyperphonated cry pattern, compared to 19 percent of the average-PI infant cry segments. When upward shifts in pitch occurred in the cries of average-PI infants, they were evident in the pain cry; however, no homogeneously high-pitched cry segments (cry pattern I) were found in the cries of average-PI infants. For low- and high-PI infants, hyperphonation was frequently found in all three cry segments, but a homogeneously high-pitched segment was found only in the pain cries and mostly in the initial segment. To the extent that the pain cry is a "maximal" response (Lind, Wasz-Hockert, Vuorenkoski, Partanen, Theorell, & Valanne, 1966) which results in more shifts to a higher pitch (Stark & Nathanson, 1975; Truby & Lind, 1965; Wasz-Hockert et al., 1968), these findings suggest that the sudden and intense stimulation of the rubber band snap may make increased demands on the biological systems of the low- and high-PI infants. The motoric activity which may produce the high pitch (Golub, 1979; Truby & Lind, 1965) appears to be accentuated in the infants of differential fetal growth, especially during the intense arousal of the initial pain cry segment.

An examination of the factor analysis of the neonatal cry features and NBAS cluster scores may provide some insight into which biobehavioral systems of the infant are related to these variations in cry sounds. Although neonatal crying, especially in response to a painful stimulus, is reflexive in nature, variations in the cry features were apparently unrelated to the dimension of behavior described by the number of abnormal reflexes the infant exhibited (factor III). Instead, the separate behavioral dimensions for the spectral (pitch) and production (threshold and duration) aspects of crying appear to parallel the conceptualization of infant cry variations as part of a complex *motor* response which is comprised of *act* plus *sound* (Truby & Lind, 1965). For example, although there was a significant motoric contribution to both the production and spectral components of crying, the act of cry production (factor II) was orthogonally related to the variations in sound produced (factor I). This suggests that the production and spectral components of infant crying may tap two different biobehavioral systems in the infant.

One model of infant cry variations hypothesizes that these two biobehavioral systems are the sympathetic and parasympathetic components of the autonomic nervous system (Lester & Zeskind, 1982). These two nervous systems act in opposition such that high sympathetic activation (arousal and excitement) is accompanied by low parasympathetic input. In order to regain homeostasis at times of high arousal, input from the parasympathetic system (inhibition of arousal) increases over time. According to this model of infant crying, fluctuations in parasympathetic activity are associated with fluctuations in the tone of the vagus nerve which affects the motoric action of the laryngeal muscles and produces variations in the cry sound. The sympathetic nervous system, which activates and arouses the infant, is hypothesized to be associated with the threshold and duration of crying (see Lester & Zeskind, 1982).

The biobehavioral loadings in the factor analysis appear to support this view. While factor IV consisted only of the spectral features of the NBAS cry, the peak pitch of that cry was most highly related to the dimensions of behavior described by the spectral features of the pain cry (factor I). This may indicate that although the NBAS cry is less intense than the pain cry, the processes associated with changes in the peak pitch are similar. The factor loadings indicate that the infants who had higher pitched cries showed poorer scores on the NBAS cluster incorporating the infant's muscle tone and motor activity (factor I). Thus infants who showed poor motor maturity, motor activity, and muscle tonus were also infants whose laryngeal and respiratory muscles might more frequently act noncontinuously, resulting in a shift of vocal registers and a hyperphonated cry sound (Golub, 1979). The contribution of the nervous system to this motoric action and resulting pitch shift may lie in vagal tone changes associated with low parasympathetic input (Lester & Zeskind, 1982).

An examination of the occurrence of hyperphonation in the different cry segments may help clarify this relation. The more frequent occurrence of hyperphonation in the pain cries than in the NBAS cries may reflect a lower level of parasympathetic input associated with the condition of high arousal (and high sympathetic activity). Changes in the amount of hyperphonation between the initial and final segments of the pain cry may also reflect the change in parasympathetic activity associated with regaining homeostasis. At the beginning of the pain cry, sympathetic activation (arousal) was high and parasympathetic input (inhibition) was low, resulting in the greater occurrence of hyperphonation in the initial cry segment. As the intensity of the arousal subsided, associated with the inhibitory effect of increased parasympathetic input, the high-pitched cry sound occurred less frequently. Similarly, among the substantial correlations between the peak dominant frequencies of three cry segments, the highest correlation was between the final pain cry and NBAS cry segments, suggesting that as the intensity of the effects of the pain stimulus were subsiding, the pain cry more consistently approximated the cry elicited by handling the infant. Previous work has shown that hyperphonation occurs more often in pain cries, especially the initial segment, than in other cries (Wasz-Hockert et al., 1968). The present study showed a similar phenomenon, but also that it occurred more often among infants with nonoptimal patterns of fetal growth and that it may be associated with other biobehavioral systems.

In addition to sharing contributions from the motoric cluster, the orientation cluster also contributed significantly to the dimensions of both the production and spectral features of infant crying. Whereas the cardiac orienting response was related to the fundamental frequency of the cries of malnourished infants (Lester, 1976), the orienting capabilities of the infants in this study were more strongly related to the dimensions of behavior incorporating the production features of the cry and the autonomic stability cluster scores on the NBAS (factor II). Infants with higher cry thresholds and a shorter crying duration obtained lower scores on the ability to orient to sights and sounds of the environment and showed more startles, tremors, and skin color changes in response to stimulation. The infant who required more stimulation to elicit a sustained cry response therefore also responded more poorly to other forms of stimulation which may reflect the nature of sympathetic activation (Lester & Zeskind, 1982). The role of this arousal system was also evident in the relation of the measures of crying activity to the range of state NBAS cluster (factor V). Infants with a less sustained cry showed lower peaks of excitement, less irritable crying, and fewer changes in states, thus reflecting a lesser overall arousal level. These results are consistent with the findings of a recent study of infants who varied in the number of rubber band snaps required to elicit a sustained cry (Zeskind & Field, 1982). Infants with higher thresholds for induced crying showed not only shorter durations of crying activity and more frequent occurrences of hyperphonation, but also greater autonomic instability as manifested in greater heart rate variation during a period of quiet resting. Spectral analysis of neonatal heart rate variability, also implicating vagal control, has also shown similar high fundamental frequencies and sudden shifts in amplitude and frequency in infants who showed signs of fetal distress (Porges, 1979).

CONCLUSION

Many years ago, Parmelee (1962) suggested that the threshold, duration, and tonal quality of crying may reflect the capacity of the central nervous system to be aroused and then to inhibit that arousal. This study provides support for a model which describes how variations in these cry features may be associated with the arousal and inhibitory functions of the autonomic nervous system (Lester & Zeskind, 1982). Whereas previous research of infants in the normal newborn nursery who show nonoptimal patterns of fetal growth has mostly focused on the average high pitch of the initial pain cry segment (Lester & Zeskind, 1978; Zeskind & Lester, 1981), this study shows that the cry sound of particular infants shifts back and forth between a nondifferentiating low-pitched cry sound and a distinguishing high-pitched one. Because underweight- and overweight-for-length infants are at higher risk that average weight-for-length infants, this cry sound may reflect individual differences in the biological functioning of infants within a risk category. The analysis of infant crying may help identify, then, which infants within the category may actually have had some change in the development of their nervous system.

Furthermore, crying is a particularly salient aspect of neonatal behavior. A high cry pitch may be one particularly distinguishing aspect of the cry sound (Ostwald, 1972; Partanen, Wasz-Hockert, Vuorenkoski,

Theorell, Valanne, & Lind, 1967) which may elicit different perceptions and responses from care givers (Zeskind, 1980; Zeskind & Lester, 1978) and thus affect the development of the infant with a nonoptimal fetal growth pattern (Zeskind & Ramey, 1978, 1981). The cry variations may then be a measure of infant behavior that taps some of the contributions to development from both the infant's biological and care-giving enviroments. By synthesizing the traditional medical and behavioral approaches to infant cry variations into a framework of normal infant development (Zeskind, in press, b), we may further clarify the biological and social significance of variations in infant crying and thus better understand the development of the infant at risk.

REFERENCES _____

Als, H., Tronick, E., Adamson, L., & Brazelton, T. B. The behavior of the full-term yet underweight newborn infant. *Developmental Medicine and Child Neurology*, 1976, *18*, 590-602.

Blinick, G., Tavolga, W. N., & Antopol, W. Variations in birth cries of newborn infants from narcotic addicted and normal mothers. *American Journal of Obstetrics and Gynecology*, 1971, *110*, 948-958.

Box, G. E. P. Non-normality and tests on variances. *Biometrika*, 1953, *40*, 318-335.

Brazelton, T. B. *Neonatal behavioral assessment scale*. London: Heinemann, 1973.

Darwin, C. *The expression of emotion in man and animals*. Chicago: University of Chicago Press, 1965. (Originally published in 1872.)

Flatau, T. S., & Gutzman, H. Die Stimme des Sauglings. *Archiv fuer Laryngologie und Rhinologie*, 1906, *18*, 139.

Gardiner, W. *The music of nature*. Boston: Wilkins & Carter, 1838.

Golub, H. L. A physioacoustic model of the infant cry and its use for medical diagnosis and prognosis. In J. J. Wolf & D. H. Klatt (Eds.), *Speech communication papers*. Presented at the 97th Meeting of the Acoustical Society of America, Cambridge, MA, June 12, 1979.

Karelitz, S., & Fisichelli, V. The cry thresholds of normal infants and those with brain damage. *Journal of Pediatrics*, 1962, *61*, 679-685.

Lester, B. M. Spectrum analysis of the cry sounds of well-nourished and malnourished infants. *Child Development*, 1976, *47*, 237-241.

Lester, B. M. A synergistic process approach to the study of prenatal malnutrition. *International Journal of Behavioral Development*, 1979, *2*, 377-393.

Lester, B. M., Als, H., & Brazelton, T. B. Regional obstetric anesthesia and newborn behavior: A reanalysis toward synergistic effects. *Child Development*, 1982, *53*, 687-692.

Lester, B. M., & Zeskind, P. S. Brazelton scale and physical size correlates of neonatal cry features. *Infant Behavior and Development*, 1978, *1*, 393-402.

Lester, B. M., & Zeskind, P. S. The organization and assessment of crying in the infant at risk. In T. M. Field, A. M. Sostek, S. Goldberg, & H. H. Shuman (Eds.), *Infants born at risk*. New York: Spectrum, 1979.

Lester, B. M., & Zeskind, P. S. A biobehavioral perspective on crying in early infancy. In H. Fitzgerald, B. Lester, & M. Yogman (Eds.), *Theory and research in behavioral pediatrics* (Volume 1). New York: Plenum, 1982.

Lind, J., Wasz-Hockert, O., Vuorenkoski, V., Partanen, T. J., Theorell, K., & Valanne, E. Vocal response to painful stimuli in newborn and young infants. *Annales Paediatriae Fenniae*, 1966, *12*, 55–63.

Miller, H. C., & Hassanein, K. Diagnosis of impaired fetal growth in newborn infants. *Pediatrics*, 1971, *48*, 511–522.

Ostwald, P. The sounds of infancy. *Developmental Medicine and Child Neurology*, 1972, *14*, 350–361.

Parmelee, A. Infant crying and neurological diagnosis. *Journal of Pediatrics*, 1962, *61*, 801–802.

Partanen, T. J., Wasz-Hockert, O., Vuorenkoski, V., Theorell, K., Valanne, E. H., & Lind, J. Auditory identification of pain cry signals of young infants in pathological conditions and its sound spectrographic basis. *Annales Paediatriae Fenniae*, 1967, *13*, 56–63.

Porges, S. W. Innovations in fetal heart rate monitoring: The application of spectral analysis for the detection of fetal distress. In T. Field, A. Sostek, S. Goldberg, & H. H. Shuman (Eds.), *Infants born at risk*. New York: Spectrum, 1979.

Stark, R. E., & Nathanson, S. N. Unusual features of cry in an infant dying suddenly and unexpectedly. In J. Bosma & J. Showacre (Eds.), *Development of upper respiratory anatomy and function*. Washington, D.C.: U.S. Government Printing Office, 1975.

Truby, H. M., & Lind, J. Cry sounds of the newborn infant. *Acta Paediatrica Scandinavia Supplement*, 1965, *163*.

Wasz-Hockert, O., Lind, J., Vuorenkoski, V., Partanen, T., & Valanne, E. *The infant cry*. London: Heinemann, 1968.

Wolff, P. H. The role of biological rhythms in early psychological development. *Bulletin of the Menninger Clinic*, 1967, *31*, 197–218.

Zeskind, P. S. Adult responses to cries of low-risk and high-risk infants. *Infant Behavior and Development*, 1980, *3*, 167–177.

Zeskind, P. S. Behavioral dimensions and cry sounds of infants of differential fetal growth. *Infant Behavior and Development*, 1981, *4*, 297–306.

Zeskind, P. S. A behavioral–pediatric synthesis of crying in the infant at risk. In M. L. Wolraich & D. K. Routh (Eds.), *Advances in behavioral pediatrics*, (Vol. 5). Greenwich, Conn: JAI Press, in press.(a)

Zeskind, P. S. A developmental perspective of the cries of the infant at risk. In B. M. Lester & C. F. Z. Boukydis (Eds.), *Infant crying: Theoretical and research perspectives*. New York: Plenum, in press.(b)

Zeskind, P. S., & Field, T. M. Neonatal cry threshold and heart rate variability. In L. P. Lipsitt & T. M. Field (Eds.), *Infant behavior and development: Perinatal risk and newborn behavior*. Norwood, N.J.: Ablex, 1982.

Zeskind, P. S., & Lester, B. M. Acoustic features and auditory perceptions of the cries of newborns with prenatal and perinatal complications. *Child Development*, 1978, *49* (3), 580–589.

Zeskind, P. S., & Lester, B. M. Analysis of cry features in newborns with differential fetal growth. *Child Development*, 1981, *52*, 207–212.

Zeskind, P. S., & Ramey, C. T. Fetal malnutrition: An experimental study of its consequences on infant development in two caregiving environments. *Child Development*, 1978, *49* (4), 1155–1162.

Zeskind, P. S., & Ramey, C. T. Preventing intellectual and inteactional sequelae of fetal malnutrition: A longitudinal, transactional and synergistic approach to development. *Child Development*, 1981, *52*, 213–218.

3

Behavioral and Psychophysiological Sequelae of Preterm Birth: The Neonatal Period

Susan A. Rose

In terms of theoretical issues about normal development and applied issues about achieving a healthy population, preterm birth has long represented a major problem. Throughout the years there has accumulated compelling evidence that large numbers of these children are at higher risk than full-term children for physical, emotional, social, and/or mental handicaps. Such handicaps include abnormalities in neurological development, poor physical growth, sustained intellectual impairment (especially in very low birth weight infants), retarded language development, learning disabilities, and a higher incidence of deviant social behavior of all sorts during early childhood and adolescence (Caputo & Mandell, 1970; DeHirsch, Jansky, & Langford, 1966; Drillien, 1964; Harmeling & Jones, 1968; Knoblock & Pasamanick, 1966; Lubchenco, 1976).

Since the early 1960s there have been extensive changes in the medical management of the preterm infant during the neonatal period (e.g., Francis-Williams & Davies, 1974; Fitzhardinge & Ramsay, 1973; Fitzhardinge, Pape, Arstikaitis, Boyle, Ashby, Rowley, Netley, & Sawyer, 1976). In particular, some of the preterm infants' disabilities have been recognized as iatrogenic, and most modern centers have eliminated those factors now known to be harmful to their development, for example, excessive use of oxygen, inadequate postnatal nutrition, hypothermia, and hyperbilirubinemia. Follow-up studies on preterm infants born in the last

Funds for the support of this work were provided by a Behavioral Sciences Research Grant from the National Foundation of the March of Dimes and by Grant HD 13810 from the National Institutes of Health.

decade suggest a brighter prognosis for them. Neonatal mortality has decreased and there has been a marked reduction in the incidence of major neurobiological abnormalities, retrolental fibroplasia, and seizures (e.g., Davies, 1976; Davies & Tizard, 1975; Fitzhardinge & Ramsay, 1973; Lubchenco, 1976; Rawlings, Reynolds, Stewart, & Strang, 1971; Stewart & Reynolds, 1974). Despite the pronounced decrease in neonatal morbidity, deficits in cognitive functioning still persist as a major problem (e.g., Fitzhardinge & Ramsay, 1973; Francis-Williams & Davies, 1974; Grellong, Vaughan, Rotkin, Daum, Kurtzberg, & Lipper, 1981; Kitchen, Ryan, Richards, McDougall, Billson, Kier, & Naylor, 1980; Rubin, Rosenblatt, & Barlow, 1973; Taub, Goldstein, & Caputo, 1977). There are continuing reports of deficits in IQ, lags in language development and academic achievement, and perceptual–motor difficulties. So although substantial gains have been made regarding the physical and neurological status of the preterm child, these infants appear to remain at higher risk for abnormal perceptual and cognitive development.

OBJECTIVES OF THIS RESEARCH

Much of this research has been directed toward gaining knowledge of the sensory and perceptual capabilities of the preterm and examining the comparability of functioning in preterm and full-term infants (Dorros, Brody, & Rose, 1979; Rose, 1980a, 1980b; Rose, Gottfried, & Bridger, 1978, 1979; Rose, Schmidt, & Bridger, 1976, 1978; Rose, Schmidt, Riese, & Bridger, 1980; Schmidt, Rose, & Bridger, 1980). These efforts have centered on the first years of life, in the hope of detecting abnormalities and dysfunctions as early as possible. Since intervention aimed at alleviating or minimizing later aberrant development is often thought to be maximally effective if introduced when the organism is young, early identification would seem to be of major importance. Knowledge of the behavioral and psychophysiological functioning of the preterm infant could also be of enormous usefulness for the monitoring and evaluation of those new techniques now being introduced into routine perinatal care.

In the past decade or two, research on development of the full-term infant has produced a wealth of information about early capabilities. For example, it has been known for some time that the healthy full-term infant comes into the world with all sensory systems functioning: the infant responds to sights, sounds, smells, and tastes in the environment and is sensitive to vestibular and tactual experience. To some extent, the infant is even able to modulate input from the environment (see Cohen & Salapatek, 1975; Osofsky, 1979). Development in this early period proceeds extremely rapidly and is thought to play an important, perhaps critical role in later functioning.

Our knowledge of the preterm infant's development, however, has lagged sadly. This situation now appears to be improving as various laboratories begin to study the emerging capabilities of these infants (see Parmelee, 1975). This increasing interest in the preterm is reflected in the recent publication of several volumes such as this one, devoted almost exclusively to the consideration of their development and outcome. In the remainder of the chapter, some of the work my colleagues and I have been doing in this area is described.

NEONATAL PERIOD

Our research during the neonatal period has been primarily concerned with comparing the sensory functioning and organization of preterm infants close to term age with that of full-term infants born after 40 weeks of gestation. The major thrust of much of this work has been to gain information about (1) infants' sensitivity and responsivity to different intensities of stimulation, (2) the interrelationship between behavior and the concomitant psychophysiological indices of responsivity, (3) autonomic lability and activation, and (4) the role of the sleep state in modulating responsivity. These studies have focused primarily on responsivity to tactile stimuli. Although the central concern of this study has been with stimulus evoked responsivity, wherever possible spontaneous base-line differences between the preterm and full-term have been examined.

The following discussion will focus on some of the principal findings. These will be preceded, however, by a brief discussion of sleep-state organization in the neonate, since there is evidence that this endogenous organization of neurophysiological activation not only plays an important role in modulating responsivity to exteroceptive stimuli, but is itself altered by pathophysiological processes. Next the subject population will be described, and then the differences we have found in what I have termed basal measures will be discussed, concentrating on spontaneous variations in the duration of sleep-state epochs, resting heart rate, and unelicited motor activation. After that, the applicability of the law of initial value to cardiac functioning in the preterm and full-term will be discussed, followed by a description of the findings obtained on cardiac and behavioral responsivity to tactile stimuli. The final section touches on some of the environmental factors found to affect the sleep-state organization and cardiac responsivity of the preterm.

THE SLEEP STATE

At the outset of this study it seemed that any effort to establish reliable assessments of responsivity would have to seriously consider the infant's state (see also Clifton & Nelson, 1976). In discussing the concept of state, Prechtl and his colleagues noted that "by the term 'state' one tries to describe constellations of certain functional patterns of physiological variables which may be relatively stable and which seem to repeat themselves" (Prechtl, Akiyama, Zinkin, & Grant, 1968, p. 1). States thus represent relatively long-term background changes in neurophysiological and behavioral activity that tend to recur in a cyclic manner and to be morphologically similar in all infants.

Actually, long before sleep states per se were defined, time-dependent changes in responsiveness within sleep were recognized. As long ago as 1891, Czerny reported that the threshold to stimulation during sleep is best described by an inverted U. In 1913 Canestrini observed that the infant is least responsive to stimulation 45–60 min after falling asleep, and in 1937 Wagner noted that the baby sleeps "deepest" when motionless and breathing regularly.

In more recent years, as a result of the resurgence of interest in sleep research, two major recurring sleep states have become widely recognized in early infancy, active sleep and quiet sleep. Active sleep is characterized by rapid and slow eye movements, ample and variable motor activity, increased and uneven functioning of the autonomic nervous system, and, in general, a low-voltage, fast electroencephalogram (EEG) pattern. Quiet sleep, on the other hand, is characterized by general quiescence, absence of eye movements and motor activity (with the exception of occasional startles), regular respiration and heart rate, and a primarily high-voltage, slow or *tracé alternant* EEG (Anders, Emde, & Parmelee, 1971). The infant's sleep generally begins with an epoch of active sleep, and then the two sleep states occur alternately. A neonatal sleep cycle consists of one epoch of active sleep and one epoch of quiet sleep (often along with some amount of indeterminate sleep); in an interfeeding period there occur anywhere from two to four such cycles. The healthy human neonate sleeps about 16 hours a day during the first 2 weeks of life, and continues to sleep as much as 15 hours a day for the next 3 months (Parmelee, Wenner, & Schultz, 1964).

The ontogeny of sleep-state development in the preterm infant has been carefully described by Dreyfus-Brisac (1970a, 1974) and Parmelee (Parmelee, Bruch, & Bruch, 1962; Parmelee, Wenner, Akiyama, Stern, & Flescher, 1966). By the time the preterm infant reaches 40 weeks conceptional age, the overall architecture of sleep has become much like that of the full-term infant. Typical active sleep becomes identifiable at about 35 weeks of gestation, and typical quiet sleep at about 37 weeks (Dreyfus-Brisac, 1970a). Once present, the two sleep states alternate during interfeeding intervals much as they do in the sleep of the full-term. However, various aspects of the parameters which define sleep continue to differ, and the two sleep states are not as well organized as they are in the full-term. As Dreyfus-Brisac (1970a) has pointed out, respiration is more irregular and faster, the cardiac rate is more rapid, and there is less low-voltage EEG activity. In speaking of the preterm at 38–41 weeks conceptional age, Dreyfus-Brisac commented, "We observe in the premature relatively few correlations between the different components of quiet sleep, a lower percentage of regular respiration, and of the low voltage EEG pattern, as well as a higher percentage of cardiac and respiratory rate" (1970, p. 115).

In my own laboratory, sleep state was continuously monitored by behavioral observations. In the studies of full-term infants, active sleep was defined as a 60-sec period with eyes closed, slow and rapid eye movements, irregular respiration, and variable motor activity. Quiet sleep was defined as a 60-sec period in which eye movements are absent, respiration is regular, and there are no body movements except for isolated startles or jerks (Anders et al., 1971). It was observed, in agreement with Dreyfus-Brisac (1970a), that even at term age the preterm infant's respiration can at times be slightly irregular in quiet sleep. The definition of quiet sleep in the preterm has therefore been modified to include semiregular respiration, provided that there are no eye movements or body movements other than isolated jerks or startles, otherwise the definitions are the same as those used for full-term children, and periods fitting neither category are labeled as transitional. Additionally, a 1-min "smoothing" period was adopted; that is, a state change has to be longer than one 60-sec rating period to be acknowledged as a new state.

SUBJECTS

The infants who served as subjects in these studies all came from the Bronx Municipal Hospital Center in New York City. The full-term samples were uniformly restricted to healthy 2- to 3-day-old infants. All had been delivered vaginally, either by normal, spontaneous, or low forcep delivery, and all had a good maternal history. Pre- and perinatal circumstances were uneventful, birth weight was always above 2500 g, and 5-min Apgar scores were always 9 or 10. Nearly all infants were bottle fed, and generally the feeding immediately preceding testing was administered by the experimenters or a research nurse. This practice tended to ensure adequate nutritional intake and to guarantee, insofar as possible, a subsequent period of undisturbed sleep.

The preterm infants who participated in these studies came from the same hospital. The preterm samples, although varying slightly from one another, had a mean gestational age at birth of around 33 weeks and a mean birth weight between 1500 and 1660 g. Individual weights at birth ranged from 820 to 2000 g, with approximately one-third of the infants in each sample weighing less than 1500 g. Generally the infants were tested as close to discharge as possible. At this time, their mean conceptional ages varied between 37.3 and 38.5 weeks (with a chronological age around 30–35 days) and their mean weight ranged from 2120 to 2300 g. About 12–15 percent of the infants in each sample were small for dates, and close to half suffered from some form of respiratory distress, often requiring several days of ventilatory assistance. None of the subjects had been on respirators, and none suffered any central nervous system damage that was obvious on neurological examination.

BASAL MEASURES

In the course of studying the infants' responsivity to stimuli, some attention was also paid to the spontaneous variations that occurred in the duration of their sleep-state epochs, resting heart rate levels, and unelicited motoric activity. Here the data will be reviewed for each in turn in order to highlight the sometimes pronounced differences found between full-term and preterm infants.

As noted above, sleep generally begins with an epoch of active sleep. In full-term infants, the duration of this first epoch of active sleep was reported to average between 17 and 19 min, and that of the subsequent epoch of quiet sleep, 16–18 min (Ashton, 1971; Murray & Campbell, 1971). In an earlier study (Schmidt & Birns, 1971), the duration of the first epoch of active sleep was found to be similar to that reported in these other studies ($\overline{X}$ = 19.1 min, SD = 8.4 min). The most complete data available bearing on the duration of individual sleep epochs come from a more recent study (Rose et al., 1980). In that study, in the hour following sleep onset the duration of the first epochs of both active and quiet sleep were examined: all 30 full-term infants tested completed the entire first sleep cycle, with the duration of the first epoch of active sleep averaging 18.7 min (SD = 7.3 min) and that of the first epoch of quiet sleep averaging 16.8 min (SD = 6.2 min). It is worth noting that the figures reported for state duration in full-term infants show a remarkable consistency across studies carried out throughout the world.

In this previous study (Rose et al., 1980) the duration of these two sleep epochs in preterm infants was also examined. Some of the differences compared to the full-term were striking. First, of the 30 preterm infants (labeled the control group in that study), only 22 completed the entire first sleep cycle. The others either awoke or stayed in the first epoch of active sleep throughout the entire session. Second, even considering just those infants who completed the entire first cycle, the duration of the first epoch of active sleep was markedly longer in the preterm ($\overline{X}$ = 30.1 min, SD = 12.8 min) than in the full-term. This difference in duration was restricted to active sleep, as the mean duration of the first epoch of quiet sleep ($\overline{X}$ = 14.3 min, SD = 4.6 min) turned out to be quite similar to that found in the full-term group ($\overline{X}$ = 16.8, SD = 6.2 min).

Clearly, a marked difference between preterm and full-term infants lies in the lengthy first epoch of active sleep of the preterm, a finding that has also been recently reported by Field et al. (1979) and which is confirmed by a reexamination of data from an earlier study with preterm infants (Rose et al., 1976). In sleep-state studies carried out on full-term infants, it has been noted that the first epoch of active sleep differs in various ways from subsequent epochs of the same state. In particular, the EEG pattern contains more high-voltage, slow waves than do later epochs, in which a low-voltage, fast EEG pattern predominates. In effect, the EEG differentiation between active and quiet sleep is less marked in early than in later sleep cycles (Dreyfus-Brisac 1970b, 1974; Roffwarg, Muzio, & Dement, 1966). According to observations in my own laboratory, this first epoch also contains more gross body movements and fewer rapid eye movement bursts than do later epochs. Polygraphic studies would probably indicate that the first epoch of active sleep is the least well-organized epoch of sleep in the preterm as well. In fact, the prolongation of this sleep epoch in preterm infants may well reflect a continuing neurophysiological immaturity which persists to term age and perhaps even beyond.

Before considering the characteristic levels of resting heart rate found in different sleep states, a word is in order as to how the heart rate data were scored. Since much of the early work here was done without the benefit of a cardiotachometer, the physiograph was generally run at a fast chart speed, 25 mm/sec or more, and then the number of cardiac cycles (R–R intervals), including fractions of a cycle, that occurred within a 5-sec period were counted and expressed as beats per minute (bpm). Infants were always tested as close to discharge as possible and all preterm infants had been out of the isolette for at least 24 hours prior to testing. Testing generally took place after the midmorning feeding in a soundproof laboratory kept at 30–31°C. Heart rate was monitored continuously throughout the testing period, but to avoid transitional periods in state change, cardiac values were sampled only after the infant had been in a particular state for at least 3 min.

To examine resting heart rate levels, cardiac values were sampled during nonstimulated periods; these were represented by the 5-sec intervals of motoric quiescence that preceded the onset of each stimulus. The base-line heart rate data from these studies are summarized in Table 3-1. Even though the infants were motorically quiescent, the heart rates were, without exception, higher in the first epoch of active sleep than in the first epoch of quiet sleep. This difference, which averages out to around 4½ beats across studies, is highly consistent for both preterm and full-term infants. It should be pointed out that when heart rate is sampled randomly, and thus not restricted to periods of motoric quiescence, the rate tends to be elevated in active sleep and the differences between the two sleep states are even more marked (e.g., Ashton & Connolly, 1971; Schmidt, Rose, & Bridger, 1974). The fact that differences are present even in the absence of gross motor movement is in keeping with what is known about state differences in autonomic activation.

The heart rate differences between the two sleep states, while highly consistent, are minor compared to the striking cardiac differences between full-term and preterm infants. We have consistently found that the basal heart rate of preterm infants is more than 30 beats higher than that of full-term infants, with very little overlap between the two groups. For example, in Rose et al. (1976), the values for full-term infants in the first epoch of active sleep ranged from 94 to 140 beats per minute (bpm), whereas those for preterm infants ranged from 134 to 164 bpm. Field et al. (1979) reported a similar difference in base level cardiac rates. The reason for these full-term–preterm differences is unclear, and to my knowledge has not been addressed in the literature. Although the preterm in our own studies and those of Field and co-workers tend to be, on the average, somewhat younger than 40 weeks conceptional age at the time of testing, this factor does not appear to account for the observed difference in heart rate. First of all, Dreyfus-Brisac (1970a) noted that the rapid, irregular cardiac rates in the preterm are not related to conceptional age; second, Rose et al. (1980) found that the correlation between the basal heart rate level and conceptional age at testing was negligible ($r = .02$). There was, however, a strong correlation between basal heart rate and both birth weight ($r = -.31$) and gestational age at birth ($r = -.31$), indicating that preterm infants who were heavier and more mature at birth had lower resting heart rate levels (an observation consistent with that of Kero, 1974). While the high heart rate of the preterm may represent immaturity in the development of the parasympathetic nervous system, with resulting low vagal tone, there is, to my knowledge, no neurophysiological evidence which bears directly on this point.

The increased autonomic activation in preterm infants is paralleled somewhat, but to a far lesser degree, by differences in motoric activation. In monitoring spontaneous, unelicited motor activity on control trials, infants were observed for 5 or 10 sec following 5 sec of motoric quiescence. On such trials, the extent of limb or gross body activation was observed in the complete absence of exteroceptive stimulation. Although there were no

Table 3-1

Basal Heart Rate Levels for Preterm and Full-Term Infants in the First Epochs of Active and Quiet Sleep Across Studies*

| | Full-Term Infants | | | | | | Preterm Infants | | | | | |
| | Active Sleep | | | Quiet Sleep | | | Active Sleep | | | Quiet Sleep | | |
Reference	n	X̄	SD	n	X̄	SD	n	X̄	SD	n	X̄	SD
Rose, Schmidt, Reise, & Bridger (1980)	30	119.3	9.8	30	113.5	8.5	20	156.8	7.6	20	153.2	9.9
Rose, Schmidt, & Bridger (1976)	20	117.4	10.9				20	155.2	9.9			
Schmidt, Rose, & Bridger (1980)							11	157.8	8.6	11	152.9	10.0
Rose, Schmidt, & Bridger (1978)†	22	123.1	8.2	22	119.8	8.4						

*In the studies cited here, heart rate was sampled only during periods of motoric quiescence.

†In this study, 8 infants were tested in the second sleep cycle as well. Mean basal heart levels in the second epochs of active and quiet sleep were 122.5 bpm (SD = 6.6 bpm) and 118.2 bpm (SD = 6.6 bpm), respectively.

significant differences between full-term and preterm infants in the mean number of limb movements, the preterm did sometimes produce less vigorous movements than the full-term (Rose et al., 1976) or show less total body activation (Rose et al., 1976, 1980). In quiet sleep, there was virtually no difference between full-term and preterm infants. As would be expected, both groups demonstrated more spontaneous motor activity in active than in quiet sleep (Rose et al., 1980), a state difference which confirms an earlier finding obtained with full-term infants (Rose, Schmidt, & Bridger, 1978).

Thus, in terms of basal measures, preterm infants exhibit a far lengthier first epoch of active sleep, a markedly elevated tonic heart rate, and a pattern of spontaneous motor movement somewhat different than that of full-term infants.

THE LAW OF INITIAL VALUE

It has often been observed that the direction and intensity of psychophysiological responses to exteroceptive stimuli can be markedly affected by preexisting levels of activation. Wilder (1967) formulated the law of initial value to characterize this relation. The law states that there is an inverse correlation between prestimulus values and the magnitude of the organismic responses that will be elicited by a given stimulus. In the case of an excitatory stimulus, the law predicts that the lower the prestimulus values, the greater will be the magnitude of the elicited response, whereas for extremely high prestimulus values, there will be either a negative change or no change at all. For a soothing stimulus, the predictions are reversed. Theoretically, the law assumes an underlying unitary arousal effect of stimulation and attempts to separate the effects attributable to prestimulus variables from those actually attributable to the stimulus itself.

Most of our studies have been done with sleeping infants, where the heart rate response to stimulation tends to be an acceleration (Graham & Jackson, 1970). This response has been generally indexed by the difference between 5-sec prestimulus and 5-sec poststimulus heart rates. The law of initial value is said to be operating when there is a significant negative correlation between prestimulus heart rate levels and these change scores.

Schmidt et al. (1974) investigated the applicability of the law of initial value for heart rate responses evoked by a nociceptive stimulus in the active and quiet sleep of full-term infants. In this study, data were combined across two or three successive epochs of each sleep state. In accordance with the law, a significant correlation was found in active sleep between the prestimulus heart rate and cardiac change scores. This relation held for virtually all infants tested during active sleep, with an average correlation of $r = -.76$ and an average slope of $\beta = -.48$. As these values indicate, the heart rate acceleration evoked by the stimulus was greater at low prestimulus levels than at higher ones. In quiet sleep, the relation was significant for only about half the infants.

A priori one anticipates that the correlations would be lower in quiet sleep simply because the characteristic autonomic quiescence and stable heart rate, hallmarks of this state, result in a restricted range of prestimulus values, and like any other correlation, the law of initial value depends on the relative variability of prestimulus and stimulus levels. The less the variability of the stimulus level and the greater the variability of the prestimulus level, the wider the range of change scores and the larger the negative correlation of change on prestimulus level (which is the law of initial value). In fact, if a stable stimulus level is obtained, there is a perfect inverse correlation between prestimulus values and change scores (Block & Bridger, 1962). While the stimulus level is generally somewhat more variable in active than in quiet sleep, this is more than compensated for by the considerably greater variability of the prestimulus level in active sleep. The law of initial value consequently tends to be stronger in active than in quiet sleep.

The importance of the prestimulus level in characterizing the individual's cardiac functioning is evident for preterm as well as full-term infants. Since the stimulus level, and consequently the range of change scores, is a function of the strength of the stimulus, the applicability of the law of initial value is best tested in conditions where there are a sufficient number of trials with any given intensity of stimulation. This condition held in the study of Rose et al. (1980), where each infant received numerous trials with the strongest of a series of stimuli in each of two sleep states. It should be noted that this study differed from that of Schmidt et al. (1974) in ways which might be expected to lessen the applicability of the law of initial value: first, instead of data from different epochs of each sleep state being combined, which serves to widen the range of prestimulus values, data obtained here were restricted to a single epoch of either state; second, the range of prestimulus values was further restricted by preselecting such periods for motoric quiescence; and finally, the stimulus, being somewhat milder, was less likely to lead to a stable stimulus level. Nonetheless, in active sleep the average correlation for preterm infants between the prestimulus heart rate and cardiac change scores was $r = -.48$, and the average slope was $\beta = -.50$; in quiet sleep, the average correlation was $r = -.35$ and the average slope was $\beta = -.36$ (Rose et al., 1980, previously unpublished analyses). The law thus seems applicable to preterm as well as full-term infants.

Consideration of the law of initial value is important when attempting to understand how state and time factors affect perceptual thresholds and discriminations. Since prestimulus heart rate levels differ from state to state (and over time) and since the magnitude of a cardiac response tends to be dependent on these prestimulus levels, seemingly state-dependent differences in the response threshold can turn out to be secondary to differences in the prestimulus level. While state and time differences may sometimes override prestimulus differences, the distinctions involved cannot be clarified without a consideration of the law of initial value.

CARDIAC AND BEHAVIORAL RESPONSIVITY

As mentioned earlier, the neonate's sensitivity and responsivity to tactile stimulation has been the focus of much of our published work. In two of these studies involving preterm infants (Rose et al., 1976; 1980) the stimuli used were plastic filaments selected from the Semmes–Weinstein aesthesiometer. These filaments differ in diameter. Those used in the first study (Rose et al., 1976) were numbered 3.84, 4.56, and 5.46, the units being the logarithm of the bending force measured in milligrams. Any excess pressure exerted when pressing these filaments against the infant's skin is taken up in the bend. We followed the practice of stimulating the infants on the abodmen, applying a single filament five times in rapid succession so that the duration of the stimulation lasted for approximately 2.5 sec; on control trials the stimulus was omitted altogether. In this first study, interstimulus intervals averaged 30 sec, with trials beginning only when the infant was quiescent. If any spontaneous movements occurred during the intertrial interval, 30 sec were allowed to elapse from that time. Trials were randomly arranged within blocks of five, with each block consisting of one trial with each of the three filaments and two control trials. Infants were tested in a neonatal soundproof laboratory following the midmorning feeding. In order to avoid periods of state transition, testing never began until the infant had been in a given sleep state for at least 3 min. In this study, infants were tested only in the first epoch of active sleep.

Preliminary beat-by-beat analyses of cardiac scores in randomly selected infants revealed that where there was a discernible response in active sleep, the response form consisted of a monophasic acceleration during the first 5 sec. This was true for both full-term and preterm infants. This being the case, the basic response measure chosen for analysis was the first 5-sec poststimulus interval. The number of cardiac cycles (R–R intervals), including fractions of a cycle, were counted for each 5-sec period before and after every trial, and then expressed in beats per minute. The difference between 5-sec prestimulus and 5-sec poststimulus heart rates constituted the measure of heart rate change used to index responsivity to the stimulus. Average change scores were computed for each subject for each level of stimulus.

Behavior responses (changes in motoric activity) were rated on a 5-point scale; ratings ranged from 0 for no limb movement to 4, which represented the movement of all four limbs, including startles and gross body movements. In addition, a minus sign represented a small movement of short duration in the respective scale, and a plus sign represented a vigorous movement. Any behavior that occurred within 5 sec after stimulation commenced was recorded. Control trials were rated similarly.

All results were analyzed by analysis of variance (ANOVA) and analysis of covariance (ANCOVA). In addition, because of the marked differences in prestimulus heart rate levels, the cardiac data of full-term and preterm infants were analyzed separately. As can be seen in Figure 3-1, whereas the full-term responded with heart rate acceleration to the stronger levels of stimulation (with the mildest stimulus, 3.84, just below significance), the preterm showed no significant heart rate response to any of the stimuli. This striking failure of the preterm to respond was confirmed by various supplementary analyses. There was no indication that averaging over the 5-sec period had obscured a response that would have otherwise been evident, and, in fact, a beat-by-beat analysis of the first 25 poststimulus beats similarly failed to reveal any significant acceleration, even with the strongest (5.46) stimulus. Other analyses discounted the possibility of habituation, since there was no evidence of any initial responsivity that waned over trials. No matter how the results were examined, there was simply no evidence of a cardiac response on the part of the preterm.

With respect to behavioral responsivity (Figure 3-2), both groups gave a significant response to the strongest stimulus (and only to that one). Even here, however, the preterm gave a decidedly weaker response than did the full-term ($\overline{X} = 2.0$ and $\overline{X} = 1.5$, respectively).*

There were two aspects of the relation between cardiac and behavioral responsivity that were perplexing. First, to the strongest level of stimulation, the full-term showed significant behavioral and heart rate responses, whereas the preterm showed only a significant behavioral response. It was puzzling as to why a cardiac response was not evoked from the preterm in the wake of these behavioral responses. In our observations of full-term infants, we had often seen cardiac responses in the absence of motoric activation, but the reverse, motor responses without cardiac acceleration, was less commonplace. Various aspects of the data were examined to better understand what might have happened. First, the nature of the relation between

---

*As can be seen in Figure 3-2, there was a sex difference for preterm infants. This difference reflects heightened motoric activation among female preterm infants to all three stimulus intensities. Although these curves might lead one to believe that the preterm females were as responsive as full-term infants to the strongest stimulus, and even more so to the weaker stimuli, there was no evidence of a triple interaction, that is, no group × sex × stimulus level interaction, and thus no statistical support for such a conclusion. The more appropriate conclusion, and the one with statistical support, simply indicates a preterm–full-term difference to the 5.46 stimulus.

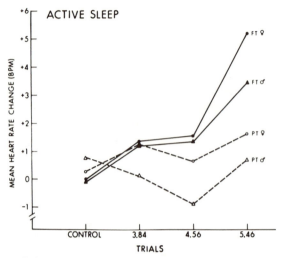

Figure 3-1

Mean heart rate change scores on control trials and in response to different intensities of tactile stimulation during the first epoch of active sleep.

behavioral and heart rate indices of responsivity was examined by computing a correlation between each particular infant's behavioral ratings and heart rate change scores across all trials. The correlations were significant ($p < .05$) in 12 of the 20 full-term infants, but in only 2 of the 20 preterm infants. The average correlation for the entire group of full-term infants was $r = .47$, whereas for the preterm it was only $r = .19$. These data suggest

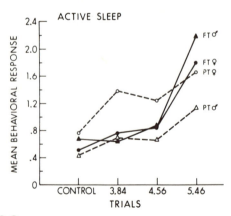

Figure 3-2

Mean behavioral response on control trials and in response to different intensities of tactile stimulation during the first epoch of active sleep.

that even at the individual level the two indices of responsivity are not conjoined in the preterm.

However, a detailed examination of the frequencies of the various types of behavioral reponses indicated that they too were different for the two groups. Even to the strongest stimulus, the preterm mostly failed to respond, and when they did respond, their movements were smaller and less vigorous than those of the full-term. Since this pattern of responsivity raises the possibility that low correlations between motor and heart rate responses may have been secondary to a reduced frequency of gross body movements, just those trials on which the infant had a large motor response were examined. Yet here to the mean heart rate change among the preterm ($\overline{X}$ = 2.42 bpm) turned out to be significantly less than that among the full-term ($\overline{X}$ = 4.35 bpm). The heart rate response of the preterm was thus smaller than that observed in the full-term, even when behavioral responses were similar and involved large muscle movements.

A second issue that puzzled us about the relation between behavioral and cardiac measures was their differential sensitivity to the responsivity of full-term and preterm infants. In full-term infants, heart rate proved to be a more sensitive index of stimulus perception than did behavior. Whereas full-term infants responded behaviorally only to the strongest stimuli, they responded with heart rate acceleration to weaker stimuli as well. This relation was anticipated, since Campos and Brackbill (1973) had earlier reported that significant cardiac changes sometimes occur even in the absence of behavioral responses. Moreover, heart rate was consistently found to be a more sensitive response measure, not only in active sleep, as seen here, but also in quiet sleep (Rose, Schmidt, & Bridger, 1978).

Yet in preterm infants the relation was just the opposite: these infants showed no significant heart rate response to any of the stimuli, but did show a behavioral response to the strongest of the three. Perhaps these differences reflect a difference in cardiovascular functioning. This is suggested by the heightened resting heart rate seen in the preterm, although this high tonic level of autonomic nervous system activation does not, in and of itself, preclude significant cardiac acceleration. Some preterm infants with high prestimulus heart rates do respond and even have as large a cardiac response as do full-term infants. A question does arise as to whether the range of cardiac activation is similar in full-term and preterm infants but simply shifted upward in the preterm, or whether the range itself is obscured among the preterm. In order to find out more about the upper limits of cardiac arousal heart rates were sampled during intervals where the infant was crying lustily. The average of 12 such 5-sec intervals was taken for each of 8 preterm infants. The mean heart rate during these periods was $\overline{X}$ = 184.8 bpm (SD = 8.55 bpm), a value quite comparable to that observed in full-term infants. Thus, while the cardiac values representing the upper limits of activation are similar in preterm and full-term infants, the lower limits are not. It remains to be determined whether the lack of cardiac responsivity in preterm infants is related to this difference in autonomic functioning, to threshold differences in sensitivity, or perhaps to a poor integration of autonomic and motor systems.

In the second study (Rose et al., 1980), the responsivity of full-term and preterm infants was examined over a longer period of time by continuing testing throughout the first sleep cycle, so that infants were tested in both active and quiet sleep. Several changes were introduced in an effort to enhance responding among the preterm. First, only the strongest stimulus (5.46) was used, since this was the only one which had evoked any response whatsoever from the preterm in the first study. Second, intertrial intervals were increased somewhat (to $\overline{X}$ = 50 sec). Third, control trials were interposed between successive stimulus trials, and the stimulus trials themselves were alternated between the right and left sides of the lower abdomen. These latter modifications were made to offset any possible response fatigue and to compensate for any lengthier refractory period that might exist among preterm infants. Additionally, because of the discovery of a biphasic response in quiet sleep, two 5-sec poststimulus periods were used and two sets of difference scores computed. One set constituted the change between the prestimulus and first poststimulus period, and the second constituted the change between the prestimulus and second poststimulus period.

Nonetheless, as can be seen in Figures 3-3 and 3-4, the results for the first epoch of active sleep were very similar to those found in the earlier study (Rose et al., 1976). Again, full-term infants responded with a significant cardiac acceleration to the stimulus, whereas preterm infants failed to respond ($\overline{X}$ = 3.5 bpm and $\overline{X}$ = 1.6 bpm, respectively). Again, both groups had a significant behavioral response, but the preterm infant's response was weaker ($\overline{X}$ = 1.3 bpm) than the full-term infant's ($\overline{X}$ = 1.8 bpm), and the correlations between behavioral ratings and heart rate change scores were also weaker.

In quiet sleep, full-term infants showed a cardiac acceleration that was significant and of similar magnitude to that seen in active sleep ($\overline{X}$ = 5.0 bpm). In fact, the actual values were quite similar to those found in an earlier study (Rose, Schmidt, & Bridger, 1978).[†] In this sleep state, preterm infants also demonstrated a cardiac response, although this response differed in several ways from that observed in the full-term. First, the acceleration, though significant, was small, averaging only about 1 beat. Second, the response form itself was different; wherever there had been a discernible

---

[†] Although there were no differences in responsivity between the first epochs of active and quiet sleep, it should be noted that full-term infants do show a marked elevation in threshold for both sleep states in the second sleep cycle (Rose, Schmidt, & Bridger, 1978). To my knowledge, comparable data for preterm infants are not available.

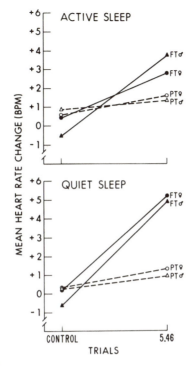

Figure 3-3

Mean heart rate change scores on control trials and in response to tactile stimulation with the 5.46 filament during the first epochs of active and quiet sleep.

response in the active sleep of either group or in the quiet sleep of the full-term, the response had taken the form of a monophasic acceleration during the first 5 sec and had then either remained on a plateau or approached base line during the next 5 sec; in the quiet sleep of the preterm, however, there was a biphasic response, with the slight cardiac acceleration during the first 5 sec followed by a deceleration below base line during the next 5 sec. This deceleration averaged close to 2 beats. Both the initial acceleration and the subsequent deceleration, while small, were significant.

As in active sleep, there was a significant behavioral response for both groups, although here too the behavioral score of the full-term ($\overline{X} = 1.5$) was significantly greater than that of the preterm ($\overline{X} = 0.6$), and the correlations between behavioral responsivity and cardiac change scores were greater too.

It should be noted that two aspects of risk, namely, birth weight and gestational age at birth, were correlated not only with basal (prestimulus) heart rate, as previously mentioned, but with cardiac responsiveness as well

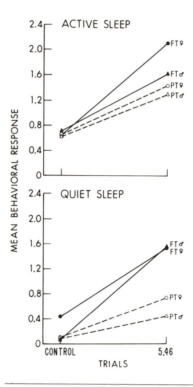

Figure 3-4

Mean behavioral response on control trials and in response to tactile stimulation with the 5.46 filament during the first epochs of active sleep and quiet sleep.

($r = .38$ and $r = .22$ in active sleep, and $r = .49$ and $r = .39$ in quiet sleep). Thus infants who were heavier and more mature at birth were more responsive during testing.

MODIFYING SLEEP AND RESPONSIVITY IN THE PRETERM

It is worth noting here that at least certain aspects of the preterm infant's functioning seem to be mutable, and even readily affected by different types of environmental interventions (see Schmidt, 1975). For example, in the 1980 study by Rose et al. we included a group of preterm infants who had been exposed to a systematic program of stimulation during their early days on the intensive care unit. This program emphasized tactile, proprioceptive, and vestibular stimulation and incorporated, but to a lesser extent, some auditory and visual components as well. A regimen of gentle

massaging and rocking formed the core of the intervention, which was initiated within the first 2 weeks after birth and was then administered daily, 5
days a week, for three 20-min periods. The regimen was terminated at least
1 day prior to testing. One of the major results of this intervention was an
increase in the preterm infant's cardiac responsivity in active sleep; in fact,
the magnitude of the cardiac response actually approached that seen among
the full-term (Rose et al., 1980).

In yet another study (Schmidt, Rose, & Bridger, 1980), half the preterm
from the sample used in the 1980 study of Rose et al. were also tested in the
presence of the tape-recorded sound of a human heartbeat (72 bpm) at
79–81 dB (C scale). This sound was turned on immediately after sleep onset,
and continued uninterruptedly throughout testing. It was introduced because several studies had shown that full-term infants respond to such a
repetitive auditory stimulus with a reduction in their own heart rate, an increased regularity of their respiration, and an increased duration of quiet
sleep (Brackbill, 1971, 1973). We were particularly intrigued by the
possibility of lowering the preterm infant's own cardiac levels with the
introduction of sound. We thought that, by virtue of a lower prestimulus
level (and in accord with the law of initial value), the magnitude of the
cardiac response evoked by superimposed tactual stimuli might then be increased. Despite these expectations, heartbeat sound turned out to have
very little effect on the base-line heart rate. Even in the presence of sound,
the preterm infant's resting heart rate remained 30 beats higher than that of
the full-term.

However, the introduction of the heartbeat sound did have a substantial impact on the preterm infant's sleep states, motility patterns, and cardiac responsiveness, with the sound bringing the functioning of the preterm
closer to the full-term norm. With sound, the lengthy first epoch of active
sleep was reduced from an average of 33 min to one of 18 min, a figure comparable to that of full-term infants. There was also a decrease in "restlessness," that is, the frequency of spontaneous motor movements in active
sleep, and an increase in the cardiac responsiveness evoked in active sleep to
the superimposed tactile stimuli. Thus the introduction of the heartbeat
sound affected cardiac responsiveness in much the same way as the intervention did, and, in addition, it affected sleep and motility. Further
observation of the infants suggested that, although heartbeat sound did not
affect cardiac rate, it did markedly reduce the irregularity of respiration in
active sleep. This observation raises the possibility that these two parameters of psychophysiological functioning may be less well coupled in the
preterm than in the full-term. Unfortunately, however, respiration was not
monitored polygraphically and thus there are no hard data which bear
directly on this issue. It would be useful to study the relation between heart
rate and respiration further, since it has important implications for understanding the psychophysiology of the preterm infant.

SUMMARY

The work with full-term and preterm neonates cited in the chapter has revealed numerous differences between the two groups, some of which are striking. These differences were present even when the preterm were close to term age. Preterm infants exhibit a far lengthier first epoch of active sleep, a markedly elevated tonic heart rate, and what could be characterized as a somewhat more "restless" pattern of spontaneous motoric activity during sleep, especially during active sleep. There are also significant differences in their cardiac and behavioral responsivity to tactile stimulation. Preterm infants showed (1) less behavioral responsiveness to tactile stimuli, (2) no discernible heart rate response in active sleep, (3) a smaller initial heart rate acceleration in quiet sleep, (4) a biphasic heart rate response during quiet sleep that is unlike the accelerative response more typically found in full-term infants, and (5) a low correlation between behavioral activation and heart rate change. It is unclear whether the dampening of behavioral responsivity is due mainly to a higher threshold for stimulation, to an inability of the organism to maintain vigorous responding even when the stimulus is perceived, or to a combination of the two. Given the same stimuli, the preterm infant more often failed to respond and often produced movements that were smaller and less vigorous than those of the full-term infant. Even when the preterm infant did have large behavioral responses, these responses were not accompanied by a heart rate acceleration as large as that seen in the full-term infant. Overall, there appear to be substantial behavioral and psychophysiological sequelae of preterm birth, even when the infant is at or close to term age.

REFERENCES

Anders, T., Emde, R., & Parmelee, A. (Eds.). *A manual of standardized terminology, techniques and criteria for scoring of states of sleep and wakefulness in newborn infants.* Los Angeles: University of California, Los Angeles, Brain Information Service, 1971.

Ashton, R. The effects of the environment upon state cycles in the human newborn. *Journal of Experimental Child Psychology*, 1971, *12*, 1–9.

Ashton, R., & Connolly, K. The relation of respiration rate and heart rate in the human newborn. *Developmental Medicine and Child Neurology*, 1971, *13*, 180–187.

Block, J., & Bridger, W. H. The law of initial value in psychophysiology: A reformation in terms of experimental and theoretical considerations. *Annals of the New York Academy of Sciences*, 1962, *98*, 1229–1241.

Brackbill, Y. Cumulative effects of continuous stimulation on arousal level in infants. *Child Development*, 1971, *42*, 17–26.

Brackbill, Y. Continuous stimulation reduces arousal level: Stability of the effect over time. *Child Development*, 1973, *44*, 43-46.

Campos, J., & Brackbill, Y. Infant state: Relationship to heart rate, behavioral responses and response decrement. *Developmental Psychobiology*, 1973, *6*, 9-19.

Canestrini, S. Uber das Sinnesleben des Neugeborenen (nach physiologischen Experimenten). *Monographien aus dem Gesamtgebiete der Neurologie und Psychiatrie*, 1913, *5*, 1-104.

Caputo, D. V., & Mandell, W. Consequences of low birth weight. *Developmental Psychology*, 1970, *3*, 363-383.

Clifton, R., & Nelson, M. N. Developmental study of habituation in infants: The importance of paradigm, response system and state. In T. Tighe & R. Leaton (Eds.), *Habituation: Perspective from child development, animal behavior and neurophysiology*. Hillsdale, N.J.: Lawrence Erlbaum, 1976.

Cohen, L. B., & Salapatek, P. (Eds.). *Infant perception: From sensation to perception* (Vols. 1 and 2). New York: Academic, 1975.

Czerny, A. Baobachtungen uber den Schlaf im Kindesalter unter physiologischen Verhaltnissen. *Jahrbuch fuer Kinderheikunde*, 1891, *33*, 1-28.

Davies, P. A. Infants of very low birthweight. In Hull, D. (Ed.), *Recent advances in pediatrics (Vol. 5)*. Edinburgh: Churchill Livingstone, 1976.

Davies, P. A., & Tizard, J. P. M. Very low birthweight and subsequent neurologist defect. *Developmental Medicine and Child Neurology*, 1975, *17*, 3-17.

DeHirsch, K., Jansky, J. J., & Langford, W. S. Comparisons between prematurely and maturely born children at three age levels. *American Journal of Orthopsychiatry*, 1966, *36*, 616-628.

Dorros, K. G., Brody, N., & Rose, S. A. A comparison of auditory behavior in the premature and fullterm infant: The effects of intervention. In H. D. Kimmel, E. H. van Olst, and J. F. Orlebeke (Eds.), *The orienting reflex in humans*. New York: Lawrence Erlbaum, 1979.

Dreyfus-Brisac, C. Ontogenesis of human sleep in human prematures after thirty-two weeks of conceptual age. *Developmental Psychobiology*, 1970, *3*, 91-121. (a)

Dreyfus-Brisac, C. Sleeping behavior in abnormal newborn infants. *Neuropaediatrie*, 1970, *3*, 351-366. (b)

Dreyfus-Brisac, C. Organization of sleep in prematures: Implication for caretaking. In H. Lewis & L. A. Rosenbaum (Eds.), *The effects of the infant on its caregiver*. New York: Wiley, 1974.

Drillien, C. M. *The growth and development of the prematurely born infant*. Edinburgh: Livingstone, 1964.

Field, T. M., Dempsey, J. R., Hatch, J., Ting, G., & Clifton, R. K. Cardiac and behavioral responses to repeated tactile and auditory stimulation by preterm and term neonates. *Developmental Psychology*, 1979, *15*, 406-416.

Fitzhardinge, P. M., Pape, K., Arstikaitis, M., Boyle, M., Ashby, S., Rowley, A., Netley, C., & Sawyer, P. R. Mechanical ventilation of infants of less than 1,501 gm birth weight: Health, growth and neurologic sequelae. *Journal of Pediatrics*, 1976, *88*, 531-541.

Fitzhardinge, P. M., & Ramsay, M. The improving outlook for the small prematurely born infant. *Developmental Medicine and Child Neurology*, 1973, *15*, 447–459.

Francis-William, J., & Davies, P. A. Very low birthweight and later intelligence. *Developmental Medicine and Child Neurology*, 1974, *16*, 709–728.

Graham, F. K., & Jackson, J. C. Arousal systems and infant heart rate response. In L. P. Lipsitt & H. W. Reese (Eds.), *Advances in child development and behavior* (Vol. 5.) New York: Academic, 1970.

Grellong, B. A., Vaughn, H. G., Rotkin, L., Daum, C., Kurtzberg, D., & Lipper, E. *Neonatal performance, cognitive and neurologic outcome to 40 months among low birthweight infants.* Paper presented at the biennial meeting of the Society for Research in Child Development, Boston, April 1981.

Harmeling, J. D., and Jones, M. B. Birthweights of high school dropouts. *American Journal of Orthopsychiatry*, 1968, *38*, 63–66.

Kero, P. Heart rate variation in infants with the respiratory distress syndrome. *Acta Paediatrica Scandinavia Supplement* 1974, *70*, 250.

Kitchen, W. H., Ryan, M. M., Richards, A., McDougall, A. B., Billson, F. A., Keir, E. H., & Naylor, F. D. A longitudinal study of very low-birthweight infants IV: An overview of performance at eight years of age. *Developmental Medicine and Child Neurology*, 1980, *22*, 172–188.

Knoblock, H., & Pasamanick, B. Prospective studies on the epidemiology of reproductive casualty: Methods, findings, and some implications. *Merrill-Palmer Quarterly of Behavior and Development*, 1966, *12*, 27–43.

Lubchenco, L. O. *The High Risk Infant.* Philadelphia: Saunders, 1976.

Murray, B., & Campbell, D. Sleep states in the newborn: Influence of sound. *Neuropaediatrie*, 1971, *2*, 335–342.

Osofsky, J. (Ed.). *Handbook of infant development.* New York: Wiley, 1979.

Parmelee, A. Neurophysiological and behavioral organization of premature infants in the first months of life. *Biological Psychiatry*, 1975, *10*, 501–502.

Parmelee, A. H., Bruck, K., & Bruck, M. Activity and inactivity cycles during sleep of premature infants exposed to neutral temperatures. *Biologia Neonatorum*, 1962, *4*, 317–339.

Parmelee, A. H., Wenner, W. H., Akiyama, Y., Stern, E., and Flescher, J. Electroencephalography and brain maturation. In A. Minkowski (Ed.), *Regional development of the brain in early life.* Oxford: Blackwell, 1966.

Parmelee, A. H., Wenner, W. H., & Schultz, H. R. Infant sleep patterns: From birth to sixteen weeks of age. *Journal of Pediatrics*, 1964, *65*, 576–582.

Prechtl, H. F. R., Akiyama, Y., Zinkin, R., & Grant, D. K. Polygraphic studies of the full-term newborn: I. Technical aspects and qualitative studies. In R. MacKeith & M. Bax (Eds.), *Studies in infancy.* London: SIMP/Heinemann, 1968.

Rawlings, G., Reynolds, E. O. R., Stewart, A., & Strang, L. B. Changing prognosis for infants of very low birthweight. *Lancet*, 1971, *1*, 516–519.

Roffwarg, H. P., Muzio, J. W., & Dement, W. C. Ontogenetic development of the human sleep-dream cycle, *Science*, 1966, *152*, 604–619.

Rose, S. A. Enhancing visual recognition memory in preterm infants. *Developmental Psychology*, 1980, *16*, 85–92. (a)

Rose, S. A. Lags in cognitive competence of prematurely born infants. In S. L.

Friedman & M. Sigman (Eds.), *Preterm birth and psychological development*. New York: Academic, 1980. (b)

Rose, S. A., Gottfried, A. W., & Bridger, W. H. Cross-modal transfer in infants: Relationship to prematurity and socio-economic background. *Developmental Psychology*, 1978; *14*, 643–652.

Rose, S. A., Gottfried, A. W., & Bridger, W. H. Effects of haptic cues on visual recognition memory in fullterm and preterm infants. *Infant Behavior and Development*, 1979, *2*, 55–67.

Rose, S. A., Schmidt, K., & Bridger, W. H. Cardiac and behavioral responsivity to tactile stimulation in premature and full-term infants. *Developmental Psychology*, 1976, *12*, 311–320.

Rose, S. A., Schmidt, K., & Bridger, W. H. Changes in tactile responsivity during sleep in the human newborn infant. *Developmental Psychology*, 1978, *14*, 163–172.

Rose, S. A., Schmidt, K., Riese, M. L., & Bridger, W. H. Effects of prematurity and early intervention on responsivity to tactual stimuli: A comparison of preterm and fullterm infants. *Child Development*, 1980, *51*, 416–425.

Rubin, R. A., Rosenblatt, M. A., & Balow, B. Psychological and educational sequelae of prematurity. *Pediatrics*, 1973, *52*, 352–363.

Schmidt, K. The effect of continuous stimulation on the behavioral sleep of infants. *Merrill-Palmer Quarterly*, 1975, *21* (2), 77–88.

Schmidt, K., & Birns, B. The behavioral arousal threshold in infant sleep as a function of time and sleep state. *Child Development*, 1971, *42*, 269–277.

Schmidt, K., Rose, S. A., & Bridger, W. H. The law of initial value and neonatal sleep states. *Psychophysiology*, 1974, *2*, 44–52.

Schmidt, K., Rose, S. A., & Bridger, W. H. The effect of heartbeat sound on the cardiac and behavioral responsiveness to tactual stimulation in sleeping premature infants. *Developmental Psychology*, 1980, *16*, 175–184.

Stewart, A. L., & Reynolds, E. O. R. Improved prognosis for infants of very low birthweight. *Pediatrics*, 1974, *54*, 724–735.

Taub, H. B., Goldstein, K. M. & Caputo, D. V. Indices of neonatal prematurity as discriminators of development in middle childhood. *Child Development*, 1977, *48*, 797–805.

Wagner, I. The establishment of the criterion of depths of sleep in infants. *Journal of Genetic Psychology*, 1937, *51*, 17–59.

Wilder, J. *Stimulus and response: The law of initial value*. Bristol: Wright, 1967.

4

Attention and Arousal in Preterm and Full-Term Neonates

Judith M. Gardner, Bernard Z. Karmel

PROBLEMS AND ISSUES

Over the past two decades medical progress in prenatal, perinatal, and postnatal care has improved the survival rate of immature and sick infants, especially those born with a very low birth weight. These advances, however, have been accompanied by certain consequences, the result of which has been unusual or abnormal growth in structural and functional organization. Although the incidence of major neurological defects such as spastic displegia (Davies & Tizard, 1975) appears to be decreasing in this group, there appears to be an increase in the incidence of more subtle cognitive and perceptual dysfunctions (Caputo, Goldstein, & Taub, 1981; Grellong, Vaughan, Rotkin, Daum, Kurtzberg, & Lipper, 1981; Kitchen, Ryan, Richards, McDougall, Billson, Keir, & Naylor, 1980; see also Rie & Rie, 1980).

This emergent human problem brought about by knowledge applied to

This research was supported, in part, by National Research Service Awards from the National Institutes of Mental Health (predoctoral MH 14280 and postdoctoral MH 15151) awarded to J. M. Gardner.

The authors wish to express their gratitude to the medical and nursery staffs of the Neonatal Intensive Care Unit and the Newborn Nursery of the Bronx Municipal Hospital Center for their cooperation. Our deep appreciation and gratitude also go to Gerald Turkewitz for his support and guidance throughout many facets of this research.

human development affects the distribution of capabilities in the population as a whole; that is, the proportion of the different forms of cognitive impairment to estimates of normality is being altered. At a minimum, this state of affairs calls for a better understanding of central nervous system function and organization. How such atypical early experiences as immaturity and illness are expressed in the altered development of brain activity and of behavior becomes even more important if the specific reasons for the more subtle effects seen in perceptual and cognitive disorders at later ages are to be understood (Karmel, Kaye, & John, 1978).

Healthy full-term infants are born with their physiological systems coordinated and well adapted for survival in the extrauterine environment. If this were true of preterm or sick infants, the problem of understanding the effects of atypical early experiences would be less difficult. Preterm infants are not just immature full-term infants to be studied as such. Direct comparisons between preterms at term age and full-term neonates may not be completely justified; that is, the nature of prematurity and early illness are such that once they occur, they alter the course and duration of subsequent developmental sequences. Thus atypical early experiences are not directly changing the organization of an already matured system; instead, because of the general plasticity present in the developing nervous system and the dynamic interactive nature of developmental processes, early experiences act both to *rearrange* functional connections in the brain undergoing change and to *reorganize* and *redirect* the development of behavior.

Moreover, what appear to be major deviations in structural and functional organization may alter the course of development but not necessarily prevent normality from eventually occurring. A case in point is the recent report of a hydrocephalic college student having a markedly reduced cortex as indicated by computerized tomography (CT) scans, but whose adult intellectual level of functioning was normal ("Research News," 1980). Additional support is found in data indicating that complete hemispherectomy in infancy may alter cognitive attainment in only very subtle ways which may not be easily detectable on standardized tests of intellectual functioning (Griffith & Davidson, 1966; McFie, 1961; Piercy, 1964).

Preterm and sick infants represent a group set apart from the rest of the population of infants. They are heterogeneous in that they differ in gestational age, birth weight, and adequacy of intrauterine growth for gestational age, in addition to other numerous prenatal, perinatal, and postnatal conditions. They have many and diverse medical problems that are treated by a variety of medical procedures which may vary from one hospital group to the next. Except for extremely adverse conditions such as severe neurological malformations or deficits, knowledge of how any of these effects or combinations of them relate to subsequent outcome, if at all, is limited. Even such neurological insults as intraventricular bleeding or hydrocephalus, which in the past were presumed to be inevitably associated with a very poor outcome, have recently been shown not to have such clear-cut negative effects (see above and Giuffre, Palma, & Fontana, 1979). In fact, depressed Bayley scores at 1 year are related only to the severest category of intraventricular bleeding, and even then it is the motor and not the mental score which is depressed (Ross & Schechner, 1980).

Increasing support for interactive or transactional processes (Sameroff & Chandler, 1975) accounts for some preterm infants having later dysfunction while others do not. For example, evidence for the ameliorating effect of social interactions comes from a recent longitudinal study by Parmelee and co-workers (Beckwith, Cohen, Kopp, Parmelee, & Marcy, 1976; Parmelee, Kopp, & Sigman, 1976; Sigman, Cohen, & Forsythe, 1981; Sigman & Parmelee, 1979) showing that outcome is only indirectly related to pre- and post-natal complications or medical problems during infancy. It is mediated by the quality of mother–infant interactions, which in turn is affected by the status of the infant at birth. These examples, as well as others, force us to conclude that conditions such as prematurity and early illness which are markedly deviant with respect to both experiential and biological factors may produce only subtle or small deviations from normal functioning in adulthood.

The converse with respect to early experiential and biological factors may also be true in that what appears to have only minor or transient effects very early in life may be amplified by development to become major difficulties later in life (Hebb, 1942; Parmelee, 1975; Schneider, 1979; also see Thoman, 1981). There are numerous "resolved" medical problems which show up later as severe medical problems or cognitive deficits. One example is the variability of bradycardia, respiration, and apnea in presumably healthy babies. These conditions may be manifestations of immaturity or disorganization in the brainstem or associated regions, the result of which could be sudden infant death syndrome, seizures, or attention disorders found at older ages. Given these alternative but not mutually exclusive possibilities, a host of developmental uncertainties arise. This chapter represents our initial attempts to address these issues.

We assume that structural and functional organization in the infant would be reflected by the processes of arousal, orientation, and attention to stimulation. Such basic characteristics are relevant to an integrated transaction between an organism and the environment throughout the organism's life-span. The subsequent series of studies were motivated by these ideas and specific assumptions. We attempted to provide both reference data for subsequent studies of preterm infants and evidence concerning early determinants of attentional behavior that could relate to structural development in the brain which could in turn influence later perceptual and cognitive organization in behavior.

Arousal as an Important Neurobiological
and Neurobehavioral Effect on Early Function

In the preterm infant, the immaturity of the nervous system and differing degrees of adaptive readiness of various subsystems appear to be manifested biologically in adverse physical problems such as intraventricular bleed, and functionally in a lack of state organization. These conditions generally are associated with a lowered functional and structural coherence or integrity within the central nervous system. The items on neonatal neurobehavioral assessments tend to bear out these differences. Most frequently, items that differentiate the preterm from the full-term infant are those that deal with interactive processes and state organization (although motoric processes are also important) (Brazelton, Als, Tronick, & Lester, 1979; Kurtzberg, Daum, Grellong, Albin & Rotkin, 1979). These types of internal mechanisms relating state organization to behavioral and central nervous system integration have been proposed to explain differences in interactions with objects and people at later ages (Field, 1979).

Modulation of state or coherent organization affecting the infant's level of arousal has been proposed by a number of investigators to explain functioning. Recently Sroufe (1979) proposed a "tension release" model in which affective behaviors such as gaze aversion and smiling help the infant modulate arousal. Field (1981) has indicated some of the problems with this model, particularly the need to include organismic variables such as state and developmental change. She has extended and combined Stroufe's model with Sokolov's (1963) model of orienting and defensive responses to propose that preterm infants exhibit a restricted range of activation or a limited range of stimulation to which they will respond optimally. They tend to show a higher threshold for response to low-intensity stimuli and a lower threshold or disorganized responding to higher intensity stimuli. Field (1979) has shown that the behavior of mothers of preterm infants can, in fact, be counterproductive in that these mothers tend to overstimulate their nonresponsive infants, who then are more likely to become overaroused. Overaroused infants avert their gaze, thereby eliciting greater efforts from their mothers to attract their attention.

In trying to select those factors which might be relevant to the level of functioning needed to perform more cognitive types of tasks at later ages, the attentional and state-modulating capacities of the neonate therefore become prime candidates. Investigators of infant behavior have repeatedly recognized the importance of internal state and arousal level factors in determining both the amount and kind of responding to stimulation (Als, Lester, & Brazelton, 1979; Parmelee, 1975; Prechtl, 1974; Thoman, 1981). There is, however, little systematic knowledge about how normal fluctuations in internal state specifically affect reactions to external stimulation.

Effects of Arousal on Responsivity _____

Changes in state or level of arousal typically refer to changes from sleep when least aroused to agitation and crying when most aroused. Between these extremes are states such as drowsiness, quiet wakefulness, and active wakefulness. Changes in arousal level have been measured in various ways such as by recording heart rate or amount of movement. Although there generally has been agreement about the types of behavior which constitute a given state of arousal (see Korner, 1972; Prechtl, 1974), researchers label effects in a variety of ways, not necessarily reflecting unidimensional phenomena. Regardless, evidence exists for a relation between both spontaneously varying and manipulated state changes and general responsiveness to stimulation as measured behaviorally and psychophysiologically (see Berg & Berg, 1979). For example, relations between state and visual attentiveness have been reported (Giacoman, 1971; Korner, 1972), and differences in response to auditory (Ashton, 1973; Berg, Berg, & Graham, 1971; Campos and Brackbill, 1973; Hutt, Lenard, & Prechtl, 1969; Korner, 1972; Pomerleau-Malcuit & Clifton, 1973; Schulman, 1970), tactile (Lewis, Bartels, & Goldberg, 1967; Pomerleau-Malcuit & Clifton, 1973), and vestibular (Pomerleau-Malcuit & Clifton, 1973) stimulation have been found to be related to infants' states of arousal as measured by heart rate. In addition, a number of investigators have found differences in scalp-recorded evoked potentials to sensory stimulation when infants were in different sleep states and therefore had different background electroencephalograms (EEGs) (Barnet & Goodwin, 1965; Akiyama, Schulte, Schultz, & Parmelee, 1969; Ellingson, 1967; Hrbek, Hrbkova, & Lenard, 1969; Monod & Garma, 1971; Weitzman & Graziani, 1968; Weitzman, Fishbein, & Graziani, 1965).

Although spontaneously varying arousal levels can be studied, arousal can be manipulated or controlled by varying factors that affect the internal state of the infant (other than by use of sensory stimulation). Empirical studies using behavioral and heart rate measures have shown both feeding and swaddling to affect the infant's level of arousal. Korner (1972) found that prandial condition affected many of the behaviors used to differentiate the various levels of arousal. For example, she reported increases in activity, crying, and the number of shifts in state and decreases in sleep before feeding as compared to after feeding. Lipton, Steinschneider, and Richmond (1965) found similar effects due to swaddling condition, as did Chisholm (1978), who found less fussing and better attention when infants were swaddled on a cradle board. Korner (1972) also reported that infants were more responsive to auditory stimuli after feeding. Giacoman (1971) reported that infants cried less and were more attentive to visual stimuli after feeding and that this effect was enhanced if they were both swaddled and fed. Turkewitz, Fleischer, Moreau, Birch, and Levy (1966) noted changes in directional finger movements as a function of feeding condition. Infants' arousal levels, as determined by prandial condition, were also found to influence eye turns in response to lateralized auditory stimuli. When infants were more aroused (i.e., before feeding), they turned their eyes in the direction of the same auditory stimulus which was ineffective when they were less aroused (i.e., after feeding) (Turkewitz, Birch, Moreau, Levy, & Cornwell, 1966). Similarly, the same tactile stimulus was more effective in eliciting head turns before rather than after feeding (Prechtl, 1958; Turkewitz, Gordon, & Birch, 1965).

Pomerleau-Malcuit and Clifton (1973) observed differential effects of feeding condition on infants' responses to stimulation. After feeding infants' heart rates tended to increase in response to stimulation, whereas prior to feeding heart rates tended to decrease in response to the same stimulation. Lipton et al. (1965) found that not only were prestimulus heart rates lower when infants were swaddled, but there was an inverse relation between infants' states of arousal, as indicated by heart rate, and responsivity to tactile stimulation.

These studies show that infants' responses are dependent not only on external stimulation from the environment, but on the internal condition of the infant as well. The infant is thus not just a passive recipient of input from the world. Inasmuch as factors such as state or level of arousal reflect the internal condition of the infant, they are therefore likely to affect responding. Thus not only would too much or too little arousal affect performance on tasks such as orienting and attending, but variations in responding to the same external stimulus would be determined, in part, by the infant's capacity to modulate arousal through these orienting and attending behaviors.

Relation Between Visual Preferences and Arousal

The classic visual preference technique, as a measure of attention, is dependent on infants looking more at one member of a pair of simultaneously presented stimuli than at the other (Berlyne, 1958; Fantz, 1958). Although arousal level affects many types of responses to stimulation, its influence on preferential looking has not been systematically established. On the other hand, the organizing effect of stimulation per se has been suggested as a major mechanism affecting attention and orienting (Berlyne, 1960; Karmel & Maisel, 1975). Because information, in the formal sense, varies with the number of items along an informational dimension (see Attneave, 1959; Karmel, 1969), variations along any visual stimulus dimension typically presented to infants could be considered to lie on an information continuum.

With respect to young infants, McGuire and Turkewitz (1979) have interpreted changes along such stimulus dimensions as quantitatively contributing to a unitary dimension related to an effective intensity variation as defined by Schneirla (1965). Schneirla's concepts provide a general approach which has served as a research framework for workers in the field. These concepts are particularly relevant when dealing with organismic as well as stimulus variables, as effective intensity is determined by both the nature of the stimulus and the nature of the organism on which it impinges. One problem with this approach, which is also true for many others that deal with organismic variables such as state, is the difficulty in specifying the quantitative contribution of each of the determinants of effective intensity.

Looking preferences as measures of early attentional mechanisms have been studied by numerous investigators, with looking generally discussed in relation to some univariate quantitative dimension of stimulation such as brightness, number of angles, size and number of elements, contour density, and spatial and temporal frequency (Brennan, Ames, & Moore, 1966; Fantz & Fagan, 1975). It has, however, become increasingly evident that variations along any single dimension cannot account for observed preferences across studies in very young infants. Most likely, dimensions interact, so that looking is determined by some combined or multivariate effect. For example, in infants younger than 2 months of age, contour density preferences can be altered by changing the brightness of the stimulus (Mc-Carvill & Karmel, 1976), and pattern preferences can be altered by changing the total pattern size (Maisel & Karmel, 1978; Ruff & Turkewitz, 1975) and/or pattern brightness (Ruff & Turkewitz, 1979). In addition to this within-modality effect on preferences, between-modality effects have also been noted. Recent studies indicate that the presence of a sound affects neonates' brightness (Lewkowicz & Turkewitz, 1981) and contour (Lawson & Turkewitz, 1980) preferences. These interactions are quite involved and depend not only upon the type of stimulus being viewed but also upon the amount and modality of extra stimulation. For example, prestimulation with 8 Hz as compared to 2 Hz produces a shift in visual temporal frequency preference away from 8 Hz and toward slower frequencies, whether the 8 Hz is presented as a visual or auditory stimulus. However, within-modality (visual) prestimulation with 8 Hz appears to produce a greater shift in preference toward slower frequencies than does between-modality (auditory) prestimulation with 8 Hz (Gardner, Lewkowicz, & Rose, 1983).

These findings support the general position that young infants' responses are dependent on the contribution of both external (exogenous) and internal (endogenous) sources of stimulation. Given some preferred or total amount of stimulation that maximizes orienting toward a particular stimulus, any changes in this amount of stimulation (from whatever sources) should alter what the baby looks at. Thus, the same physical stimulus which is preferred when the baby is in a quiet attending state might not be preferred when his or her arousal is altered. Moreover, because the system is biologically self-limiting, the combined effects of external and internal factors must reach some maximal limit (Karmel & Maisel, 1975), thereby producing a directional relation such that when levels of arousal (and internal activity) are higher, the baby might orient toward a less intense stimulus and when levels of arousal (and internal activity) are lower, the baby might orient toward a more intense stimulus (see Field, 1981; Gardner, 1979). Whether this "maximal" level is also the "optimal" level (Dember & Earl, 1957) is a separate issue.

If our interest is in understanding and promoting active, awake involvement of the infant with the environment, investigation within the more restricted range of awake levels of arousal might be one specific goal. Experimentation involving arousal within this restricted range can be conducted nonintrusively by taking advantage of normally occurring arousal changes during the infant's day, as when the infant is fed or swaddled. The effects of arousal on preferential looking can thus be studied by testing infants before and after feeding and when they are unswaddled and swaddled.

STUDIES OF AROUSAL INFLUENCES ON VISUAL PREFERENCE FUNCTIONS

Studies 1 and 2: Initial Studies

Our initial studies related arousal levels, as modified by feeding and swaddling, to the visual preferences of preterm infants (Gardner, 1979; Gardner & Turkewitz, 1982). Because organized coherent functioning seemed to be a major problem with preterm and sick infants, even when they were assumed to be medically stable, these studies were conducted to (1) see whether either or both these manipulations would produce greater functional organization of the preterm infant's looking behavior, (2) serve as information indicating the present level of functioning against which subsequent levels of functioning might be compared, and (3) serve as a methodological exploration of optimal behavioral methods that could be subsequently used in evoked potential studies of the preterm. Feeding and swaddling effects on arousal were assumed to be cumulative. Infants were thus considered to be in the least aroused condition when tested after feeding while swaddled, in the most aroused condition when tested before feeding while unswaddled, and in two intermediate conditions when tested before feeding while swaddled or after feeding while unswaddled.

Two studies involving 16 preterm infants each were conducted. In each study, infants were tested just prior to their discharge from the Neonatal Intensive Care Unit (ICU) of Jacobi Hospital of the Bronx Municipal Hospital Center. All infants were from either black or Hispanic families of primarily lower socioeconomic status. Prematurity was defined as being born at or before 37 weeks of gestation as estimated by the Dubowitz method (Dubowitz, Dubowitz, & Goldberg, 1970). The infants varied with regard to their age at birth, the basis for their prematurity, and the medical procedures they received in the ICU. At testing, however, all weighed more than 2100 g and were considered medically stable. The mean estimated gestational ages at birth for the groups were 33.7 and 34.1 weeks, the mean birth weights were 1675.3 and 1799.1 g, and the mean postconceptional ages at the time of testing were 38.3 and 37.5 weeks.

The infants were tested twice within 1 hour before feeding and once within 1 hour after feeding on two successive days. On the second day, they were swaddled during the postfeeding test and during the second of the pre-feeding tests. This fixed sequence of arousal manipulations was established in order to provide a constant base line for all infants for future reference. Although it was recognized that sequence testing effects were confounded in this initial study, subsequent controls for sequential effects in the administration of arousal conditions indicated no significant effects of order of arousal manipulation either within or across days.

During testing, infants sat in a semireclining position on the lap of an assistant facing the back panel of a three-sided looking chamber modeled after one described by Fagan (1970). Stimulus presentations were initiated only when infants had their eyes open and were not crying. All infants were thus tested in a quiet, alert state (state 3 or 4 of the Prechtl scale; Prechtl, 1965). Between trials, a number of tactics were used to maintain this state, including talking, patting, stroking, and rocking.

The first group of infants (9 males and 7 females) viewed stimuli that varied in the size and in the number of elements. The stimuli were black cubes symmetrically arranged in rows and columns on white cards. They were chosen for their potential three-dimensional contrast salience and were patterned after those used by Jones-Molfese (1972). They consisted of one 2-inch cube, four 1-inch cubes, sixteen ½-inch cubes, and an unpatterned white stimulus card (zero cubes). Although the number of cubes is used here to describe the stimulus dimension, this description is recognized to covary with other dimensions, such as contour density and spatial frequency. The stimuli were presented in the following pairs: 0 and 1 cube, 1 and 4 cubes, and 4 and 16 cubes. Each of the six test sessions involved two 30-sec presentations of these three pairs of stimuli (with right–left positions reversed). The procedure replicated that of Jones-Molfese (1972) in order to allow cross-laboratory validation of preference effects as a function of stimulation, while at the same time introducing the added conditions related to arousal levels.

For the second group of infants (8 males and 8 females), the procedure was basically the same except that during the prefeeding–unswaddled condition, all infants were given a pacifier during and between trials. The introduction of the pacifier served to both facilitate maintenance of the head in the midline position and reduce bodily movement and fussiness. It was done, however, with the recognition that the pacifier might itself act to reduce arousal, but, in so doing, could then only act to decrease the magnitudes of the differences between the conditions.

These infants viewed stimuli that varied in frequency of illumination. The stimuli were homogeneous fields of light having square-wave-modulated frequencies of 0.5, 1, 2, and 4 Hz, with 100 percent depth of modulation and a 50 percent duty cycle. Thus they had equal on and off durations of 1000, 500, 250, and 125 msec. They were presented in the following pairs: 0.5 and 1 Hz, 1 and 2 Hz, and 2 and 4 Hz. These frequencies were selected because previous research indicated that 14-week-old infants showed both maximized evoked-potential signal strength and attentional responses to stimuli between 4 and 6 Hz (Karmel, Lester, McCarvill, Brown, & Hofmann, 1977). If the mechanisms controlling looking at temporal and spatial frequencies acted in a similar fashion, it was assumed likely that these younger babies would prefer stimuli of slower frequencies (i.e., about 2 Hz); that is, because young infants in general tend to look at larger spatial frequency pattern stimuli and a suspected relation between spatial and temporal effects had been reported at least for evoked potentials (Maffei, 1968), the range from 0.5 to 4 Hz was selected for evaluating preferences on both sides of an assumed curvilinear frequency preference function.

The duration of fixation for each of the stimuli was measured by an observer who looked through a centrally located peephole and recorded the direction of eye gaze. The heart rate of the infants viewing the frequency stimuli was recorded to provide a test of the assumption that feeding and swaddling affect arousal.

The data were analyzed with regard to three levels of arousal. The infant was considered to be most aroused when tested before feeding while unswaddled, least aroused when tested after feeding while swaddled, and at some intermediate level of arousal when tested either after feeding while unswaddled or before feeding while swaddled.

Similar systematic relations between the distribution of looking at the stimuli and the level of arousal were found regardless of the stimulus dimension used. The proportion of time directed at the stimulus having more cubes or a higher frequency increased from the most aroused condition (prefeeding–unswaddled) to the least aroused condition (postfeeding–swaddled). The mean proportions of time spent looking at the stimulus with more cubes were .51 (SD = .07) for the most aroused condition, .57

(SD = .08) for the intermediate aroused condition, and .60 (SD = .12) for the least aroused condition (see Fig. 4-1). For the lights, the mean proportions of time spent looking at the stimulus of higher frequency were .48, .54, and .61 (SD = .06, .10, and .10) for the three levels, from the most aroused to the least aroused condition (see Fig. 4-2). These differences were reflected in a significant treatment effect using repeated-measures analysis of variance (ANOVA) [for the cubes, $F(2,30) = 4.88$, $p < .02$; for the lights, $F(2,30) = 12.47$, $p < .01$].

The effects of arousal on looking behavior were not due to different amounts of attention in different states of arousal; that is, infants spent

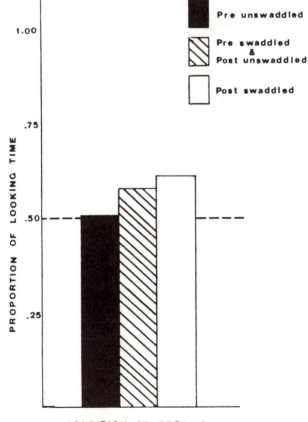

Figure 4-1

The proportion of time infants spent looking at the stimulus having more cubes as a function of the level of arousal (all pairs combined).

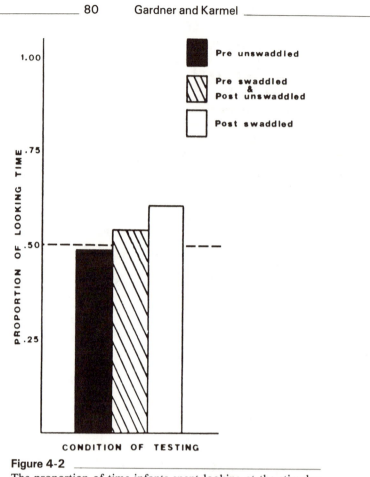

Figure 4-2

The proportion of time infants spent looking at the stimulus
having a faster frequency as a function of the level of arousal
(all pairs combined).

equivalent amounts of time looking when in different conditions. From the
most aroused to the least aroused condition, the mean looking times per
30-sec trial were 19.9, 22.1, and 23.3 sec for the cubes, and 20.6, 21.4, and
20.8 sec for the lights.

The assumption that feeding and swaddling influences arousal level
was supported by the finding that the infants' base heart rates differed as a
function of arousal condition. The base heart rate in a particular condition
was taken as the mean rate for 7 beats prior to each stimulus presentation in
that condition. As expected, the infants' heart rates were highest when they
were unswaddled prior to feeding, and lowest when they were swaddled
after feeding. Of 15 infants, 12 had their highest heart rates during the most
aroused condition, and only 1 infant had his lowest heart rate during this

condition. Their mean heart rates were 176.8 bpm (SD = 9.5), 172.1 bpm (SD = 6.7), and 166.2 bpm (SD = 6.7), and 166.2 bpm = 6.7) for the high, intermediate, and low levels of arousal, respectively ($p < .001$, Friedman one-way analysis of variance of ranks).

In summary, babies preferred looking at stimuli having higher spatial and temporal frequencies when they were fed and swaddled. However, when in the prefeeding–unswaddled condition, although the overall amount and variability of looking did not differ from other arousal conditions, babies showed no preferential responding. This observation suggests that there may be a disruption in looking with high levels of arousal, rather than a shift in preference from more intense to less intense or less informative stimuli. It is possible that if a broader range of stimulus conditions had been used, a preference for less intense or less informative stimuli may have been found at the highest arousal levels.

Study 3: Experimental Refinements and Extension of the Stimulus Range

This study was designed to examine whether the failure to obtain a preference for less intense or less informative stimuli at higher arousal levels stemmed from the restricted range of stimuli used, or whether it reflected a disruption of looking. Furthermore, methodological refinements were made to increase the possibility of detecting a shift in preference as a function of arousal conditions (Gardner & Turkewitz, 1982).

A total of 12 preterm infants (5 males and 7 females) were tested. The infants' mean estimated gestational age was 34.2 weeks, their mean birth weight was 1905 g, and their mean postconceptional age at the time of testing was 38.0 weeks. Infants were tested under only two arousal conditions: once unswaddled before feeding and once swaddled after feeding, the previous conditions which produced the largest differences in preferences. All possible pairings of stimuli were presented in order to obtain stimulus preference functions with which to evaluate shifts along the stimulus dimension, rather than simply changes in the relative amounts of looking between stimuli in each pair. The 1-, 4-, and 16-cube stimuli were the same as previously used; in addition, a stimulus having 64 ¼-inch cubes was included and the unpatterned stimulus was eliminated. The order of test condition was counterbalanced across infants. In each condition, infants were presented with different random sequences of the 12 pairs of stimuli according to a modified Graeco-Latin square in which each of the 6 possible pairs was presented with right–left positions reversed in half of each sequence, with no stimulus following itself in the same position.

As can be seen in Figure 4-3, visual preference functions were found at each level of arousal. In addition, a difference in the shape of the functions

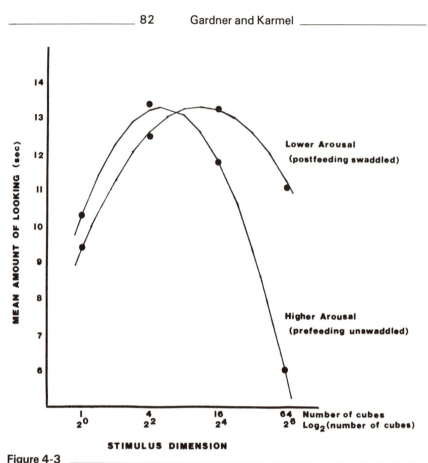

Figure 4-3

Looking preference functions (to cube stimuli) for infants at higher and lower levels of arousal. Data points are for observed means.

was found between the two levels. Looking in both conditions was best described by inverted U-shaped curves. Separate repeated-measures trend analyses on the amount of time each infant looked at the stimuli indicated significant quadratic components for each condition [for prefeeding-unswaddled, $F(1,11) = 15.09, p < .003$; for postfeeding–swaddled, $F(1,11) = 9.21, p < .02$]. Infants looked most at stimuli of intermediate value, and looked less at those of higher or lower value. The quadratic equations describing the preference functions are $Y = 10.29 + 2.59X - 0.55 X^2$ and $Y = 9.37 + 2.30X - 0.33 X^2$ for the more aroused and less aroused conditions, respectively. As can also be seen in Figure 4-3, there was a marked reduction in the amount of time infants looked at the most intense stimulus when they were more aroused, with no such marked reduction when they were less aroused. This resulted in the function for the more aroused condition being skewed and containing a significant linear component [$F(1,11) =$

7.32, $p < .02$], with no such significant linear component in the function for the less aroused condition. These differences between conditions in the characteristics of the response to stimuli were revealed by a significant condition × stimulus interaction between linear trends [$F(1,11) = 12.53$, $p < .005$] and an overall condition × stimulus interaction [$F(3,33) = 2.83$, $p < .05$].

The data suggest an inverse relation between arousal level and preferred visual stimulus, with infants looking longest at the 16-cube stimulus when less aroused, and at the 4-cube stimulus when more aroused. This was supported by the results of the regression analyses, which indicated maxima of 11.3 and 5.3 cubes, respectively, for the functions of the less aroused and more aroused conditions. Thus, in this study, a significant preference was obtained in the higher as well as in the lower arousal condition, indicating that the effects of arousal on preferential looking cannot be understood simply in terms of disruption of differential looking with increasing arousal. Rather, an explanation which considers shifts in preference with shifts in arousal level is required.

Discussion of Studies 1, 2, and 3

The results of these studies are clear in indicating that the visual attention of preterm infants is influenced by their state. The interaction between visual preference and internal state suggests that attention to features of the world is, in part, determined by the infant's internal organization at the time of stimulation. The direction of the shift in preference is such that more "intense" or "informative" stimuli are preferred when infants are less aroused, and less "intense" or "informative" stimuli are preferred when infants are more aroused. This relation between level of arousal and level of stimulation appears fairly obvious for marked state differences. Sleeping infants thus respond only to relatively intense stimuli, and highly aroused infants close their eyes or turn away from almost all incoming stimuli. The fact that this relation exists within the restricted range of arousal levels encompassed within the present studies reinforces the importance of the influence of the state of arousal on the type of environmental information being attended to by the infant. Furthermore, a self-limiting assumption when endogenous and exogenous stimulation factors interact could now be unambiguously and directly inferred from the data.

There are several possible explanations for these findings. Not only are babies responsive to within- and between-modality variations in stimulation, but there appears to be a relation among these features such that looking is determined by their combination. One implication of this finding is that, as postulated by Schneirla (1965), for the neonate specific dimensional variations are not responded to as such, but only as they contribute to some combined or multivariate effect that can be understood only as a unitary or wholistic phenomenon. The finding of similar patterns of arousal effects when stimuli vary in spatial or temporary frequency is consistent with Schneirla's view in that it makes it likely that features of both types of stimuli were being responded to as varying along some common dimension. That is, the effect of stimulation was contributed to by the amount of stimulation from both endogenous and exogenous sources, regardless of whether the external source came from cubes or lights.

An explanation of the neural mechanisms mediating the activating properties of stimulation in determining infant attentional behavior has been hypothesized by Karmel (see Karmel & Maisel, 1975). This position contends that visual preferences are related to the activating properties of the stimuli, specifically to the degree to which visual stimuli produce coherence in neural activity. Preferred spatial patterns produce the greatest component amplitudes in visually evoked potentials (VEPs) recorded over occipital regions in older infants (Karmel, Hoffmann, & Fegy, 1974) and over widely distributed regions in younger infants (occipital, parietal, and posterior temporal; Hoffmann, 1978). It was assumed that the greater the magnitude of VEP components elicited, the greater the neural synchrony produced at some source generator level within the brain by the stimulus (Karmel & Maisel, 1975). Indeed, the distribution of these components across the scalp provided some evidence as to the generators or neuronal sources that were potentially involved. This stimulus-dependent correlation to "neural activity" was offered as a general guide to understanding the mechanisms relating infant attention to developing neuronal systems. As such, it relied only on the degree to which stimulation produced organized activity in visually related cortical and subcortical centers. Moreover, this position was supported by the large degree to which magnitudes of particular VEP components covaried with measures of behavioral attention (Karmel et al., 1974, 1977).

Because general arousal levels in preterm infants alter basic stimulus-dependent preferences as shown, we would extend this stimulus-specific neuronal activity hypothesis to suggest that whatever specific activating properties produce orientation to specific stimuli, these properties must be expanded to include input from the nonspecific (or tonic or gate-modulating) arousal systems that control central nervous system integrity as reflected by the general arousal implied by manipulations of feeding and swaddling. Our data indicate that at a minimum, these two systems (specific and nonspecific) interact in a reciprocal way. This finding suggests some general self-limiting or channel capacity features of the processing of both exogenous and endogenous sources of stimulation.

We would thus like to extend the more specific visually dependent neuronal activity hypothesis to cover internally generated arousal as well by suggesting that manipulation of arousal independent of stimulation interacts with the arousal effects produced by stimulation itself. More generally then, the amount of coherent neural activity, independent of the manner in which it is achieved, is an important determinant of infant attention. Given this conclusion, there would be a relation between the level of arousal of the infant and amount of external stimulation, with preferential looking determined by the extent to which this combination approached some "maximal" or "optimal" level of coherent neural activity directed toward some integrated behavioral state.

The mechanisms mediating this effect are not well understood. Regardless, they would likely involve at least the actions of the reticular formation on subcortical mechanisms controlling the young infant's visual behavior (Bronson, 1974; Hoffmann, 1978; Karmel & Maisel, 1975, Salapatek, 1975; Woodruff, 1978). The infant's lack of cortical inhibitory influences over lower brain regions (Gerrity & Woodruff, 1979; Lindsley & Wicke, 1974; McGraw, 1943) probably contributes to this effect. The exact degree of specificity of developing cortical inhibitory influences and their involvement in specific behavioral actions, however, remain to be determined. In theory, however, when infants were in the most aroused condition, that is, prefeeding–unswaddled, stimulation of the reticular formation from both specific and nonspecific sources, without concomitant inhibitory influences, could have produced high levels of self-perpetuating neuronal activity. When the amount of endogenous stimulation was reduced by feeding and swaddling, and possibly made more organized by low-intensity synchronous firing of the reticular formation through action of the intestines via afferent projections of the vagus nerve through the solitary tract of the medulla (Beckstead & Norgren, 1979; Magnes, Moruzzi, & Pompeiano, 1961; Morest, 1967; Sessle, 1973), the overall level of neural activity could have been decreased or at least made more coherent (Anokhin & Shuleikina, 1977; Kukorelli & Juhasz, 1977), resulting in increased looking at higher intensity stimuli.

A channel capacity explanation from an information-theoretic perspective therefore is concordant with these hypotheses in that high levels of internally produced neural activity could create preferences for stimuli having fewer additional activating properties, and lower levels of internally produced activity could allow for attention directed at more activating external stimuli.

How such a capacity itself could be dynamically altered with broader or more diverse fluctuations of state and stimuli remains to be detailed empirically, as does the developmental course of these events. The involvement of other modalities of stimulation that affect arousal levels is also of major theoretical interest. Regarding the neonate, it remains to be demonstrated that these effects require cortical systems for their functional organization.

An expansion of the temporal frequency aspects of our previous study addresses these issues.

TEMPORAL FREQUENCY PREFERENCE FUNCTIONS

Whatever the mechanisms underlying the relation between infant state and visual preference, they are likely to change, even during early stages of development. There is evidence that by 2–3 months of age, infants become less responsive to quantitative aspects of spatial visual stimuli, such as size and brightness, and more responsive to qualitative aspects of visual stimuli, such as form and configuration. It would be reasonable to hypothesize that developmental changes in response to temporal as well as spatial changes in stimulation are likely to occur. For spatial patterns, this has been interpreted as a generalized shift in preference toward stimuli with higher spatial frequencies (Brennan et al., 1966; Fantz & Fagan, 1975; Karmel, 1969).

Study 4: Preference Functions for Temporal Frequencies in Preterm Infants

In this study, we (Gardner & Karmel, 1981) evaluated the responses of a subset of the infants (of study 2) shown the frequency stimuli with an extended set of stimulus pairings presented after the original stimulation sequence had been fulfilled. A total of 11 infants (5 males and 6 females) viewed all possible pairings of the stimuli after feeding on two successive days. On the first day, they were unswaddled, and on the second day they were swaddled.

As can be seen in Figure 4-4, the amount of time spent looking at each stimulus increased with stimulus frequency. Figure 4-4 shows the observed mean amount of time infants looked at each of the four stimuli postfeeding–unswaddled and postfeeding–swaddled, and the power function describing the best-fitting curve for both arousal conditions combined. An arousal (2) × stimulus (4) repeated-measures ANOVA found both main effects to be significant [$F(1,10) = 9.07$ and $p < .01$ for the arousal factor, $F(3,30) = 6.27$ and $p < .002$ for the stimulus factor]. Examination of the stimulus effect revealed a significant linear trend between the amount of time spent looking and the stimulus frequency when the data from the two arousal levels were combined [$F(1,10) = 20.94$, $p < .001$], as well as for each arousal level separately [$F(1,10) = 5.88$ and $p < .04$ for postfeeding–unswaddled, $F(1,10) = 8.86$ and $p < .01$ for postfeeding–swaddled].

Of particular interest in this analysis and extension was the contrast of the present findings with what we might have anticipated from our knowledge of age-related shifts in preferential looking at spatial patterns. That is, we expected very young infants to show a preference shift toward lower temporal frequencies as they do with spatial frequencies, assuming

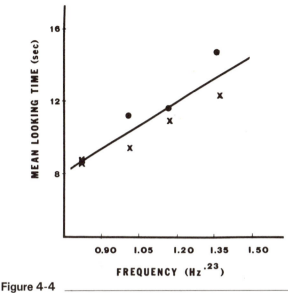

Figure 4-4

The amount of time infants spent looking at each stimulus plotted as a power function, $R = 9.55 \times S^{0.23}$, where $R =$ mean-looking time in sec combined for both days and $S =$ frequency in Hz. Data points are for observed means ($\times$, day 1; $\bullet$, day 2).

that the development of preferences to spatial and temporal frequencies is controlled by the same mechanisms. Consequently, because 3-month-olds had shown the most attention to stimuli between 4 and 6 Hz (Karmel et al., 1977), we assumed that preterm infants would prefer frequencies below 4 Hz. We found, however, that these infants preferred the highest frequency used in testing (4 Hz). Therefore the preterm infants did not show a shift to lower temporal frequencies as might have been inferred from younger infants' shifts in attention to lower spatial frequencies as compared to older infants. Another study was therefore designed to investigate the preference function to a wider range of temporal frequencies.

Study 5: Preference Functions for Temporal Frequencies in Full-Term Infants

In this study (Gardner & Karmel, 1982), we examined the influence of arousal on looking preferences to frequency stimuli up to 8 Hz in 12 full-term healthy neonates (5 males and 7 females). Procedures were identical to those discussed for study 2, except for the additional experimental controls subscribed to in study 3. The stimuli, however, were square-wave-modulated luminance frequencies of 1, 2, 4, and 8 Hz.

As seen in Figure 4-5, the infants looked most at the 8-Hz stimulus when they were fed and swaddled, and looked most at slower frequencies when prior to feeding and unswaddled. Separate repeated-measures trend analyses on the amount of time each infant looked at the stimuli indicated significant linear components for both the more aroused and the less aroused conditions [$F(1,11) = 5.00$ and $p < .05$, $F(1,11) = 12.32$ and $p < .005$, respectively], and a tendency toward a significant cubic component for the more aroused condition [$F(1,11) = 3.73$, $p < .08$]. The cubic and linear equations describing the preference functions are $Y = 12.22 + 17.17X - 6.76X^2 + 1.37X^3$ and $Y = 7.65 + 2.53X$ for the more aroused and less aroused conditions, respectively. These differences between conditions were revealed by a significant condition × stimulus interaction between linear trends [$F(1,11) = 13.00$, $p < .004$] and an overall condition × stimulus interaction [$F(3,33) = 7.22$, $p < .001$].

In summary, frequency preferences within the awake state interact with

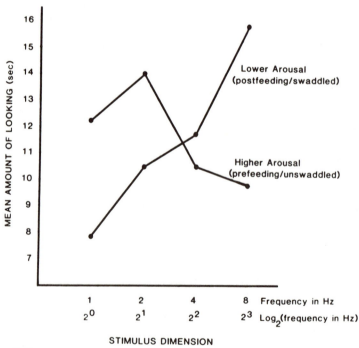

Figure 4-5

The amount of time infants spent looking at temporal frequency stimuli as a function of level of arousal.

arousal level such that an inverse relation exists between the level of arousal and the stimulus temporal frequency. As arousal increases, a shift in preference toward slower temporal frequency occurs, and as arousal decreases, a shift in preference toward faster temporal frequency occurs.

Discussion of Temporal Frequency Effects _____

These data are in agreement with recent evidence from evoked-potential studies which have expanded the temporal stimulus dimension previously reported by Karmel et al. (1977). Moskowitz and Sokol (1980) have indicated that at least two peaks or "optima" for evoked-potential amplitudes can be obtained in infants, one in the 4–6 Hz (in terms of pattern alternations/sec) range and one in the 8–10 Hz range. The former appears to be contrast dependent and the latter appears to be related to luminance effects. Spekreijse (1981) has indicated that luminance effects were reflected in the higher alternation rates discussed by Moskowitz and Sokol (1980). Because we used square-wave-modulated homogeneous fields of illumination in our studies, our data appear to be in line with these findings with the added influence of the interactive nature of stimulus effects and arousal. Moreover, preliminary analyses of data from a recent study (Karmel, Gardner, & Lewkowicz, 1983) also are in line with these findings and, in addition, reinforce our ideas about the interactive nature of stimulation in determining neonates' visual preferences. In this study, we evaluated the influence of spatial, temporal, or combined spatial and temporal frequencies. Comparisons of the preference functions obtained when each dimension was varied separately to those obtained when both dimensions were varied simultaneously indicated that spatial preferences were affected by the presence of different temporal frequencies but temporal preferences were less affected by the presence of different spatial frequencies. The strong systematic influences of arousal on such effects, however, as documented in the studies reported in this chapter, would argue that arousal mechanisms cannot be dismissed and must be systematically controlled if the mechanisms underlying the early processing of stimulus information are to be adequately understood. Further study is required if age-dependent changes in visual preferences and evoked-potential findings are to be integrated.

GENERAL DISCUSSION _____

The effects reported here and elsewhere allow us to speculate from an empirical basis as to the determinants of attentional behavior, both with regard to the structural development of the brain and the perceptual and cognitive organization of behavior. The well-documented shift in attentional responses to spatial stimuli shown by infants at about 2 months of age may be related to the development of contrast-sensitive neurons in the occipital cortex. These must in some way interact with developed subcortical systems connected to the retina, such as the lateral geniculate nucleus, superior colliculus, pretectum, reticular activating system, and/or limbic system.

VEP data provided by Hoffmann (1978) indicated that in 4-week-old infants a late negative component (after 500 msec), which was widely dispersed over the scalp and presumed subcortical in origin, was isomorphic with preference behavior at that age, even though an early-occurring positive component (primarily occipital) was clearly present. Although at birth projections to the visual cortex from at least one type of retinal ganglion cell appear to be well developed, projections to subcortical components of the specific sensory visual system as well as other nonspecific sensory systems such as the reticular system are, in general, more developed than cortical ones. However, even if the system is fairly mature, considerably more development takes place in the cortical neurons, myelination of thalamocortical tracts, and receptor field sizes and representations. One example (of many) is that cortical excitatory processes from the geniculate may develop prior to inhibitory projections which extend centrifugally both intra- and interhemispherically (Vaughan & Kurtzberg, 1981).

One explanation which has been proposed for understanding the mechanisms underlying the development of visual attention stems from data showing differential rates of development of two types of retinal cells and their pathways. Maurer and Lewis (1979) proposed that prior to 2 months of age, the infant's visual behavior is controlled by one set of receptors and their projections to the cortex, and changes that occur at about 2 months are due to the development of another set of projections to the cortex (see Maurer & Lewis, 1979, for a review of visual system development and behavioral correlates). A second explanation is that prior to 2 months of age, spatial and temporal preferences are predominantly controlled by subcortical mechanisms. Support for this position comes from anatomical and electrophysiological studies, as well as behavioral studies indicating that almost all of the visual behavior observed in the neonate prior to about 2 months of age can be accounted for on the basis of subcortical systems. Further evidence is provided by studies demonstrating that cortically lesioned animals and human neonates respond similarly to visual stimuli (Meyer, 1963; Pasik, Pasik, Nolan, & Solomon, 1976; Schilder, Pasik, & Pasik, 1972).

However, there is anatomical evidence of developed neurons and pathways to area 17 of the visual cortex (Purpura, 1975), even though various levels of the system in general are quite immature and a great deal of further change occurs in the systems subsequent to the neonatal period. For example, in neonates the macular region of the retina which contains the primary receptors involved in fine acuity and pattern discrimination has cones which are very immature as compared to receptors in more peripheral parts of the retina (Abramov, Gordon, Hendrickson, Hainline, Dobson, & LaBoissiere, 1981). On the other hand, there is electrophysiological evidence indicating a potential for cortical involvement with respect to some aspects of visual behavior (Harter, Deaton, & Odom, 1977; Moskowitz & Sokol, 1980). That is, VEPs with some components traced to cortical laminae can be obtained from infants as young as 26 weeks gestational age (Vaughan, 1975). However, in the studies of Moskowitz and Sokol and Harter et al., distributions of stimulus-dependent components over wider cortical regions as in Hoffman's (1978) study have not been generally studied, and their linkage to the data from Vaughan's studies is not clear. In addition, Harter and co-workers did not find that attentional responses were related to the early "cortical" components.

Evidence for cortical functioning does not mean that subcortical systems are not responsive, or that if cortical function is present it predominates in controlling behavior. We wish to emphasize that although at the stage of development with which we are concerned some cortical systems may be functional and interacting with other components of the nervous system, the cortex is still not highly developed. Indeed, it seems more likely that as the cortex matures, arousal effects such as those reported here would be reduced. That is, as the role of the cortex vis-à-vis other systems is largely inhibitory, we would anticipate that a subcortical focus for the mediation of behavior and arousal would be of lesser consequence for the functioning of the organism. Therefore, in view of the relative immaturity of the cortex during the neonatal period, an explanation of the observed effects in terms of cortical functioning seems both unnecessary and unlikely. We believe it more parsimonious to propose that subcortical systems (including the reticulomesencephalic projections of the specific and nonspecific tracts of the sensory systems, as well as the lateral geniculate, superior colliculus, pretectum, and limbic system) have the capacity to mediate the functional aspects of visual behavior observed in neonates, without postulating cortical control at a time when it is in such transition. As stated previously, we are not proposing that the cortex is nonfunctional, but that the system determining neonates' temporal and spatial behavioral preferences is dominated primarily by more mature subcortical mechanisms of neuronal integration and behavioral control.

In general, it appears that infants prefer more intense or informative stimulation when they are less aroused, and less intense or informative stimulation when they are more aroused. It would seem that the identification of any influences or experiences that would affect this interdependence in

some permanent or precedent-setting way would be extraordinarily important if the subsequently altered structural and functional features of the central nervous system are to be organized in a healthy, productive manner.

In addition to the different stimulus preferences observed for different
arousal conditions in the present studies, our findings might also reflect the
importance and contribution of internal activity to responding when comparisons between studies are attempted. That is, the 3-month-old infants
who looked at a flashing optimal spatial frequency might also have been in
variable states during testing, and therefore the function obtained for them
might reflect this variability by yielding a curve other than what would have
been found had state been more vigorously controlled.

It is also possible that the use of manipulations that simultaneously affect both endogenous and exogenous sources of stimulation might provide
an indication of the present status of the infant. Infants who do not have
the capacity to modulate their own states in the context of stimulation might
be at some risk for poor developmental outcome. As a group, preterm infants are notoriously deficient in this capacity; however, most will not
appear to present problems later in life. It is therefore possible that differentiation of these infants in terms of whether they are responsive to externally
imposed modulation effects will be more predictive of future structural and
functional states than simply evaluating responses to series of univariate
stimulus manipulations.

REFERENCES

Abramov, I., Gordon, J., Hendrickson, A., Hainline, L., Dobson, V., & LaBois-
    siere, E. The retina of the newborn human infant. *Science*, 1982, *217*, 265–267.
Akiyama, Y., Schulte, F. J., Schultz, M. A., & Parmelee, A. H. Acoustically de-
    termined responses in premature and full term newborn infants. *Elec-
    troencephalography and Clinical Neurophysiology*, 1969, *26*, 371–380.
Als, H., Lester, B. M., & Brazelton, T. B. Dynamics of the behavioral organization
    of the premature infant: A theoretical perspective. In T. Field, A. Sostek, S.
    Goldberg, & H. H. Shuman (Eds.), *Infants born at risk: Behavior and develop-
    ment*. New York: Spectrum, 1979.
Anokhin, P. K., & Shuleikina, K. V. System organization of alimentary behavior in
    the newborn and the developing cat. *Developmental Psychobiology*, 1977, *10*,
    385–419.
Ashton, R. The state as variable in neonatal research. *Merrill-Palmer Quarterly*,
    1973, *19*, 3–20.
Attneave, F. *Applications of information theory to psychology: A summary of
    basic concepts, methods, and results*. New York: Holt, Rinehart, & Winston,
    1959.
Barnet, A. B., & Goodwin, R. S. Averaged evoked electroencephalographic
    responses to clicks in the human newborn. *Electroencephalography and Clinical
    Neurophysiology*, 1965, *18*, 441–450.

Beckstead, R. M., & Norgren, R. Autoradiographic examination of the central distribution of the trigeminal, facial, glossopharyngeal, and vagal nerves in the monkey. *Journal of Comparative Neurology*, 1979, *184*, 455–472.

Beckwith, L., Cohen, S. E., Kopp, C. B., Parmelee, A. H., & Marcy, T. G. Caregiver–infant interaction and early cognitive development in preterm infants. *Child Development*, 1976, *47*, 579–587.

Berg, K. M., & Berg, W. K. Psychophysiological development in infancy: State, sensory function, and attention. In J. Osofsky (Ed.), *Handbook of infant development*. New York: Wiley, 1979.

Berg, K. M., Berg, W. K., & Graham, F. K. Infant heart rate response as a function of stimulus and state. *Psychophysiology*, 1971, *8*, 30–44.

Berlyne, D. The influence of the albedo and complexity of stimuli on visual fixation in the human infant. *British Journal of Psychology*, 1958, *56*, 315–318.

Berlyne, D. *Conflict, arousal and curiosity*. New York: McGraw-Hill, 1960.

Brazelton, T. B., Als, H., Tronick, E., & Lester, B. M. Specific neonatal measures: The Brazelton Neonatal Behavior Assessment Scale. In J. Osofsky (Ed.), *Handbook of infant development*. New York: Wiley, 1979.

Brennan, W. M., Ames, E. W., & Moore, R. W. Age differences in infants' attention to patterns of different complexities. *Science*, 1966, *151*, 354–356.

Bronson, G. The postnatal growth of visual capacity. *Child Development*, 1974, *45*, 265–276.

Campos, J. J., & Brackbill, Y. Infant state: Relationship to heart rate, behavioral response and response decrement. *Developmental Psychobiology*, 1973, *6*, 9–19.

Caputo, D. V., Goldstein, K. M., & Taub, H. B. The development of prematurely born children through middle childhood. In S. Friedman & M. Sigman (Eds.), *Preterm birth and psychological development*. New York: Academic, 1981.

Chisholm, J. S. Swaddling, cradleboards and the development of children. *Early Human Development*, 1978, *2*, 255–275.

Davies, P. A., & Tizard, J. P. M. Very low birthweight and subsequent neurological defect (with special reference to spastic diplegia). *Developmental Medicine and Child Neurology*, 1975, *17*, 3–17.

Dember, W. N., & Earl, R. W. Analysis of exploratory, manipulatory, and curiosity behavior. *Psychological Review*, 1957, *64*, 91–96.

Dubowitz, L. M. S., Dubowitz, V., & Goldberg, C. Clinical assessment of gestational age in the newborn infant. *Journal of Pediatrics*, 1970, *77*, 1–10.

Ellingson, R. J. The study of brain electrical activity in infants. In L. Lipsitt & C. C. Spiker (Eds.), *Advances in child development and behavior* (Vol. 3). New York: Academic, 1967.

Fagan, J. F. Memory in the infant. *Journal of Experimental Child Psychology*, 1970, *9*, 217–226.

Fantz, R. L. Pattern vision in young infants. *Psychological Record*, 1958, *8*, 43–47.

Fantz, R. L., & Fagan, J. F. Visual attention to size and number of pattern details by term and preterm infants during the first six months. *Child Development*, 1975, *46*, 3–18.

Field, T. Interaction patterns of high-risk and normal infants. In T. Field, A. Sostek, S. Goldberg, & H. H. Shuman (Eds.), *Infants born at risk: Behavior and development*. New York: Spectrum, 1979.

Field, T. Infant arousal, attention, and affect during early interactions. In L. Lipsitt & C. Rovee-Collier (Eds.), *Advances in infancy research* (Vol. 1). Norwood, N.J.: Ablex, 1981.

Gardner, J. M. *Determinants of attention in premature infants.* Unpublished Ph.D. thesis, City University of New York, 1979.

Gardner, J. M., & Karmel, B. Z. Preferential looking at temporal frequencies by preterm infants. *Child Development*, 1981, *52*, 1299–1302.

Gardner, J. M., & Karmel, B. Z. *Neonates' arousal level and visual attention to temporal frequencies.* Paper presented at the International Conference on Infant Studies, Austin, Texas, March 1982.

Gardner, J. M., Lewkowicz, D. J., & Rose, S. A. *Effects of prestimulation on visual preferences in neonates.* Paper presented at the biennial meeting of the Society for Research in Child Development, Detroit, April 1983.

Gardner, J. M., & Turkewitz, G. The effect of arousal level on visual preferences in preterm infants. *Infant Behavior and Development*, 1982, *5*, 369–385.

Gerrity, K. M., & Woodruff, D. S. *Central nervous system maturation and infant visual development.* Paper presented at the biennial meeting of the Society for Research in Child Development, San Francisco, March 1979.

Giacoman, S. L. Hunger and motor restraint on arousal in visual attention in the infant. *Child Development*, 1971, *42*, 605–614.

Giuffre, R., Palma, L., & Fontana, M. Extracranial CSF shunting for infantile non-tumoral hydrocephalus—A retrospective analysis of 360 cases. *Clinical Neurology and Neurosurgery*, 1979, *81*, 199–210.

Grellong, B., Vaughan, H., Rotkin, L., Daum, C., Kurtzberg, D., & Lipper, E. *Neonatal performance, cognitive and neurologic outcome to 40 months among low birthweight infants.* Paper presented at the biennial meeting of the Society for Research in Child Development, Boston, April 1981.

Griffith, H., & Davidson, M. Long-term changes in intellect and behavior after hemispherectomy. *Journal of Neurological Psychiatry*, 1966, *29*, 571–576.

Harter, M. R., Deaton, F. K., & Odom, J. V. Maturation of evoked potentials and visual preference in 6–45-day-old infants: Effects of check size, visual acuity, and refractive error. *Electroencephalography and Clinical Neurophysiology*, 1977, *42*, 595–607.

Hebb, D. O. The effect of early and late brain injury upon test scores and the nature of normal adult intelligence. *Proceedings of the American Philosophical Society*, 1942, *85*, 275–292.

Hoffmann, R. Developmental changes in human infant visual-evoked potentials to patterned stimuli recorded at different scalp locations. *Child Development*, 1978, *49*, 110–118.

Hrbek, A., Hrbkova, M., & Lenard, H. G. Somatosensory, auditory and visual evoked responses in newborn infants during sleep and wakefulness. *Electroencephalography and Clinical Neurophysiology*, 1969, *26*, 597–603.

Hutt, S. J., Lenard, H. G., & Prechtl, H. F. R. Psychophysiological studies in newborn infants. In L. Lipsitt & H. W. Reese (Eds.), *Advances in child development and behavior* (Vol. 4). New York: Academic, 1969.

Jones-Molfese, V. Individual differences in neonatal preferences for planometric and stereometric visual patterns. *Child Development*, 1972, *43*, 1289–1296.

Karmel, B. Z. The effect of age, complexity, and amount of contour on pattern preferences in human infants. *Journal of Experimental Child Psychology*, 1969, *7*, 339–354.

Karmel, B. Z., Gardner, J. M., & Lewkowicz, D. J. *Spatial-temporal interactions in neonates' visual preferences.* Paper presented at the biennial meeting of the Society for Research in Child Development, Detroit, April 1983.

Karmel, B. Z., Hoffmann, R. F., & Fegy, M. J. Processing of contour information by human infants evidenced by pattern-dependent evoked potentials. *Child Development*, 1974, *45*, 39–48.

Karmel, B. Z., Kaye, H., & John, E. R. Developmental neurometrics. In W. A. Collins (Ed.), *Minnesota symposia on child psychology* (Vol. 11). Hillsdale, N.J.: Lawrence Erlbaum, 1978.

Karmel, B. Z., Lester, M. L., McCarvill, S. L., Brown, P., & Hofmann, M. Correlation of infants' brain and behavior response to temporal changes in visual stimulation. *Psychophysiology*, 1977, *14*, 134–142.

Karmel, B. Z., & Maisel, E. B. A neuronal activity model for infant visual attention. In L. Cohen & P. Salapatek (Eds.), *Infant perception: From sensation to cognition* (Vol. 1). New York: Academic, 1975.

Kitchen, W. H., Ryan, M. M., Richards, A., McDougall, A. B., Billson, F. A., Keir, E. H., & Naylor, F. D. A longitudinal study of very low-birthweight infants. IV: An overview of performance at eight years of age. *Developmental Medicine and Child Neurology*, 1980, *22*, 172–188.

Korner, A. F. State as variable, as obstacle, and as mediator of stimulation in infant research. *Merrill-Palmer Quarterly*, 1972, *18*, 77–94.

Kukorelli, T., & Juhasz, G. Sleep induced by intestinal stimulation in cats. *Physiology and Behavior*, 1977, *19*, 355–358.

Kurtzberg, D., Vaughan, H., Daum, C., Grellong, B., Albin, S., & Rotkin, L. Neurobehavioral performance of low birthweight infants at 40 weeks conceptional age: Comparison with normal full term infants. *Developmental Medicine and Child Neurology*, 1979, *21*, 590–607.

Lawson, K. R., & Turkewitz, G. Intersensory functions in newborns: Effect of sound on visual preferences. *Child Development*, 1980, *51*, 1295–1298.

Lewis, M., Bartels, B., & Goldberg, S. State as a determinant of infants' heart rate response to stimulation. *Science*, 1967, *155*, 486–488.

Lewkowicz, D. J., & Turkewitz, G. Intersensory interaction in newborns: Modification of visual preferences following exposure to sound. *Child Development*, 1981, *52*, 827–832.

Lindsley, D. B., & Wicke, J. D. The electroencephalogram: Autonomous electrical activity in man and animals. In R. F. Thompson & M. M. Patterson (Eds.), *Bioelectric recording techniques*. New York: Academic, 1974.

Lipton, E. L., Steinschneider, A., & Richmond, J. B. Swaddling, a child practice: Historical, cultural, and experimental observations. *Pediatrics*, 1965, *35*, 521–567.

Maffei, L. Spatial and temporal averages in retinal channels. *Journal of Neurophysiology*, 1968, *31*, 283–287.

Magnes, J., Moruzzi, G., & Pompeiano, O. Synchronization of the EEG produced by low-frequency electrical stimulation of the region of the solitary tract. *Archives Italiennes de Biologie*, 1961, *99*, 33–67.

Maisel, E. B., & Karmel, B. Z. Contour density and pattern configuration in visual preferences of infants. *Infant Behavior and Development*, 1978, *1*, 127–140.

Maurer, D., & Lewis, T. L. A physiologic explanation of infants' early visual development. *Canadian Journal of Psychology*, 1979, *33*, 232–252.

McCarvill, S. L., & Karmel, B. Z. A neural activity interpretation of luminance effects on infant pattern preferences. *Journal of Experimental Child Psychology*, 1976, *22*, 363–374.

McFie, J. The effects of hemispherectomy on intellectual functioning in cases of infantile hemiplagia. *Journal of Neurology, Neurosurgery and Psychiatry*, 1961, *24*, 240–249.

McGraw, M. *The neuromuscular maturation of the human infant.* New York: Hafner Press, 1943.

McGuire, I., & Turkewitz, G. Approach–withdrawal theory and the study of infant development. In M. Bortner (Ed.), *Cognitive growth and development: Essays in memory of Herbert G. Birch.* New York: Brunner/Mazel, 1979.

Meyer, P. M. Analysis of visual behavior in cats with extensive neocortical ablations. *Journal of Comparative and Physiological Psychology*, 1963, *56*, 397–401.

Monod, N., & Garma, L. Auditory responsivity in the human premature. *Biology of the Neonate*, 1971, *17*, 292–316.

Morest, D. K. Experimental study of the projections of the nucleus of the tractus solitarius and the area postrema in the cat. *Journal of Comparative Neurology*, 1967, *130*, 277–300.

Moskowitz, A., & Sokol, S. Spatial and temporal interaction of pattern-evoked cortical potentials in human infants. *Vision Research*, 1980, *20*, 699–707.

Parmelee, A. H. Neurophysiological and behavioral organization of preterm infants in the first month of life. *Biological Psychiatry*, 1975, *10*, 501–512.

Parmelee, A. H., Kopp, C. B., & Sigman, M. Selection of developmental assessment techniques for infants at risk. *Merrill-Palmer Quarterly*, 1976, *22*, 177–199.

Pasik, P., Pasik, T., Nolan, J. T., & Solomon, S. J. Bar orientation discrimination in normal and destriated monkeys. *Neuroscience Abstracts*, 1976, *2*, 1130.

Piercy, M. The effects of cerebral lesions on intellectual functioning: A review of current research trends. *Annual Review of Psychology*, 1964, *110*, 310–322.

Pomerleau-Malcuit, A., & Clifton, R. K. Neonatal heart rate response to tactile, auditory, and vestibular stimulation in different states. *Child Development*, 1973, *44*, 485–496.

Prechtl, H. F. R. The directional head turning response and allied movements of the human body. *Behavior*, 1958, *13*, 212–242.

Prechtl, H. F. R. Problems of behavior studies in the newborn infant. In D. S. Lehrman, R. A. Hinde, & E. Shaw (Eds.), *Advances in the study of behavior* (Vol. 1). New York: Academic, 1965.

Prechtl, H. F. R. The behavioral states of the newborn infant. *Brain Research*, 1974, *76*, 185–212.

Purpura, D. P. Morphogenesis of visual cortex in the preterm infant. In M. A. B. Brazier (Ed.), *Growth and development of the brain.* New York: Raven Press, 1975.

Research news: Is your brain really necessary? *Science*, 1980, *210*, 1232–1234.

Rie, H. E., & Rie, E. D. *Handbook of minimal brain dysfunctions. A critical review.* New York: Wiley, 1980.

Ross, G., & Schechner, S. *Developmental follow-up of infants with intraventricular hemorrhage*. Paper presented at the International Conference on Infant Studies, New Haven, April 1980.

Ruff, H. A., & Turkewitz, G. Developmental changes in the effectiveness of stimulus intensity on infant visual attention. *Developmental Psychology*, 1975, *11*, 705–710.

Ruff, H. A., & Turkewitz, G. Changing role of stimulus intensity as a determinant of infants' attention. *Perceptual and Motor Skills*, 1979, *48*, 815–826.

Salapatek, P. Pattern perception in early infancy. In L. Cohen & P. Salapatek (Eds.), *Infant perception: From sensation to cognition* (Vol. 1). New York: Academic, 1975.

Sameroff, A. J., & Chandler, M. J. Reproductive risk and the continuum of caretaking casualty. In F. D. Horowitz, E. M. Hetherington, S. Scarr-Salapatek, & G. M. Siegel (Eds.), *Review of child development research* (Vol. 4). Chicago: University of Chicago Press, 1975.

Schilder, P., Pasik, P., & Pasik, T. Extrageniculostriate vision in the monkey: III. Circle vs triangle and "red vs green" discrimination. *Experimental Brain Research*, 1972, *14*, 436–448.

Schneider, G. C. Is it really better to have your brain lesion early? A revision of the "Kennard Principle." *Neuropsychologia*, 1979, *17*, 557–583.

Schneirla, T. C. Aspects of stimulation and organization in approach/withdrawal processes underlying vertebrate behavioral organization. In D. S. Lehrman, R. A. Hinde, & E. Shaw (Eds.), *Advances in the study of behavior* (Vol. 1). New York: Academic, 1965.

Schulman, C. A. Effects of auditory stimuli on heart rate in premature infants as a function of level of arousal, probability of CNS damage, and conceptual age. *Developmental Psychobiology*, 1970, *2*, 172–183.

Sessle, B. J. Excitatory and inhibitory inputs to single neurons in the solitary tract nucleus and adjacent reticular formation. *Brain Research*, 1973, *53*, 319–331.

Sigman, M., Cohen, S. E., & Forsythe, A. B. The relation of early infant measures to later development. In S. Friedman & M. Sigman (Eds.), *Preterm birth and psychological development*. New York: Academic, 1981.

Sigman, M., & Parmelee, A. H. Longitudinal evaluation of the preterm infant. In T. Field, A. Sostek, S. Goldberg, & H. H. Shuman (Eds.), *Infants born at risk: Behavior and development*. New York: Spectrum, 1979.

Sokolov, E. N. *Perception and the conditioned reflex*. New York: MacMillan, 1963.

Spekreijse, H. *Development of the visual evoked potential*. Paper presented at the New York Academy of Sciences Conference on Evoked Potentials, New York, June 1981.

Sroufe, A. L. Socioemotional development. In J. Osofsky (Ed.), *Handbook of infant development*. New York: Wiley, 1979.

Thoman, E. B. A biological perspective and a behavioral model for assessment of premature infants. In L. A. Bond & J. M. Joffee (Eds.), *Primary prevention of psychopathology* (Vol. 6). Hanover, N.H.: University Press of New England, 1981.

Turkewitz, G., Birch, H. G., Moreau, T., Levy, L., & Cornwell, A. C. Effect of intensity of auditory stimulation on directional eye movements in the human neonate. *Animal Behavior*, 1966, *14*, 93–101.

Turkewitz, G., Fleischer, S., Moreau, T., Birch, H. G., & Levy, L. Relationship between feeding condition and organization of flexor-extensor movements in the human neonate. *Journal of Comparative and Physiological Psychology*, 1966, *61*, 455-460.

Turkewitz, G., Gordon, E. W., & Birch, H. G. Head-turning in the human neonate: Effect of prandial condition on lateral preference. *Journal of Comparative and Physiological Psychology*, 1965, *59*, 189-192.

Vaughan, H. Electrophysiologic analysis of regional cortical maturation. *Biological Psychiatry*, 1975, *10*, 513-526.

Vaughan, H., & Kurtzberg, D. *ERPs in the developing brain: Perceptual and cognitive processes.* Paper presented at EPIC VI, Chicago, June 1981.

Weitzman, E. D., Fishbein, W., & Graziani, L. J. Auditory evoked responses obtained from scalp electroencephalogram of the full-term human neonate during sleep. *Pediatrics*, 1965, *35*, 458-462.

Weitzman, E. D., & Graziani, L. J. Maturation and topography of the auditory evoked response of the prematurely born infant. *Developmental Psychobiology*, 1968, *1*, 79-89.

Woodruff, D. Brain electrical activity and behavior relationships over the life span. In P. Baltes (Ed.), *Life span development.* New York: Academic, 1978.

5

Behavioral and Cardiac Responses to Sound in Preterm Neonates Varying in Risk Status: A Hypothesis of Their Paradoxical Reactivity

Elizabeth E. Krafchuk
Edward Z. Tronick, Rachel K. Clifton

The infant's reactivity affects the quality of his or her interaction with the social and physical world. Reactivity has a strong influence upon the type of care the infant will receive and on how the infant approaches new situations (Brazelton, 1969; Escalona & Heider, 1959; Thomas, Chess, Birch, Hertzig, & Korn, 1963). In regard to preterm infants, Goldberg (1978) has suggested that differences in reactivity might be at the base of their deviant patterns of later social interaction. Field (1977) has observed that mothers of preterm infants tend to be more active in face-to-face play than mothers of full-term babies, and has hypothesized that these mothers are attempting to compensate for their baby's lack of expressiveness. Cognitive deficits in preterm populations have also been noted, in association with hyperactivity, learning disabilities, attentional deficits, and other behavior problems, even in the absence of gross physical or neurological involvement (Caputo &

The authors would like to thank the nursing staff of the Baystate Medical Center for their willingness to incorporate our testing into their caregiving routine. Doctors B. Shah, C. Dabiri, and J. Mendosa were extremely helpful in guiding our selection of infants and in helping us integrate psychological and medical evaluations. Elizabeth Shea and Steve Winn helped immeasurably in implementing this project. John Kulig was a tireless colleague who helped in many ways, from actual testing to numerous discussions of habituation/sensitization theory. And of course we wish to thank the many parents and infants who willingly participated with the hope that this research would aid those yet unborn. This research was supported primarily by a grant from the March of Dimes to E. Z. Tronick and by grants from the National Institutes of Health (HD-06753) and the National Institute of Mental Health (No. 00332) to R. K. Clifton. Our report is dedicated to Dr. Thomas Teree.

Mandel, 1970; Drillien, 1964; Knobloch & Pasamanick, 1963). Each of the diverse behavioral outcomes associated with premature birth might be an expression of inherent extremes in reactivity. Indeed, clarification of the reactivity of the preterm in the newborn period might suggest appropriate interventions that would mitigate the negative outcomes frequently found.

In an attempt to characterize the reactivity of preterm infants and to relate it to the degree of perinatal stress, this study examined the preterm neonate's behavioral and cardiac responses to repeated auditory stimuli. In characterizing "reactivity," we focused upon three components of an individual's response: (1) readiness to become aroused (as in sensory threshold), (2) the magnitude of arousal, and (3) the ease with which response is inhibited (as in the response duration for a given stimulus event and habituation over successive events).

Available data indicate that preterm neonates do differ from full-term neonates in their readiness to respond, or sensitivity to stimulation, and in their magnitude of response; however, reports of these differences vary widely. In a study examining cardiac and behavioral responses to three levels of tactile stimulation, Rose, Schmidt, and Bridger (1976) characterized the preterm as hyporesponsive. They observed a lack of cardiac responding among preterm infants, even to their strongest stimulus. There were, however, increases in overt activity, although the magnitude of responding was less than in full-term infants. The report of Rose and coworkers was consistent with the behavioral observations of weak reflexive responding made by Howard, Parmelee, Kopp, and Littman (1976). In contrast, Bench and Parker (1971) noted a high base rate of overt activity among the preterm; when preterm babies were stimulated, the authors found it difficult to judge whether changes in activity were spontaneous or stimulus specific. They interpreted this as a high false alarm rate in responding, and described the infants as hyperresponsive.

The pattern of hyporesponsivity might result from a deficit in either the sensory perceptual apparatus or the efferent motor system. Rose and her colleagues (1976) hypothesized a deficit on the sensory rather than the effector side. This conclusion was congruent with the finding of Graham, Matarazzo, and Caldwell (1956), that full-term newborns who had experienced perinatal insult had higher pain thresholds than healthy term newborns. Another study (Field, Dempsey, Hatch, Ting, & Clifton, 1979) supports this interpretation. Using two auditory stimuli (a buzzer and a rattle) presented at a high decibel level (i.e., 90 dB) and a tactile stimulus comparable to the strongest stimulus of Rose and co-workers, Field and her colleagues found that the magnitude of cardiac responding in preterm infants was comparable to that in full-term infants. The Field study implied that with sufficient sensory input the efferent response of preterm babies was the same as in full-term babies. There has been little work on and no suggestions as to the possible mechanism accounting for the hyperresponsive tendency described by Bench and Parker.

The study of Field et al. (1979) reported an additional characterization of the preterm infant's reactivity. They found that the preterm was unable to habituate to repeated presentations of stimuli. Lack of habituation in the preterm neonate has been found in other laboratories as well (Eisenberg, Coursin, & Rupp, 1966; Martinius & Papousek, 1970; Rose et al., 1976). This finding is intriguing in terms of the varying characterizations of the preterm. An infant who cannot ignore redundant input from the environment is at the mercy of external stimulus events. Continued responsiveness is extremely costly to the infant, causing a disruption of homeostatic functioning, sleep-wake cycling, digestive functioning, and other normal processes of growth and development (Gellis, 1978). Also note that an infant who did not habituate would look hyperresponsive once a stimulus exceeded even an elevated threshold.

To further explore these qualities of preterm infants' sensory threshold and capacity for habituation, the present project examined their sensitivity to two intensities of auditory stimulation. Testing at two intensity levels provided an opportunity to determine if the hyporesponsive pattern observed by Rose et al. (1976) would be repeated using a mild auditory stimulus. Additionally, the work of Sokolov (1963) and Thompson, Groves, Teyler, and Roemer (1973) has indicated that habituation is inversely associated with intensity, such that the more intense the stimulus, the less likely it is for an organism to habituate to that stimulus. We chose an intensity level that was below that used by Field et al. (1979), reasoning that the compromised infant might habituate to a mild or moderately intense stimulus if not to a strong one.

Both behavioral and cardiac systems were examined, as each has proved valuable in different contexts. The two response systems do not always parallel one another in the preterm neonate. Rose et al. (1976) observed significant change in overt activity in the absence of reliable cardiac change. Similarly, Field et al. (1979) found that preterm neonates showed habituation of behavioral but not of cardiac responses.

The overt behaviors observed during testing were based on the behaviors typically scored in the Neonatal Behavioral Assessment Scale (NBAS). Brazelton (1973) and his colleagues have documented a set of responses that sleeping babies demonstrate, for example, startles, activity, and color change. These behaviors are typically observed during the NBAS habituation series and were confirmed in pilot work on this study.

Cardiac activity was monitored to replicate and extend the findings of Rose et al. (1976) and Field et al. (1979). Cardiac change has proven its usefulness over the past two decades as an index of responding to many variations in stimuli (Berg & Berg, 1979; Clifton, 1974; McCall, 1971).

Several investigators have reported that the heart rate acceleration associated with active sleep in response to auditory stimulation is subject to habituation in full-term human neonates (Graham, Clifton, & Hatton, 1968; Field et al., 1979; Berg & Berg, 1979; Kulig & Clifton, 1980), but little work has been done on habituation and cardiac responding in the preterm.

Infants were tested in repeated sessions to evaluate the stability of individual response patterns both within a day and over a 24-hour period. A demonstration of stability in reactivity would suggest the usefulness of reactivity as an assessment of individual functioning. Behavioral studies have found that the propensity to become aroused and upset in the face of aversive stimulation was moderately stable over days (Bell, Weller, & Waldrop, 1971; Birns, 1965; Sameroff, Krafchuk, & Bakow, 1978). Similarly, babies who were very difficult to arouse and flat in their responses showed consistency in this pattern over time (Sameroff et al., 1978). Studies examining the consistency of cardiac arousal to auditory stimulation have met with limited success. Again, measures of extremes—lowest base level cardiac rate and unadjusted individual peak response—were among the most stable (Clifton, and Graham, 1968). To the best of our knowledge, no one has reported stability of behavioral or cardiac responding to stimulation within a particular state of arousal.

A major problem with previous reports of the premature neonate has been a tendency to treat babies of varying gestational ages and perinatal condition as if they were a homogeneous group. Such treatment is inappropriate. Healthy preterm infants tend not to show as severe deficits as those preterm infants who sustained illness or complications at delivery (Douglas, 1960; Sostek, Quinn, & Davitt, 1979). The deleterious effects of prematurity generally increase as gestational age decreases (Caputo & Mandel, 1970; Lubchenco, Bard, Goldman, Coyer, McIntyre, & Smith, 1974). A substantial literature suggests that the small-for-gestational age infant has a unique set of problems (Fitzhardinge & Steven, 1972; Schulte, Hinze, & Schrempf, 1972; Als, Tronick, Adamson, & Brazelton, 1976). Each of these factors must be considered in characterizing the infant at risk.

The present study sought to clarify the effects of prematurity per se from those of prematurity complicated by illness. Three groups of premature neonates were selected (see Table 5-2). Two groups consisted of infants born at 29–35 weeks gestation. One group, designated as high risk, suffered substantial illness in the perinatal period; the second group, designated as moderate risk, represented healthy prematures. The third group, born at 36–38 weeks gestation and designated as low risk, was recruited for control comparison purposes. Typically premature neonates are maintained in the hospital until their medical problems have resolved and their weight has increased to 5 pounds. For a large portion of infants this is accomplished by the time the baby is 36–38 weeks of conceptional age. Available reports of the preterm compared their behavior to that of infants born at term, that is, at 40 weeks gestation (Rose et al., 1976; Field et al., 1979). Such control groups were 2–4 weeks older in conceptional age than the preterm group, which might produce biased comparisons in unknown ways. The low risk comparison group of the present study was considered a more appropriate comparison than full-term newborn, since they were matched with the conceptional age of the other preterm groups at the time of testing.

The design of the study is presented in Table 5-1. Each infant was seen on three separate sessions: twice on day 1 and once on day 2. On day 1 behavioral and cardiac responses to an 85-dB and a 75-dB rattle were noted, with order of intensity presentation counterbalanced within each group. This provided a within-subjects comparison of responding to each intensity level. The stimulus series that had been presented first on day 1 was repeated on day 2, allowing for an examination of the stability of reaction tendencies and habituation over a 24-hour period. The rattle was chosen for the habituation trials and the startle response for the dishabituation stimulus in an effort to replicate the series used by Field et al. (1979).

Within each session, 10 rattle presentations were made, followed by a dishabituation stimulus and succeeded by 4 more rattle trials. The dishabituation stimulus was included to control for sensory fatigue effects (Thompson et al., 1973). Additional rattle trials were presented after the dishabituation trial to ascertain whether response recovery occurred following the dishabituation stimulus.

Our hypotheses concerning their responses were the following:

1. Moderate and high risk preterm infants would be hyporesponsive in their behavioral and cardiac responses in comparison to low risk infants (Rose et al., 1976; Howard et al., 1976).
2. Low risk infants would habituate their behavioral and cardiac responses, whereas moderate and high risk groups would not (Field et al., 1979).
3. Magnitude of responses and habituation would be affected by stimulus intensity such that greater responding (Bartoshuk, 1964) and less habituation (Thompson et al., 1973) would occur for the more intense stimulus.
4. Severity of perinatal insult would affect hypotheses 1 and 2, such that the hyporesponsive tendency and inability to habituate would be exaggerated in the most compromised group.
5. Magnitude of response and habituation would be stable characteristics over days in all groups.

Table 5-1
Experimental Design (N = 43)

		Low Risk (n = 14)		Moderate Risk (n = 14)		High Risk (n = 15)	
		Order 1	Order 2	Order 1	Order 2	Order 1	Order 2
Day 1	Session 1	85 dB (n = 7)	75 dB (n = 7)	85 dB (n = 7)	75 dB (n = 7)	85 dB (n = 7)	75 dB (n = 8)
	Session 2	75 dB (n = 7)	85 dB (n = 7)	75 dB (n = 7)	85 dB (n = 7)	75 dB (n = 5)	85 dB (n = 6)
Day 2	Session 3	85 dB (n = 6)	75 dB (n = 6)	85 dB (n = 6)	75 dB (n = 6)	85 dB (n = 7)	75 dB (n = 6)

METHOD _____

Subjects _____

Infants were recruited from the newborn nurseries at the Baystate Medical Center in Springfield, Massachusetts. Table 5-2 presents a medical description of the three risk groups. The low risk (LR) sample consisted of 14 healthy infants born at 36–38 weeks gestation. These infants, while born at the lower bound of what is generally considered a term gestation, were treated as full-term infants by the medical staff.

The second group, designated as moderate risk (MR), represented healthy prematures. These neonates, born at 31–35 weeks gestation,* experienced a relatively smooth transition to extrauterine life and failed to develop illness prior to their discharge. No infant in this group demonstrated true respiratory distress, although three infants were identified as having transient tachypnea. Those receiving oxygen required assistance for 24–48 hours only. None were intubated or put on respirators. Four infants experienced brief periods of hypocalcemia. High bilirubin counts were noted in 78 percent of the infants, with one infant requiring an exchange transfusion. In general, the group gained weight quickly in the preterm nursery setting.

The third group of infants, designated as high risk prematures (HR), experienced relatively more medical difficulties in the first weeks of life. This group consisted of 15 infants born at 29–34 weeks gestation. Two-thirds of the sample suffered from perinatal anoxia, with two cases requiring intubation at delivery. Two-thirds of this sample developed hyaline membrane disease. Metabolic disorders common to prematures such as hypocalcemia, anemia, and hypoglycemia occurred in 11 of the 15 babies; 2 cases were exposed to placental infarction; another 2 babies developed pneumonia, while 2 cases of pneumothorax occurred. A total of 7 infants suffered from prolonged difficulties with apnea and bradycardia. All high risk infants were treated for hyperbilirubinemia.

These two preterm groups did not differ in maternal age or previous childbearing history. The moderate risk group, however, appeared to be composed primarily of cases whose mothers had had some warning of early termination of their pregnancy and who had obtained medical assistance prior to the baby's arrival. Of the 14 moderate risk mothers, 9 developed

---

*Gestational age for all groups was determined by the date of the mother's last menstrual period. These dates were confirmed by the Dubowitz Newborn Maturity Rating and Classification Exam (1977), performed routinely by the hospital personnel. In cases where there was a discrepancy between these two estimates, the mother's dates were used for determining selection, provided that she was confident of the time of conception. If she was not and there was more than a 2-week discrepancy between the estimate of gestational age as determined by the Dubowitz exam and the mother's dates, the infant was not included in the study.

Table 5-2
Medical Description of Infants

	Low Risk Mean (Range)	Moderate Risk Mean (Range)	High Risk Mean (Range)
Gestational age (weeks)	37.7 (36–38)	32.9 (31–35)	31.6 (29–34)
SD	0.64	1.34	1.76
Conceptional age at testing (weeks)	37.9	35.9	37.2
SD	0.64	0.86	1.08
Birth weight (grams)	3011.7 (2608–3614)	1805 (1261–2310)	1555 (1077–2400)
SD	377.9	270.9	374.2
Ponderal index	2.3 (1.94–3.01)	2.14 (1.78–2.54)	2.08 (1.51–2.47)
SD	0.32	0.24	0.30
Apgar (1 min/5 min) Number of subjects with ratio of:			
0–3	0/0	0/0	6/0
4–6	0/0	3/1	3/4
7–9	14/14	11/13	6/11
Respiratory distress	none	3 transient tachypnea 2 oxygen assisted 9 no problems	2 severe 6 moderate 3 mild 1 transient tachypnea 3 oxygen assisted

Metabolic disorder	none	4 yes 10 no	11 yes 4 no
Hyperbilirubinemia	2 yes 12 no	11 yes 3 no	15 yes
Highest count	14.0	20.0	14.4
Mean days phototherapy	0	4	7
Maternal age	24.9 (18–37)	24.6 (16–36)	25.7 (18–38)
SD	5.82	5.89	6.19
Percentage receiving steroids—maternal	0	50	20
Obstetric medication (anesthesia; analgesia)	30 mg; 50 mg	35 mg; 27 mg	18 mg; 25 mg
Delivery route—vaginal	14	10	9
C Section	0	4	6
Gender	8M; 6F	9M; 5F	7M; 8F

premature rupture of the membranes (PROM), with 5 of these cases receiving corticosteroids to accelerate their fetus' lung maturation. Two additional cases in this group also received corticosteroids prior to delivery, but without PROM. In contrast, only 3 mothers of the high risk sample received corticosteroids and there were 5 cases of PROM.

All preterm infants were tested at a time when their condition was stable and they required no special medical care. Testing was done at 36–38 weeks of conceptional age. In a sense our sample was biased, representing infants who were able to overcome perinatal difficulties relatively quickly. The samples do not represent infants requiring prolonged intensive care. Although infants were excluded when the Dubowitz exam or maternal history provided evidence of intrauterine growth retardation, one can see from the ponderal indexes that some of the more compromised infants did fall into the lowest 10 percent range of length/body weight ratios at birth (Lubchenco et al., 1966).

Apparatus

Illumination of the testing room was kept low (5.84 fl (foot lamberts) at the site of the infant's head). Such lighting was maintained to encourage sleep (Ashton, 1971b).

The habituation stimulus consisted of a rattle, constructed of a 2 × 2 × 3-inch plastic box one-third full of popcorn kernels (Brazelton, 1973). Each rattle presentation consisted of 4–6 shakes over a 2- to 2.5-second epoch. The stimulus was played on a Revox tape recorder, type A77, amplified by a Realistic amplifier, model number SA-100B, and fed through a Grundig Microbox (#320). The intertrial interval (ITI) ranged from 32 to 39 sec, with an average ITI of 36 sec. The ITI was variable to preclude the possibility of temporal conditioning. The rattle trials were presented at either 75 or 85 dB, with the source located about 12 inches from the baby's ear. Background noise was 50–54 dB. Intensity was measured with a General Radio Sound Level Meter (type 1565-D, A scale, re = 0.0002 dynes/cm²) placed at the site of the infant's head.

The dishabituation stimulus consisted of raising the head end of the infant's bassinet 2–3 inches from the supporting cart base and releasing it. This manipulation produced a Moro response on 80 percent of the trials on which it was administered.

Raw electrocardiogram (ECG) was amplified on a Hewlett-Packard 7702B polygraph and recorded with a Vetter Model-A FM tape recorder. Beckman miniature electrodes were applied to the infant's chest in a triangular array: one active lead was applied high on the sternum, the second active lead to the left costal margin, and the ground electrode to the right costal margin.

For statistical analyses, the recorded heart rate signal was converted from analog to digital form by a Hewlett-Packard 2100A computer. The computer timed the interval between each beat, weighting the interbeat interval with the proportion of the 1-sec period it occupied. These second-by-second weighted average heart periods were converted to heart rate in beats per minute. For each trial 5 prestimulus and 20 poststimulus seconds were extracted from each subject's record on each of the three sessions.

Procedure

Written consent from each mother was obtained for her newborn's participation, and the attending pediatrician was also contacted for his or her consent. Testing was conducted in a room close to the newborn nurseries. The ECG electrodes were applied to the infant's chest and he or she was swaddled. Two experimenters independently monitored the infant's state. The stimulus series was initiated when both examiners judged the baby to have been in active sleep for 2 min. Active sleep was evidenced by eye movements, shallow, irregular respiration, and occasional body movements (Brazelton, 1973).

Each session consisted of 10 rattle trials followed by 1 dishabituation trial and 4 rattle trials. These presentations were fixed across infants: the same stimulus order and ITI were maintained, regardless of the infant's activity.

The series was terminated if the infant changed state prior to trial 5 (1 infant moved to quiet sleep, while 7 woke up). The series was reinitiated from trial 1 only if the baby was judged to have returned to a sustained bout of active sleep, operationally defined by the demonstration of active sleep characteristics for a minimum of 2 min (4 babies were retested). The 5-trial criterion was established in an effort to control for spontaneous swings in state without excluding infants who might have moved into quiet sleep as a means of coping with the stimulation. The procedure was also terminated if the infant became fussy at a later point in the stimulus series. Whenever possible, an effort was made to initiate the series at the beginning of an active sleep epoch; however, it was not always possible to begin testing at that time. The 5-trial criterion was therefore used to allow for variability in the time of test onset within the sleep bout. Table 5-3 provides a summary of the attrition rate within each group.

A second habituation series on day 1 was initiated either when the infant remained in active sleep throughout the first series and for at least 5 min once the series was over ($n = 18$) or at the beginning of a new bout of active sleep ($n = 21$). Tables 5-4 and 5-5 provide a description of prandial condition at testing and the time between sessions. The reader will note that the moderate and high risk groups generally had less time between sessions on day 1. These groups tended to display longer bouts of active sleep and it was usually possible to complete both sessions within one state epoch.

Table 5-3
Summary of Attrition

	Early Discharge	Technical Failure	Experimenter Error	Failed Settle into Sleep	Woke up Prior to Trial 5	
					Discontinued	Retest
Low risk	2	0	0	1	1	3
Moderate risk	2	2	0	1	1	0
High risk	0	0	2	0	1	1

Table 5-4
Prandial Condition at Time of Testing

Time Elapsed Since Last Meal (Hours)	Low Risk			Moderate Risk			High Risk		
	S_1	S_2	S_3	S_1	S_2	S_3	S_1	S_2	S_3
Mean	1.71	2.09	.91	1.15	1.40	1.09	1.23	1.43	1.39
SD	0.81	0.89	0.73	0.67	0.69	0.83	0.87	0.86	0.80
Range	0.5–3.00	0.5–3.00	0.25–2.5	0.25–2.25	0.25–2.50	0.25–3.00	0.25–2.25	0.25–3.50	0.5–2.50

Table 5-5
Amount of Time Elapsed Between Sessions

Time Elapsed Between Sessions (Hours)	Low Risk			Moderate Risk			High Risk		
	S_1 to S_2	S_2 to S_3	S_1 to S_3	S_1 to S_2	S_2 to S_3	S_1 to S_3	S_1 to S_2	S_2 to S_3	S_1 to S_3
Mean	1.43	20.62	22.43	0.34	21.67	22.47	0.28	22.08	22.44
SD	1.47	2.53	2.53	0.28	3.92	3.88	0.30	3.18	3.12
Range	0.1–4.0	0.28–0.43	18.5–29.0	0.08–0.83	14.5–28.0	15.0–28.25	0.12–1.17	18.0–29.0	18.25–29.25

Independent observations of the infants' behavioral responses were made by both experimenters. The behaviors chosen were deemed to be the most frequently occurring responses that could be assessed with better than 90 percent reliability between observers. Infants were observed for 60 sec prior to introduction of the rattle to assess spontaneous behavior. On rattle trials, the behaviors were recorded if they occurred within 5 sec of the stimulus event. The behavioral checklist consisted of the following reactions: (1) intensity of activity, rated on a 4-point scale designating absent, slight, moderate, or high intensity of activity; (2) startles; (3) irritable crying; (4) other vocalizations; (5) grimaces or blinks; (6) hand-to-mouth contacts; (7) sucking or mouthing; (8) color changes; and (9) state of arousal (Brazelton, 1973; Prechtl, 1977).

RESULTS

Examination of the behavioral responses indicated that certain categories were consistently observed in response to stimulation, while others were associated with the spontaneous behavior of active sleep. Startles, body activity, and color changes occurred reliably in response to stimulation and served as the major dependent variables. For various reasons all other behaviors were excluded from analysis. Grimacing and sucking had a high frequency during dense rapid eye movement (REM) activity and did not seem to be systematically associated with stimulus presentations. Vocalizations and crying occurred with low frequency, except when the sleep state was disrupted. Blinks appeared relatively late in the trial series, subsequent to the suppression of startles and body activity, being apparently associated with other factors, like response inhibition, rather than with perception of the stimulus per se. All significance levels for the between-groups comparisons of the behavioral data was based upon the Bonferonni distribution, with K, the number of planned comparisons, equal to 3 (Myers, 1972).

Cardiac data for the 10 habituation trials were reduced to 5 trial blocks, each block consisting of the average of two adjacent trials. For analyses, 1 prestimulus and 10 poststimulus seconds were included, except where otherwise indicated.

Base Level Responding

Behavior. There were virtually no group differences in base level activity, startles, or color change. The single exception was base level activity in session 3, in which HR infants demonstrated greater activity than LR infants [$t(25) = 2.75$, $p < .05$].

Heart rate. Resting heart rates of both the MR and HR groups were generally a full 30 bpm higher than the LR control subjects. Average heart rates for the 5-sec period prior to stimulation in session 1 were 124, 151, and 157 bpm for the LR, MR, and HR groups, respectively. These data were consistent with reports by Rose and co-workers (Rose et al., 1976; Rose, Schmidt, Riese, & Bridger, 1980) and Field et al. (1979). The moderate and high risk infants also exhibited more variability in cardiac rate prior to stimulation than did low risk infants. Standard deviations for 5 sec immediately preceding the first stimulus presentation were 10.9, 17.3, and 15.6 bpm for the low, moderate, and high risk infants, respectively. Separate analyses were performed for each group's cardiac data except where otherwise indicated.

Reactivity Differences Among the Groups _____

Group differences in reactivity were assessed using data from session 1, that portion of our experiment which is most comparable to reports by Rose et al. (1976) and Field et al. (1979). Habituation results were evaluated both within session 1 and across sessions 1 and 2 and sessions 1 and 3. Stability of individual differences was examined by comparing data from session 1 with session 2 and 3. Behavioral and cardiac results will be presented in each of the following sections.

Four separate approaches to the data were used to explore reactivity among the risk groups. Initially behavioral and cardiac responses on trial block 1 were noted. Subsequent analyses were made of responses on all 5 trial blocks, followed by an examination of intensity differences and response to the dishabituation stimulus.

Trial Block 1 _____

Behavior. There were no group differences in the amount of activity or in the incidence of startles and color changes on trial block 1.

Heart rate. Low risk infants showed a significant cardiac acceleration on trial block 1 [seconds, $F(10, 120) = 4.23$, $p < .001$] that was quadratic in form [quadratic trend, $F(1,12) = 6.58$, $p < .05$]. However, both moderate and high risk infants failed to demonstrate reliable cardiac change to the initial rattle presentation.

Response over 10 Trials _____

Behavior. The sum of activity and of the number of instances of startles and color changes for the first 10 trials were tabulated for each of the groups (see Table 5-6). Comparison of the three groups revealed the following differences:

1. LR babies demonstrated more activity in response to the rattle than MR babies, while LR and HR groups were comparable in activity.
2. LR infants exhibited more frequent instances of startling than either MR or HR groups.
3. LR subjects exhibited fewer color changes than HR infants.

Heart rate. Low and moderate risk groups responded to the rattle stimuli with reliable cardiac acceleration, as indicated by a significant seconds effect in both groups [$F(10,120) = 10.60$ and $3.81, p < .001$, in low and moderate risk groups, respectively]. The LR infants' response contained a significant quadratic and cubic trend [$F(1,12) = 19.01$ and 19.43, respectively, $p = .001$], while a significant cubic trend was shown in the MR infants' response [$F(1,12) = 7.43, p < .025$]. HR infants failed to show reliable heart rate change in the first session. Figure 5-1 illustrates the three groups' cardiac responses to the rattle on session 1, collapsed over trials and intensity. Note that behavioral activity and cardiac change were congruent for the LR infants, but showed a lack of consistency in the HR group.

Response to Two Intensity Levels _____

Behavior. There were no instances in which behavioral responding differed with intensity level during the 10 habituation trials.

Heart rate. While there was no effect of intensity in LR infants, the MR prematures showed a prolonged increase in heart rate to the 85-dB stimulus relative to the 75-dB condition, seconds × intensity [$F(10,120) = 2.90, p < .005$, and seconds (linear) × intensity, $F(1,12) = 16.59, p < .005$] (see Fig. 5-2). Acceleration to the 85-dB stimulus reached a peak 3–5 sec after the stimulus presentation and remained high for 10 sec [linear trend on seconds, $F(1,6) = 17.4, p < .01$]. In contrast, responding to the 75-dB series had "recovered," that is, returned to base level, in the same amount of time [cubic trend on seconds, $F(1,6) = 22.46, p = .005$].

In summary, the cardiac data demonstrated that HR infants were less responsive than their MR and LR counterparts. Low risk babies responded readily to stimulation and were equally responsive to the two intensity levels. Moderate risk infants showed prolonged cardiac arousal to the louder intensity.

Table 5-6

Average Sum of Behavioral Ratings in 10 Trials on Session 1

	Activity		Startles		Color Changes	
	$\overline{X}$	SD	$\overline{X}$	SD	$\overline{X}$	SD
Low risk ($n = 14$)	10.43	3.10	2.64	1.41	0.93	1.44
Moderate risk ($n = 14$)	7.36	3.0	0.64	0.84	2.14	1.29
High risk ($n = 15$)	9.70	3.81	0.36	0.61	2.57	1.70
Group differences	LR > MR		LR > MR		HR > LR	
	$t = 2.65$, $df = 26$		$t = 3.42$, $df = 26$		$t = 2.78$, $df = 27$	
	$p < .05$		$p < .01$		$p < .05$	
			LR > HR			
			$t = 4.48$, $df = 27$			
			$p = .01$			

115

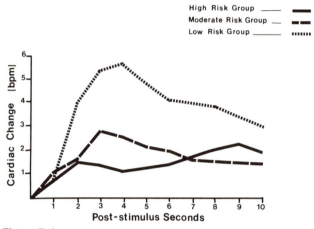

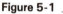

Figure 5-1 _____

Cardiac change to rattle stimulus in three groups averaged over trials and intensity on session 1.

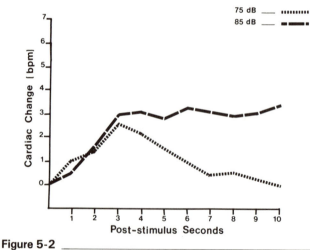

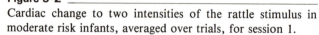

Figure 5-2 _____

Cardiac change to two intensities of the rattle stimulus in moderate risk infants, averaged over trials, for session 1.

Response to the Dishabituation Trial

Behavior. Pairwise comparisons failed to reveal any significant differences between the groups in their activity levels or in the incidence of startles and color change during the dishabituation trial.

Heart rate. The crib manipulation elicited large cardiac accelerations in all groups [seconds, $F(10,120) = 4.38$, $p < .001$, and seconds quadratic, $F(1,13) = 32.51$, $p < .001$ for LR; seconds, $F(10,120) = 19.10$, $p < .001$, and seconds linear and quadratic, $F(1,13) = 32.92$ and 10.98, $p < .01$ in MR; seconds, $F(10,140) = 13.37$, $p < .001$, and seconds linear, $F(1,14) = 44.58$, $p < .001$ in HR]. Figure 5-3 depicts heart rate change to the dishabituation stimulus among the three risk groups. Although HR infants did reliably respond to the stimulus, they failed to show as great a magnitude of responding as the other neonatal groups (peak acceleration was 12 beats, versus 14 and 13 beats in LR and MR groups, respectively). Comparison of peak acceleration indicated that the HR group was significantly less responsive than both MR [$F(1,27) = 5.06$, $p < .05$] and LR [$F(1, 27) = 4.65$, $p < .05$] subjects. There was no difference in peak acceleration between moderate and low risk babies.

The MR group's peak acceleration lasted longer than that of LR babies, extending a full 9–10 sec, with return to base level reached at 20 poststimulus seconds. The HR group, however, showed a different pattern in which the peak response was not reached until 10 poststimulus seconds.

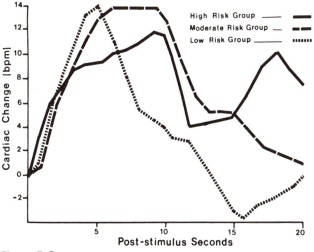

Figure 5-3

Cardiac change to dishabituation stimulus in three groups on session 1.

The response began to diminish, but returned again between 14 and 18 sec, when the other groups had for the most part returned to base level. Given that the curve represented the average of 15 infants' data, the possibility existed that its shape was due to an averaging artifact, that is, a reflection of early responders who recovered fairly quickly, mixed with infants whose response was delayed in its onset. Alternatively, it could be that HR babies really did perseverate in their responses, apparently having difficulty inhibiting their initial reaction.

An examination of individual cases indicated that each type of response was represented, but that the latter was most frequent. Defining a response as an acceleration of at least 5 beats within 5 poststimulus seconds, four patterns of response were readily identifiable: (1) *normative responders*, who showed an immediate response which rapidly recovered; (2) *flat responders*, who failed to show any immediate identifiable acceleration (delayed accelerations were not counted); (3) *perseverators*, whose response pattern was labile, showing an initial heart rate acceleration that reversed direction for 2–4 sec but accelerated subsequently for 5 or more seconds; and (4) *hyperresponders*, whose heart rate increased and failed to approach base level within 15 secs.

Table 5-7 lists the distribution of cases among the response types in each of the risk groups. As one can see, the perseveration tendency was the modal pattern among HR infants.

If one were to characterize the hyperresponders and perseverators as having difficulty inhibiting their initial reaction tendencies, then 67 percent of the high risk sample could be so described. The moderate risk group had strikingly fewer hyperresponders (14%) and perseverators (36%), while the low risk group had only one perseverator (7%).

Thus the degree of risk was reflected in the individual's inability to inhibit responding to a strong stimulus. A chi-square test was performed to ascertain whether membership in a risk group and type of response were independent phenomena. For the purposes of this analysis, hyperresponders and perseverators were collapsed together. This test was significant ($\chi^2 = 15.6$, $df = 4$, $p < .005$), indicating that risk status and quality of response to a strong stimulus were in fact related.

Table 5-7

Response to Dishabituation Stimulus on Session 1 — Distribution of Cases Among Four Response Types

	Hyperresponder	Perseverator	Flat	Normative
Low risk ($n = 14$)	0	1 (7%)	2 (14%)	11 (78%)
Moderate risk ($n = 14$)	2 (14%)	5 (36%)	4 (28%)	3 (21%)
High risk ($n = 15$)	3 (20%)	7 (47%)	2 (13%)	3 (20%)

Habituation

Response Across Trials on Session 1

Behavior.   Activity and startle ratings were used to describe overt responses over trials. There was no evidence of an orderly decrement in these data. It appeared, rather, that most infants showed spontaneous fluctuations in responding over trials.

It should be noted that using the criteria for a behavioral shutdown formulated by Brazelton (1973), that is, cessation of motor or startle activity for a minimum of two trials, we did observe response inhibition in the risk groups (78, 86, and 60 percent of LR, MR, and HR infants, respectively). However, few infants were able to maintain inhibition of responding over the remaining trials (7, 36, and 27 percent of LR, MR, and HR respectively). Furthermore, patterns of behavioral response decrement did not differ significantly among the three risk groups. This result is consistent with the report by Field et al. (1979), which noted behavioral inhibition using Brazelton's criteria in both preterm and full-term infants.

Heart rate.   Three separate analyses of variance (ANOVAs) were performed to evaluate the cardiac data for habituation effects: session 1 was first considered, followed by sessions 1 and 2 combined, and finally sessions 1 and 3. The data were parsed in this manner to assess within-sessions habituation and possible retention across sessions.

An ANOVA of the data for session 1 treated trial blocks (5) × seconds (11) in a repeated-measures design. This analysis failed to provide statistical support for an interpretation of habituation or any orderly change associated with trial blocks.

Habituation over Sessions and Days: Cardiac Responses

Data from sessions 1 and 2 were combined in a blocks (5) × sessions (2) × seconds (11) ANOVA with order of intensity presentation as the between-subjects variable. While all three groups showed significant responding in this analysis [seconds, $F(10,120) = 10.65$, $p < .001$ in LR; $F(10,120) = 3.27$, $p < .001$ in MR; $F(10,90) = 2.52$, $p < .01$ in HR], there was no evidence of systematic change in responding over trials.

When cardiac data were examined for order effects, it was found that the sequence of the two intensity series had a significant influence on the LR group. LR babies showed a seconds × order interaction [$F(10,120) = 2.50$, $p < .01$, and seconds (cubic × order, $F(1,12) = 7.02$, $p < .025$] that is illustrated in Figure 5-4. Responsiveness to the 85- and 75-dB stimuli were comparable when first encountered during session 1. The differential impact of the two intensities became apparent with the second testing session.

Infants who had been exposed to the 75-dB series earlier demonstrated large accelerations, the magnitude of which was comparable to the first session. However, infants who had been exposed to the stronger stimulus series first were less reactive in their subsequent response to the lower intensity. There were no significant order effects for the five trial blocks in either the moderate or high risk groups.

To assess carry-over effects from day 1 (session 1) to day 2 (session 3), ANOVAs for each group were performed comparing days (2) × blocks (5) × seconds (11) with intensity as the between-subjects variable. Again, LR and MR infants showed reliable cardiac acceleration [seconds, $F(10,100)$ = 15.10, p < .001 in LR; $F(10,90)$ = 2.99, p < .003 in MR], while the HR group did not. The MR group again showed differential responding to the two intensity levels [$F(10,90)$ = 3.32, p < .001, for seconds × intensity] as they had on day 1. However, there was no habituation either within sessions or across sessions for any group, nor were there any consistent carry-over effects across days. The trials following the dishabituation stimulus were not analyzed for response recovery, as there was no habituation during the first 10 trials.

Stability of Individual Differences over Sessions

Behavior. The percentage of infants demonstrating consistency in their pattern of behavioral decrement across sessions was unremarkable.

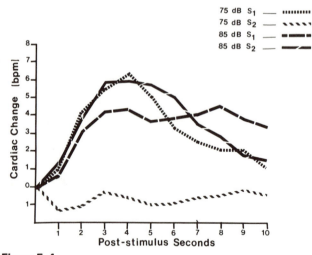

Figure 5-4

Carry-over effects on low risk infants' heart rate responses, sessions 1 to 2.

Heart rate.   Stability of reactivity on trial block 1 was assessed by computing Spearman rho correlations on initial peak heart rate acceleration. LR infants maintained significant stability in rank order over days (r_s = .532, t = 1.94, df = 10, p < .05), while MR and HR infants did not. This relation appeared to be carried by LR subjects receiving the 75-dB series (r_s = .77, t = 2.42, df = 4, p < .05). Infants in the 85-dB series were not stable, as a subgroup, over days (r_s = .14, t = .29, df = 4, NS).

The peak heart rate acceleration for all 5 trial blocks on sessions 1 and 3 were considered on a case-by-case basis to determine if the pattern of response over trials was consistent in individual infants; no consistency was found in any group.

The dishabituation stimulus elicited cardiac acceleration in all three groups, although the shape and latency of the response differed. Magnitude of peak acceleration failed to capture those response characteristics, yielding unreliable Spearman rho correlations across sessions. Cardiac responses to the dishabituation trial on sessions 2 and 3 were classified into the typologies used for session 1. The consistency of these response patterns over sessions was examined by determining the number of matches from session 1 to session 2 and from session 1 to session 3 for each group. A match was defined as maintaining the same typology across two sessions, or shifting from the hyperresponder to the perseverator category. The percentage of cases that maintained a similar response typology across sessions was unremarkable. Thus even qualitative, general characterizations of reactivity to a strong stimulus failed to maintain stability over time in the three risk groups.

The HR infants demand some attention in this regard. This group was expected to be stable in their style of responding. If these babies were consistently flat and hyporesponsive, they would look worrisome indeed. However, a shift toward greater normalcy in responding was seen upon examination of their response typologies. Table 5-8 presents the distribution of the HR infants' classifications over the three sessions.

The percentage of cases showing an inability to inhibit responses decreased by more than half across the two days. When we compared the HR samples' distribution relative to the other groups, they looked much more similar on the third session than they did on the first. A chi-square test

Table 5-8 _____
High Risk Infant's Response to Dishabituation Stimulus on Three Sessions

	Perseverator or Hyperresponsive	Normative	Flat
Session 1	67%	20%	13%
Session 2	54%	18%	27%
Session 3	31%	46%	23%

was performed to evaluate the distribution of cases; in fact, perinatal risk classification and response type were unrelated in session 3.

DISCUSSION

In examining three risk groups in an habituation paradigm, we found little evidence of behavioral or cardiac habituation, even in the normative control sample. Major group differences emerged in the infants' abilities to organize a coherent response to stimulation. The patterning of these differences is summarized below by group, with a discussion following.

Tested in active sleep, LR infants responded with cardiac acceleration to both intensities of the rattle sound. Startles and other motor activity were observed during the session. Intensity did not influence behavioral responding, but an order effect across sessions 1 and 2 was apparent in heart-rate responding. Specifically, the magnitude of responding to the 75-dB series was less when it followed the 85-dB series than when it preceded it. This effect occurred despite the fact that LR infants had the longest time interval between these sessions of any group. The dishabituation stimulus elicited cardiac acceleration that returned to base line more quickly than in the other groups. Overall, LR infants displayed little stability in behavioral or cardiac responses over the 24-hour period. However, LR infants who showed large responses to the rattle on trial block 1 on day 1 tended to do so on day 2; stability was greatest in the 75-dB condition.

MR infants also responded consistently to both intensities of the rattle, but showed several differences compared to the LR group. Behaviorally, the MR group was less active and showed fewer startles. Additionally, cardiac change was less stable, being reliable only when all five trial blocks were considered. Cardiac acceleration was prolonged to the 85-dB stimulus relative to the 75-dB condition. The dishabituation stimulus elicited a heart rate response with magnitude comparable to LR infants, but responding took longer to return to base level.

The most compromised group of infants failed to show reliable cardiac change to the rattle, confirming the hypothesis that severe perinatal insult is associated with hyporesponsivity. This lack of response was not due to their elevated base-line heart rate (Wilder, 1967), because MR infants had similar high base rates but were responsive. Furthermore, HR infants did show reliable cardiac acceleration on the dishabituation trial, which featured a stronger stimulus than the rattle. The magnitude of change was smaller than in the other groups and some infants tended to perseverate once an acceleration was initiated. The HR group was comparable to the other groups in activity level, but had fewer startles and more color changes compared to the

LR group. In data reported elsewhere, this group also tended to show more sleep disruptions during the session (Krafchuk, Shea, & Tronick, 1982). Like the MR infants, this group showed no stability in maintaining response patterns over days.

As noted above, base-line heart rate in the two preterm groups was elevated compared to the LR infants, a group difference noted by previous investigators (Field et al., 1979; Rose et al., 1976). Since all groups were matched for conception age, but differed in how close testing followed birth, the lower basal heart rate appears to be a depression associated with birth itself rather than due to maturation. Increasing base levels have been reported for full-term newborns retested over the first 5 days of life (Graham et al., 1968), a change which can now be interpreted as a rise back to normal levels. Medication administered during labor and delivery is known to depress fetal and postnatal heart rate, but probably was not a major contributing factor in the present sample, as none of the mothers of LR infants received large doses of anesthesia or analgesia. The physiological stress of birth itself may be primarily responsible, but further research is needed to clarify the source of change in this important indicator of neonatal health.

The lack of habituation in these infants is consistent with previous characterizations of the premature (Eisenberg et al., 1966; Field et al., 1979; Martinius & Papousek, 1970). Habituation in the full-term newborn to a similar rattle stimulus presented for 10 trials has been demonstrated (Field et al., 1979; Kulig & Clifton, 1980), which suggests that even the LR infants in this study were qualitatively different from the 40-week-old healthy newborn. Rapid habituation to a nonsignal stimulus has been associated with increasing maturity of the central nervous system, a view based primarily on the finding that habituation is progressively easier to demonstrate in older as compared to younger infants (for critical reviews, see Clifton & Nelson, 1976; Graham, Anthony & Zeigler, in press). Preterm infants may be capable of habituation with additional trials. If the rattle were presented 20–30 times or more, response decrement might well occur. Group differences would then be expressed in rate of habituation rather than by presence versus absence of response decrement. However, lengthening the test session inevitably increases the probability of a state change, which can mimic habituation (Clifton & Nelson, 1976). Despite these methodological problems, habituation is an important tool to explore behavioral functioning, as evidence mounts that insults to the central nervous system affect infants' responses to repeated stimulation (for a review, see Lipsitt & Werner, 1981).

Lack of habituation in the preterm infants' cardiac acceleration may indicate a qualitatively different response that originated in a different system from that controlling the full-term infants' response. Graham (Graham, 1979; Graham et al., in press) has differentiated two types of acceleratory cardiac responses: (1) a component of the startle response which is elicited by stimuli with sharp transient onsets, habituates rapidly, and functions as an "interrupt system" and (2) a defense response, akin to Sokolov's (1963) description of a global, nonspecific response, which is elicited by strong stimulation, habituates slowly, and functions to reduce sensitivity. Graham described the startle interrupt system as serving to halt ongoing activities when a rapid-onset signal has been detected. In the traditional view of Sokolov (1963), the defense response protects the organism by limiting the effects of stimulation by raising threshold sensitivity. The development of these two response systems during infancy has not been charted, but our data suggest that the defense response is present earlier and may be a more primitive response.

The lack of stability in behavior and heart rate over sessions in high and moderate risk groups argues against reactivity as a stable individual characteristic in the more at-risk groups. However, there was a shift towards "normalcy" in the HR group's response over sessions. These results support Brazelton's formulation (Brazelton, 1978) that the shape of the recovery curve is a better indicator of later functioning than performance at any single point in time. The data also illustrate a point made by Emde (1978), that variability and range in behavior, rather than stability, are likely to be more adaptive for further development, particularly in the newborn infant.

Specific reactivity measures probably stabilize only after homeostatic regulation is achieved. That the LR group evidenced some stability in the magnitude of heart rate acceleration to the rattle suggests that it is appropriate to use reactivity as a descriptor of individual differences in the healthy newborn. Thus assessment in terms of future outcome could be a two-step process: first, the monitoring of the infant's capabilities for achieving homeostatic regulation, and second, the assessment of the infant's specific reactivity patterns. Such a two-stage process would be consistent with the formulations of Sander (1962) and Brazelton (1978).

Implications

How, then, do we characterize these infants? We think that our data support a paradoxical description of the preterm infant, especially the more stressed infant, as hypo- and hyperreactive (Tronick, 1979). Furthermore, we believe that this paradox arises out of the underlying functioning of these infants. The data have suggested a characterization that might serve as a working hypothesis in subsequent research.

Tronick's (1979) hypothesis of paradoxical reactivity has four dimensions (see also, Krafchuk, Tronick and Clifton, 1980, and Krafchuk, Shea and Tronick, 1982). First, preterm infants, in contrast to older infants, have an elevated sensory threshold that functions protectively and makes them less reactive. This is the concept of the stimulus barrier (Freud, 1957; Spitz, 1965; Spitz, Emde & Metcalf, 1970), which finds support in our cardiac data and the data of others (Rose et al., 1976). Second, following Sokolov (1963), the preterm infant has a lower response threshold for making defense reactions to stimuli that are strong enough to pass the sensory threshold. These two characteristics combine to produce a very narrow range of receptivity in which the preterm will evidence optimal and organized responding. Third, the preterm infant either cannot or does not readily habituate (Eisenberg et al., 1966; Rose et al., 1976; Field et al., 1979); this too makes the infant appear more reactive once responding is initiated. Finally, the preterm infant's reaction patterns are global and diffuse. In combination, these functional qualities produce an infant who is less available to stimulation but more reactive once a response is initiated. Perinatal stress has the effect of exacerbating all of these characteristics. We suspect that the relation holds true regardless of gestational age, and that it in fact has its analog among adults experiencing illness or environmental stress.

The data now available on preterm infants begin to indicate how severely compromised the high risk and even healthy preterm neonate may be. While the infant appears to have an elevated sensory threshold that functions protectively, it is not adequate to ward off all input, and once the baby is stimulated sufficiently to respond, he or she is particularly vulnerable. The infant is not able to habituate and responds in a costly global fashion. While we have been describing qualities inherent in the infant, it is the quality of the infant's transactions with the environment that will determine just how overwhelmed the infant will be. The care-giving environment must make special efforts to provide the infant with the protection his or her own central nervous system does not provide. But it is also clear just how difficult it might be for the care giver to find the compromised infant's optimal range of responsivity.

REFERENCES

Als, H., Tronick, E., Adamson, L., & Brazelton, B. The behavior of the full-term but underweight newborn infant. *Development Medicine and Child Neurology*, 1976, *18*, 590–602.

Ashton, R. The effects of the environment upon state cycles in the human newborn. *Journal of Experimental Child Psychology*, 1971, *12*, 1–9.

Bartoshuk, A. Newborn cardiac reaction to sound. *Psychonomic Science*, 1964, *1*, 151–152.

Bell, R. Q., Weller, G. M., & Waldrop, M. F. Newborn and preschooler: Organization of behavior and relations between periods. *Monographs of the Society for Research in Child Development*, 1971, *36*(2, Whole No. 142).

Bench, J., & Parker, A. Hyper-responsivity to sound in the short-gestation baby. *Developmental Medicine and Child Neurology*, 1971, *13*, 15–19.

Berg, W. K., & Berg, K. M. Psychophysiological development in infancy: State, sensory function and attention. In J. D. Osofsky (Ed.), *Handbook of infant development*. New York: Wiley, 1979.

Birns, B. Individual differences in human neonates' responses to stimulation. *Child Development*, 1965, *36*, 249–256.

Brazelton, T. B. *Infants and mothers*. New York: Delta, 1969.

Brazelton, T. B. *Neonatal behavioral assessment scale*. London: Heinemann, 1973.

Brazelton, T. B. Introduction. In A. J. Sameroff (Ed.), Organization and stability of newborn behavior: A commentary on the Brazelton Neonatal Behavior Assessment scale. *Monographs of the Society for Research in Child Development*, 1978, *43*, 1–13.

Caputo, D. V., & Mandell, W. Consequences of low birthweight. *Developmental Psychology*, 1970, *3*, 368–383.

Clifton, R. K. Cardiac conditioning and orienting in the infant. In P. A. Obrist, A. H. Black, J. Brener, & L. V. DiCara (Eds.), *Cardiovascular psychophysiology: Current issues in response mechanisms, biofeedback and methodology*. Chicago: Aldine, 1974.

Clifton, R. K., & Graham, R. K. Stability of individual differences in heart activity during the newborn period. *Psychophysiology*, 1968, *5*, 37–50.

Clifton, R. K., & Nelson, M. N. Developmental study of habituation in infants: The importance of paradigm, response system, and state. In T. J. Tighe & R. N. Leaton (Eds.), *Habituation: Perspectives from child development, animal behavior and neurophysiology*. Hillsdale, N.J.: Lawrence Erlbaum, 1976.

Drillien, C. M. *The growth and development of the prematurely born infant*. Baltimore: Williams and Wilkins, 1964.

Douglas, J. W. B. "Premature" children at primary schools. *British Medical Journal*, 1960, *1*, 1008–1013.

Dubowitz, L. Newborn Maturity Rating and Classification Exam. Scoring system from J. L. Ballard. A simplified assessment of gestational age. *Pediatric Research*, 1977, *11*, 374. [Figures from A. Y. Sweet. Classification of the low birth-weight infant. In M. H. Klaus & A. A. Fanaroff (Eds.), *Care of the high risk infant*. Philadelphia: Saunders, 1979.]

Eisenberg, R. B., Coursin, D. B., & Rupp, N. R. Habituation to an acoustic pattern as an index of differences among human neonates. *Journal of Auditory Research*, 1966, *6*, 239–248.

Emde, R. N. Commentary. In A. J. Sameroff (Ed.), Organization and stability of newborn behavior: A commentary on the Brazelton Neonatal Behavior Assessment Scale. *Monographs of the Society for Research in Child Development*, 1978, *43*, 135–138.

Escalona, S. K., & Heider, G. *Prediction and outcome: A study of child development*. New York: Basic Books, 1959.

Field, T. M. Effects of early separation, interactive deficits, and experimental manipulations on infant–mother face-to-face interaction. *Child Development*, 1977, *48*, 763–771.

Field, T. M., Dempsey, J. R., Hatch, J., Ting, G., & Clifton, R. K. Cardiac and behavioral responses to repeated tactile and auditory stimulation by preterm and term neonates. *Developmental Psychology*, 1979, *15*, 406–416.

Fitzhardinge, P. M., & Steven, E. M. The small-for-date infant: Later growth patterns. *Pediatrics*, 1972, *49*, 671.

Freud, S. Beyond the pleasure principle (1920). In J. Rickman (Ed.), *A general selection from the Works of Sigmund Freud*. Garden City: Doubleday, 1957.

Gellis, S. S. The newborn. In S. S. Gellis (Ed.), *Yearbook of pediatrics*. Chicago: Yearbook Medical Publishers, 1978.

Goldberg, S. Prematurity: Effects on parent–infant interaction. *Journal of Pediatric Psychology*, 1978, *3*, 137–144.

Graham, F. K. Distinguishing among orienting, defense, and startle reflexes. In H. D. Kimmel, E. H. van Olst, & J. F. Orlebeke (Eds.), *The orienting reflex in humans*. Hillsdale, N.J.: Lawrence Erlbaum, 1979.

Graham, F. K., Anthony, B. J., & Zeigler, B. L. The orienting response and developmental processes. In D. Siddle (Ed.), *The orienting response*, Sussex, England: Wiley, in press.

Graham, F. K., Clifton, R. K., & Hatton, H. M. Habituation of heart rate response to repeated auditory stimulation during the first five days of life. *Child Development*, 1968, *39*, 35–52.

Graham, F. K., Matarazzo, R. G., & Caldwell, B. M. Behavioral differences between normal and traumatized newborns: II. Standardization, reliability, and validity. *Psychological Monographs*, 1956, *70*, 121.

Howard, J., Parmelee, A. H., Kopp, C. B., & Littman, B. Neurologic comparison of preterm and full term infants at term conceptual age. *Journal of Pediatrics*, 1976, *88*, 995–1102.

Knobloch, H., & Pasamanick, B. Predicting intellectual potential in infancy. *American Journal of Diseases of Children*, 1963, *106*, 43–51.

Krafchuk, E. E., Shea, E. M., & Tronick, E. Z. *Prematurity, perinatal trauma and coping with stimulation*. Paper presented at the biennial meetings of the International Conference on Infant Studies in Austin, March 1982.

Krafchuk, E. E., Tronick, E. Z., & Clifton, R. K. *Perinatal risk and habituation: Limitations in information processing capacity*. Paper presented at the annual meeting of The American Psychological Association, Montreal, September 1980.

Kulig, J. W., & Clifton, R. K. Habituation and sensitization of heart rate responses in newborn infants. Paper presented at the annual meeting of The American Psychological Association, Montreal, September 1980.

Lipsitt, L. P., & Werner, J. S. The infancy of human learning processes. In E. S. Gollin (Ed.), *Developmental plasticity*. New York: Academic, 1981.

Lubchenco, L. D., Bard, H., Goldman, A. L., Coyer, W. E., McIntyre, C., & Smith, D. M. Newborn intensive care and long-term prognosis. *Developmental Medicine and Child Neurology*, 1974, *16*, 421.

Lubchenco, L. D., Hansman, C., & Boyd, E. Intrauterine growth in length and head circumference as estimated from live births at gestational ages from 26 to 42 weeks. *Pediatrics*, 1966, *37*, 403.

Martinius, J., & Papousek, H. Responses to optic and exteroceptive stimuli in relation to state in the human newborn. *Neuropaediatrie*, 1970, *1*, 452–460.

McCall, R. B. Attention in the infant: Avenue to the study of cognitive development. In D. N. Walcher & D. L. Peters (Eds.), *Early childhood: The development of self-regulatory mechanisms*. New York: Academic, 1971.

Myers, J. L. *Fundamentals of experimental design*. Boston: Allyn and Bacon, 1972.

Prechtl, H. *The neurological examination of the full-term newborn infant*. London: Heinemann, 1977.

Rose, S., Schmidt, K., & Bridger, W. H. Cardiac and behavioral responsivity to tactile stimulation in premature and fullterm infants. *Developmental Psychology*, 1976, *12*, 311–320.

Rose, S. A., Schmidt, K., Riese, M. L., & Bridger, W. H. Effects of prematurity and early intervention on responsivity to tactile stimuli: A comparison of preterm and full term infants. *Child Development*, 1980, *51*, 416–425.

Sameroff, A. J., Krafchuk, E., & Bakow, H. A. Issues in grouping items from the neonatal behavioral assessment scale. In A. J. Sameroff (Ed.), Organization and stability of newborn behavior: A commentary on the Brazelton Neonatal Behavior Assessment Scale. *Monographs of the Society for Research in Child Development*, 1978, *43*, 46–59.

Sander, L. Issues in early mother–child interaction. *Journal of the American Academy of Child Psychiatry*, 1962, *1*, 141–166.

Schulte, F. J., Hinze, G., & Schrempf, G. Maternal toxemia, fetal malnutrition, and bioelectrical brain activity of the newborn. In C. Clemente, D. Purpura, & F. Mayer (Eds.), *Sleep and the maturing nervous system*. New York: Academic Research, 1972.

Sokolov, E. N. *Perception and the conditioned reflex*. New York: MacMillan, 1963.

Sostek, A., Quinn, P., & Davitt, M. K. Behavior, development, and neurological status of premature and full-term infants of varying medical complications. In T. Field, A. M. Sostek, S. Goldberg, & H. H. Shuman (Eds.), *Infants born at risk*. New York: Spectrum, 1979.

Spitz, R. *The first year of life; Normal and deviant object relations*. New York: International Universities Press, 1965.

Spitz, R., Emde, R. N., & Metcalf, D. R. Further prototypes of ego formation: A working paper from a research project on early development. *The Psychoanalytic Study of the Child*, 1970, *24*, 417–441.

Thomas, A., Chess, S., Birch, H. C., Hertzig, M. E., & Korn, S. *Behavioral individuality in early childhood*. New York: New York University Press, 1963.

Thompson, R. F., Groves, P. M., Teyler, T. J., & Roemer, R. A. A dual-process theory of habituation: Theory and behavior. In H. V. S. Peeke & M. J. Herz (Eds.), *Habituation* (Vol. 2). New York: Academic, 1973.

Tronick, E. Sensory and defensive thresholds in preterm neonates. Grant funded by the National Foundation March of Dimes, September 1979.

Wilder, J. *Stimulus and response: The law of initial value*. Bristol: Wright, 1967.

6

Nonnutritive Sucking Opportunities:
A Safe and Effective Treatment
for Preterm Neonates

*Gene Cranston Anderson
Arlene K. Burroughs, Carol Porter Measel*

Data from three studies will be reported in this article. However, to integrate these three studies some background information and a theoretical framework are needed first. The primary research concern began with infant crying. As a staff nurse on a general obstetrical unit back in 1968, the senior author became aware of a great deal of crying in full-term infants, particularly prior to the first feeding. The first feeding was not given until

The first research was conducted by Gene Cranston Anderson with the assistance of Melen McBride, Janet Dahm, Marla Ellis, and Dharmapuri Vidyasagar. It was supported by Grants NU00673 (Gene Cranston Anderson, projector director), PHSNU500 (Gladys Courtney and Lois Malasanos, project directors), and NU01548 (Harriet Werley, project director) from the Division of Nursing, Health Resources Administration. The second research was conducted by Gene Cranston Anderson and Arlene K. Burroughs with the assistance of Dharmapuri Vidyasagar, Udochukwu Asonye, and Minu Patel; it was supported by Grants NU01548 and NU000673 from the Division of Nursing, Health Resources Administration. These first two studies took place at the University of Illinois at the Medical Center in Chicago. The third research was conducted at Wayne State University by Gene Cranston Anderson and Carol Porter Measel and was supported by the National Institutes of Health Biomedical Research Grant BR070511 (Jean Johnson, project director) and by the Grant NU00673 from the Division of Nursing, Health Resources Administration. The authors wish to express their appreciation to the co-investigators, the obstetric and nursery staffs, and the mothers and their newborn infants for their participation and cooperation.

Paper presented in T. M. Field (Chair), *Sucking, crying, and stimulation in preterm neonates*. Symposium presented at the Second Biennial International Conference for Infancy Studies, New Haven, April 1980; paper presented at the Southern Perinatal Association meeting, New Orleans, January 1981.

12 hours postbirth in this hospital. During these 12 hours the infants were not only fasted, but separated from their mothers as well. This meant that the stimulation inherent in mother–newborn interaction was unavailable to the newborn and the mother.

Two very helpful acronyms developed out of the concern for this lack of mother-newborn interaction. The first acronym is SMYLI (smi'lē)—self-regulatory mother–young (fetus or newborn) longitudinal (uninterrupted by birth) interaction. This level of interaction is considered to be ideal. The mother and her newborn are mutual care givers, physiologically dependent on each other and mutually adapted to provide each other with the care they need, provided they are permitted to continue to interact in a self-regulatory fashion during the first few hours postbirth. The SMYLI level of interaction is proposed to have survival value for our species. In addition, mother–newborn attachment should be enhanced during SMYLI, because the mother and her newborn are experiencing an increased sense of well-being in association with each other. The antithesis of SMYLI is ASMYLI, or absence of SMYLI (Anderson, 1977).

At any rate, early feedings were not allowed, and the infants could not be with their mothers. How else might these crying infants be quieted? Helpful knowledge was shared by Florence Blake (personal communication, 1967), a famous pediatric nurse, who reported that William Kessen and his colleagues had demonstrated that nonnutritive sucking was an effective settling technique. First these investigators conducted a study with restless newborn infants who had already been fed. The activity level of these infants decreased when they were provided with 2 min of nonnutritive sucking on a pacifier, and their activity level increased again when the pacifier was withdrawn (Kessen & Leutzendorff, 1963). However, critics suggested that the infants may have quieted down because of an association between sucking and relief of hunger, not because of sucking. A second study was then conducted with infants who had not received their first feeding. Sucking quieted these infants also (Kessen, Leutzendorff, & Stoutsenberger, 1967). This study ruled out the possibility that the soothing effect of the pacifier derived from the association of sucking with food. This was intriguing, especially because sucking, both nutritive and nonnutritive, is a major component of self-regulatory mother–young longitudinal interaction. Clinically, the settling effect of nonnutritive sucking was dramatic and unmistakable.

Prior to their first feeding, the senior author began letting these restless infants suck to satiety, that is, until they stopped sucking. This was easy to do while caring for other babies, because the infants, placed prone or on their sides, would hold the nipple in their mouths themselves. Often they sucked for as long as an hour. Based on these observations, it was hypothesized that sucking not only settled, but that sucking to *satiety* resulted in *prolonged* settling. This hypothesis has been substantiated since (Anderson & Grant, 1983).

In addition to this settling effect, other effects seemed beneficial. First, respiration became deep and even, relative to what it had been before. Second, the arousal level was strikingly improved; infants either began to sleep deeply or became alert and responsive. Third, frequently the passage of meconium, material filling the infant's gastrointestinal tract, occurred during or shortly after the sucking opportunities. Fourth, neuromuscular coordination improved. And fifth, infants given sucking opportunities, even though on a commercial bottle nipple, seemed to nurse well at the breast.

These observations led to questions about *why* sucking settled, and the proposal that a parasympathetically governed organic set (cf. Moltz, 1960, 1963) results from sucking. In other words, sucking may result in generalized cholinergic stimulation; put still another way, sucking may have a vagal effect. The resultant deep and regular respirations would allow venous blood to return to the heart under less pressure. This, in the transitional newborn, allows more venous blood to reach the lungs for proper oxygenation, which would in turn facilitate the necessary circulatory adaptations postbirth. Crying would have the opposite effect (Anderson, 1983).*

Sucking, which is one of the first experiences following natural birth, may trigger the onset of certain physiological regulations (cf. Adolph, 1968; Anderson, 1975). Sucking, which has the obvious function of bringing nutrient into the body, may also result in a generalized peristalsis, which would promote glandular secretion, mixing of secretions with nutrients, propulsion and absorption of secretions and nutrients, and expulsion of waste products. This would mean that sucking not only initiates the gastrointestinal cycle, but facilitates its completion.

These ideas were also useful when working as a staff nurse in a neonatal intensive care unit. Many similarities were apparent in the behavior of full-term infants (Anderson, 1976) and preterm infants. Both rooted actively, were restless and cried frequently (although preterm infants

---

*Crying and hard crying, during which the glottis is partially or almost closed, is a modified Valsalva maneuver. The Valsalva maneuver (more accurately called the Valsalva procedure) occurs when an expiratory effort is made against a closed glottis. Everyone is familiar with this procedure, which is frequently used in defecation, parturition (McKay, 1981; McKay & Roberts, in press), coughing, lifting, and other types of strenuous physical exertion (Jones, 1965). Commonly the face reddens. Venous return is obstructed during the prolonged expiratory effort, which when released allows the blood to rush into the right atrium of the heart under high pressure. In the newborn, about two-thirds of this blood is channeled so that it hits the foramen ovale, where a flap of tissue should lie closed and eventually seal along the inner wall of the left atrium after birth. If this tissue has not sealed tightly, the high pressure of the blood is sufficient to allow the blood, which is poorly oxygenated and should go to the lungs, to pass through the foramen ovale and back into the systemic circulation instead (cf., Lind, Stern, & Wegelius, 1964, pp. 37–40; Walsh, Meyer, & Lind, 1974, pp. 90–93). This poorly oxygenated blood may delay anatomic closure of the ductus arteriosus. Moss, Emmanouilides, Adams, and Chuang (1964) report that a functionally closed ductus arteriosus may reopen up to the third day postbirth if arterial PO_2 decreases.

often cry silently), engaged in hand–mouth activity, and responded similarly when given sucking opportunities.

Observations of these similarities added support to the theoretical framework and prompted the rather colloquial thought that if infants seem to want to suck so much, perhaps they need to. This idea seems logical enough. We have learned from Hooker (1942), Kohn, Nelson, and Weiner (1980), Liley (1965), Nilsson, Furujhelm, Ingelman-Sundberg, and Wirsen (1976, pp. 124–125), and Nilsson, Ingelman-Sundberg, and Wirsen (1965, p. 92) that the fetus not only thumb and finger sucks, but does so frequently.

Flanagan (1962) has republished a series of film clips by Hooker (1942) in which a newly delivered 6½-month-gestation fetus is seen engaging in hand-mouth and rooting activity just as older preterm and full-term infants do. In each film clip the position of the right hand changes, moving away from and toward, and sometimes touching, the mouth and perioral area. The mouth opens and closes several times as well.

Figure 6-1 shows sucking lesions on the back of the wrists of a healthy full-term infant. These lesions were present at birth and were assumed to be caused by fetal sucking.†

Thus, fetuses suck in utero. Yet preterm infants, who really are would-be fetuses and who would be sucking often if still in utero, receive few, if any, sucking opportunities during their first days postbirth. The premature infant is truly an infant who experiences absence of self-regulatory mother–newborn interaction, that is, ASMYLI. Indeed, maternal kinds of stimulation are virtually absent.

These observations and ideas led the senior author to the suggestion that nonnutritive sucking be given to preterm infants in order to test the effect of these treatments on subsequent clinical course. Invariably this suggestion prompted three questions, even from the medical directors of the intensive care nurseries: Are small, weak premature infants able to suck, even nonnutritively? Is nonnutritive sucking safe? Is nonnutritive sucking beneficial? Three studies were conducted to answer these questions and will be reported briefly here.

CAN SMALL PREMATURE INFANTS SUCK NONNUTRITIVELY?

To answer this first question, 27 premature infants were studied from birth (Anderson, 1983). These infnats had a mean gestational age by exam

---

†The photograph was contributed by Murdina Desmond, the pediatrician who studied the transitional newborn in great detail (Desmond, Franklin, Vallbona, Hill, Plumb, Arnold, & Watts, 1963) and who founded the transitional newborn nursery (Desmond, Rudolph, & Phitaksphraiwan, 1966).

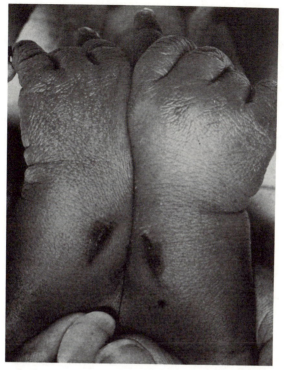

Figure 6-1
Lesions on the back of wrists of a healthy newborn infant.
These lesions were assumed to be caused by fetal sucking.
(Reprinted with permission from Murdina Desmond, M.D.).

(Dubowitz, Dubowitz, & Goldberg, 1970), of 36.5 weeks and a mean birth weight of 1986 g. Fourteen of the infants weighed less than 2000 g.

Two instruments were used in this research. The first was a small portable electronic suckometer with a research nipple adapted from the works of Kron, Stein, & Goddard (1963) and Sameroff (1965). These instruments are described elsewhere (Anderson & Vidyasagar 1979). The nipple measures both components of sucking: the suction, or negative component, and the expression, or positive pressure component. The second instrument was a feeding scale used to evaluate bottle feedings. This scale has a scoring system similar to the Apgar score (Apgar, 1953). Possible scores range from 0 to 24, and a score of 17 represents an acceptable feeding. This feeding scale has been described by Anderson, McBride, Dahm, Ellis, and Vidyasagar (1982). Nonnutritive suction and expression pressures were measured 30 times in each of the 27 preterm infants from 5 min to 7 days postbirth. Pressures were measured for 2 min each time, 12 times from birth to 8 hours, and 3 times daily during days 1–7. Also, pressures were measured just before the first feeding. This feeding was evaluated with the feeding scale.

Mean sucking pressures are plotted in Figure 6-2. The data are expressed in units of torr (mmHg). Sucking was present in 11 preterm infants at 5 mins. Suction pressures peaked at 57 torr at 90 min postbirth, but dropped to 33 torr by 8 hours. Pressures varied considerably during days 1–7 ($\overline{X}$ = 56 Torr), reaching the 90-min peak only 7 out of 18 times. Interestingly, this same 90-min peak (103 torr) and subsequent decline (67 torr at 4 hours) was seen in 30 full-term infants, as shown in Figure 6-3 (Anderson et al., 1982). Two additional very small infants were studied anecdotally. A 520-g infant sucked at 10 torr at 5 min postbirth, and a 590-g, 25-week-gestation infant sucked at 25 torr on day 6.

Feeding scores for the first feeding averaged a satisfactory score of 16.9 on the day of birth and were as strong then as during the next 6 days. The correlations between sucking pressures and feeding scores were not significant at the first feeding. Clinically, the full-term infants and even many of the premature infants seemed ready to feed at 90 min postbirth. In fact, they seemed more organized at this time, or sooner, than they did at 4 or 8 hours.

Also, in this research factors were explored which might be related to the ability to suck; that is, to answer a secondary question, why did premature infants suck at some times, but not at others? Sucking pressures were positively correlated with gestation and birth weight. Pressures were weaker with increasing temperature, heart rate, and breathing rate and with delayed voiding and stooling. These findings indicate that sucking strength is related to condition, as well as to maturity and size. The correlations were not strong, however, and did not occur at all times of measurement, so these findings are best considered as only trends. However, further suckometer refinements using new microcomputer technology are now in progress. The new suckometer will measure cumulative pressure every 15 sec instead of only the maximum pressure. This more sensitive instrument, no larger or more expensive than the first, may yield more useful correlations in future studies and hopefully will allow us to predict when a preterm infant is able to begin oral feeding safely.

One finding was strong and consistent: time after time, we saw adequate suction pressures drop to 0 following prolonged activity, invasive therapy, and/or a crying episode. Logically, invasive therapy and vigorous procedures such as chest percussion would be done prior to feedings. To do this between feedings would disturb the infant's rest; to do this after a feeding would invite regurgitation; however, to do this before a feeding, as is commonly done for the reasons mentioned, appears to compromise the infant's sucking ability, and thus the feeding. This important finding remains to be studied systematically.

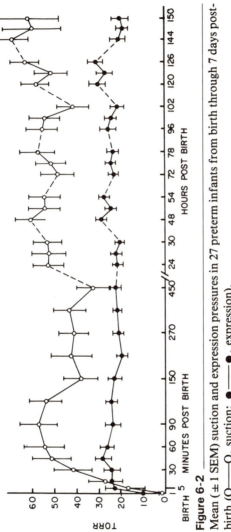

Figure 6-2
Mean (± 1 SEM) suction and expression pressures in 27 preterm infants from birth through 7 days postbirth (O———O, suction; ●——————●, expression).

135

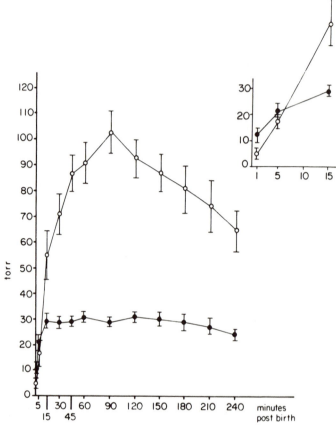

Figure 6-3

Mean (± 1 SEM) suction and expression pressures in 30 term infants from birth through 4 hours postbirth (O——O, suction; ● — ●, expression). (Reprinted with permission from Anderson, G. C., McBride, M. R., Dahm, J., Ellis, M. K., & Vidyasagar, D. Development of sucking in term infants from birth to four hours postbirth. *Research in Nursing and Health,* 1982, *5,* 21–27.)

The conclusion to be drawn from this research is that small, ill premature infants can suck.

IS NONNUTRITIVE SUCKING SAFE FOR ILL PREMATURE INFANTS?

To answer this question, the effect of nonnutritive sucking on transcutaneous oxygen tension was studied with noncrying preterm infants (Burroughs, Asonye, Anderson-Shanklin, & Vidyasagar, 1978). This research was needed because of the fear that the energy cost of sucking might cause problems for the premature infant. Clinically, we knew that premature infants responded favorably to sucking opportunities, but this had never been documented. The plan was to study the effect of non-nutritive sucking with the noncrying infant first, in order to demonstrate that sucking is a safe activity. The second study which remains to be conducted would document the effect of nonnutritive sucking on transcutaneous oxygen tension in the crying infant.

Three instruments were used in this research. The first was an activity scale adapted from the one reported by Parmelee, Kopp, and Sigman in 1976. The adapted scale ranged from 0 through 12, in contrast to the 9 levels used by Parmelee and co-workers. Activity with eyes closed was scored from 0 through 3 and ranged from no movement to total body movement. Eyes opening and closing with no other movement was scored 4. Activity with eyes open was scored from 5 through 9 and ranged from no movement and alert inactivity to total body movement. A score of 10 represented fussing, 11 crying activity, and 12 extreme agitation. The second instrument was the suckometer and research nipple.

We were tremendously fortunate to have the third instrument, the transcutaneous oxygen monitor. This instrument measures transcutaneous oxygen tension, which is referred to as $tcPo_2$. The $tcPo_2$ monitor is an extremely important technological breakthrough: it uses an electrode attached to the skin to measure oxygen tension transcutaneously, continuously, noninvasively, and *without artifact*. This last point is emphasized because the validity of heel stick Po_2 is very poor, running 18 torr below intra-arterial readings (Dinwiddle, Patel, Kumar, & Fox, 1979). However, the validity of the $tcPo_2$ monitor is well established. Numerous investigators have reported correlations ranging from .93 to .97 for $tcPo_2$ and intra-arterial catheter readings (Huch, Huch, & Lucey, 1979). The $tcPo_2$ monitor makes it possible to study the effects on $tcPo_2$ of the infant's own activity, whatever is happening to him or her, or whatever is happening in the environment. For example, Jerold Lucey and his colleagues at the University of Vermont have found that $tcPo_2$ drops precipitously when the telephone rings. Most importantly, $tcPo_2$ is generally accepted now as a marker of infant condition. An example of the type of data which can be obtained with the $tcPo_2$ monitor is presented in Figure 6-4: Huch and Huch (1976), the developers of the $tcPo_2$ monitor, published this record of a healthy term infant who was crying intermittently. The dotted portions are periods of crying. The vertical axis represents $tcPo_2$ expressed in torr, and the horizontal axis represents the time expressed in minutes. Note how the line representing $tcPo_2$ drops during each cry. We have documented this phenomenon in preterm infants (see Fig. 6-5). In addition, the typical effect of sucking following crying can be seen (Burroughs et al., 1978).

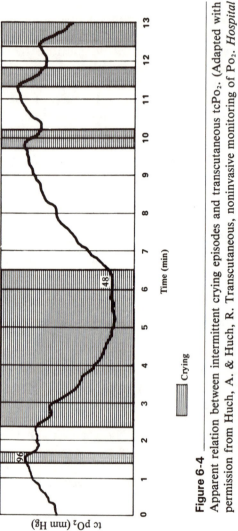

Figure 6-4

Apparent relation between intermittent crying episodes and transcutaneous $tcPo_2$. (Adapted with permission from Huch, A. & Huch, R. Transcutaneous, noninvasive monitoring of Po_2. *Hospital Practice*, 1967, *38*, 43–52.)

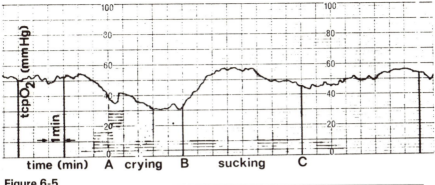

Figure 6-5 _____

Typical tcPo₂ recording of a premature infant during crying (A to B) and sucking (B to C). (Reprinted with permission from Burroughs, A. K., Asonye, U. O., Anderson-Shanklin, G. C., & Vidyasagar, D. The effect of nonnutritive sucking on transcutaneous oxygen tension in noncrying preterm neonates. *Research in Nursing and Health*, 1978, *1*, 69–75).

A pretest–post-test design was used to document the effect of sucking on tcPo₂ in noncrying infants. This design consisted of 24 min divided into three equal time periods: pretreatment, sucking treatment, and posttreatment. The tcPo₂ and activity were recorded continuously throughout these 24 min. Each infant was in the supine position, in either an incubator or a radiant heat bed. Activity scores were assigned based on observation during the first 20 sec of each minute. Data collection was completed only when an infant did not fuss or cry (an activity score of < 10) during the pretreatment period. Sucking was given during the treatment period. All infants sucked and most began immediately after nipple insertion.

A total of 26 sets of measurements were completed on 11 preterm infants (mean gestational age, 31 weeks; mean birth weight, 1594 g). No infant was measured more than three times. An example of the raw data for each set of measurements can be seen in Figure 6-6. The three means of tcPo₂ for each time period were significantly different at the < .01 level. During sucking tcPo₂ rose and continued to rise following sucking (see Fig. 6-7). Also, infants with a tcPo₂ above 50 Torr had significantly stronger suction pressures ($p < .01$) than infants with tcPo₂ at or below 50 Torr (Burroughs, Anderson, Patel, & Vidyasagar, 1981).

The following conclusions can be drawn from this study: (1) Sucking pressures appear to be, at least in part, a function of infant condition, and (2) nonnutritive sucking is a safe, and apparently beneficial, activity for ill, noncrying, premature infants. Whatever the energy cost of sucking, it appears to be, somehow, well reimbursed.

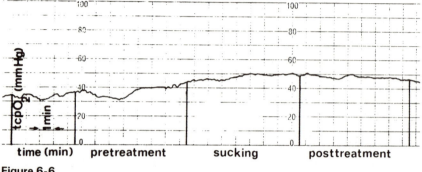

time (min)   pretreatment   sucking   posttreatment

Figure 6-6 _____

Typical tcPo₂ recording of a premature infant receiving assisted ventilation during pretreatment, sucking, and post-treatment. (Reprinted with permission from Burroughs, A. K., Asonye, U. O., Anderson-Shanklin, G. C., & Vidyasagar, D. The effect of nonnutritive sucking on transcutaneous oxygen tension in noncrying preterm neonates. *Research in Nursing and Health*, 1978, *1*, 69–75.)

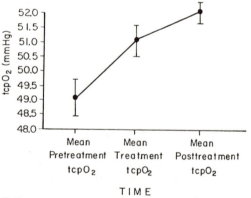

Figure 6-7 _____

Effect of nonnutritive sucking on tcPo₂ level as demonstrated by 26 sets of measurements on premature infants. Values (mean ±1 standard error) are the averaged readings for each 8-min observation period. (Reprinted with permission from Burroughs, A. K., Asonye, U. O., Anderson-Shanklin, G. C., Vidyasagar, D. The effect of nonnutritive sucking on transcutaneous oxygen tension in noncrying preterm neonates. *Research in Nursing and Health*, 1978, *1*, 69–75).

IS NONNUTRITIVE SUCKING AN EFFECTIVE TREATMENT? _____

To answer this question, nonnutritive sucking treatments were given to 59 premature infants during tube feedings and for 5 min postfeeding (Measel & Anderson, 1979). The purpose was to test the effect of this treatment on the subsequent clinical course of these infants, who are commonly troubled with gastric retention and intestinal distention. The infants were between 28 and 34 weeks gestation ($\overline{X}$ = 32.3 weeks), and between 1000 and 2000 g ($\overline{X}$ = 1420 g). They were assigned by alternate sequential series to a treatment group and a control group.

A commercial bottle nipple (Ross Laboratories, Columbus, Ohio) was used to give the sucking treatment. The plunger from a 20-cc syringe was inserted into the base of the nipple to make it airtight, to use for propping, and, as it turned out, for the infant to hold (see Fig. 6-8). A feeding scale described in Measel and Anderson (1979) was used to assess performance during the first bottle feeding. The sucking treatment began when an infant could tolerate room air and 10 cc of full-strength formula by tube, and ended when the infant was totally bottle fed. Data collection continued until hospital discharge.

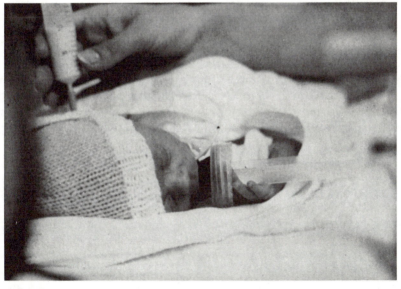

Figure 6-8 _____
Treatment infant sucking on a pacifier during tube feeding. (Reprinted with permission from Measel, C. P., & Anderson, G. C. Nonnutritive sucking during tube feedings: Effect on clinical course in premature infants. *Journal of Obstetric, Gynecologic and Neonatal Nursing*, 1979, *8*, 265–272.)

Prior to treatment, the sample was statistically similar, except for three variables. Two of these variables appeared to favor the control group. First, 14 percent of the treatment group consisted of second-born twins, the twin known to be at greater risk, in contrast with 0 percent of the control group. Second, 24 percent of the treatment group had exchange transfusions, a treatment thought to predispose infants to the dread condition of necrotizing enterocolitis (Hodson, 1975, pp. 20 and 27–28), in contrast with 7 percent of the control group. The third variable which differed was that 40 percent of the infants in the treatment group were delivered by cesarean section, in contrast with 20 percent of the control group. The effect this difference may have had is less clear.

Feeding scores at first bottle feeding were statistically similar for both groups. This supports the clinical judgment of the nursery staff in determining an infant's readiness to begin bottle feeding. The important difference is that treated infants showed this readiness for bottle feeding 3.4 days earlier, that is, with 27 fewer tube feedings each ($p < .05$). From study entry to discharge home, the treated infants were discharged 4 days sooner ($p < .025$). These findings have implications for cost effectiveness, as well as for improved health.

Infants were excluded from the study if they developed complications that were treated by eliminating feedings and water by mouth. Here the differences between groups are worth noting. From the perspective of the theoretical framework presented earlier, fewer and less severe complications had been predicted for the treatment group. This prediction was upheld. Although patent ductus arteriosus was diagnosed in 3 infants in each group, 2 of the 3 control infants required surgical ligation of the ductus. All 3 treatment infants and 1 control infant received minimal medical therapy and remained in the study. A total of 1 control infant and 2 treatment infants developed necrotizing enterocolitis; 1 treatment infant recovered with medical management. Ileostomies were performed on 1 control infant and 1 treatment infant; the treatment infant lived, but the control infant died.

Another control infant required a surgical shunt for hydrocephalus. This difference had not been predicted. Recently, however, new evidence has resulted in the awareness that hydrocephalus can result from intraventricular hemorrhage (Mantovani, Pasternak, Mathew, Allan, Mills, Casper, & Volpe, 1980; Volpe, 1979). From this standpoint, increased frequency of hydrocephalus in the control group could have been predicted by another portion of the theoretical framework discussed elsewhere briefly (Burroughs et al., 1978) and in detail (Anderson, 1983). Crying, straining, and other intense activity involving the Valsalva maneuver, probably would raise intracranial pressure. Crying in preterm infants resembles the Valsalva maneuver in adults (Dinwiddie, Pitcher-Wilmott, Schwartz, Shaffer, & Fox, 1979). If sucking quiets restless infants, then sucking

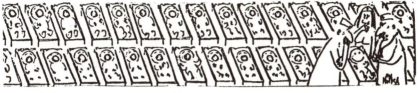

Figure 6-9
Why is this nursery staff so concerned about the different infant, the smiling one? Perhaps the crying infant is common, but the smiling infant is normal. (Reprinted with permission from *Look Magazine*, 1969.)

should decrease intracranial pressure. This hypothesis can be tested now with a new instrument which noninvasively and continuously measures intracranial pressure.

To sum the differences in complications, 4 control infants, but only 1 treatment infant required major surgery; 1 control infant died, but all treatment infants survived. With only 59 infants studied, the differences in complication rate reported here can only be considered suggestive, but these findings are supported by replication–extension research (Bernbaum, Pereira, Watkins, & Peckham, 1983; Field, Ignatoff, Stringer, Brennan, Greenberg, Widmayer, & Anderson, 1982). At any rate, this study suggests that nonnutritive sucking during and following tube feedings improved clinical course and can be considered beneficial.

SUMMARY

To summarize the results of all three studies reported here, weak premature infants sucked nonnutritively when the opportunity was provided, and this activity appeared to be safe and beneficial.

In closing, here is one final thought. For a long time, most of us have assumed that newborn crying is normal, because it is so common. Perhaps that is why the nursery staff in the cartoon in Figure 6-9 is so concerned about the different infant, the smiling one. Recall that the crying newborn can be settled with sucking opportunities, an inherent component of natural mother–newborn interaction postbirth. Then consider the possibility that the crying infant is common, but the smiling infant is normal.

REFERENCES

Adolph, E. F. *Origins of physiological regulations.* New York: Academic, 1968.
Anderson, G. C. A preliminary report: Severe respiratory distress in two newborn lambs with recovery following nonnutritive sucking. *Journal of Nurse-Midwifery*, 1975, *20*, 20–28.

Anderson, G. C. *The transitional newborn (hand-mouth activity: Intention to suck?).* Chicago: Aldine, 1976 (and instructional guide).

Anderson, G. C. The mother and her newborn: Mutual caregivers. *Journal of Obstetric, Gynecologic and Neonatal Nursing,* 1977, *6,* 50–57.

Anderson, G. C. *Relation of self-regulatory sucking from birth to oxygenation and clinical course in premature infants: A theoretical framework.* Unpublished manuscript, 1983.

Anderson, G. C. *Development of sucking in low-birth-weight infants from birth through seven days postbirth.* Manuscript in preparation, 1983.

Anderson, G. C., & Grant, A. R. *Effects of self-regulatory nonnutritive sucking on behavioral state in restless newborn infants.* Manuscript in preparation, 1983.

Anderson, G. C., McBride, M. R., Dahm, J., Ellis, M. K., & Vidyasagar, D. Development of sucking in term infants from birth through four hours postbirth. *Research in Nursing and Health,* 1982, *5,* 21–27.

Anderson, G. C., & Vidyasagar, D. Development of sucking in premature infants from 0–7 days postbirth as measured with a suck scoring system. In G. C. Anderson & B. Raff (Eds.), *Newborn behavioral organization: Nursing research and implications.* New York: Liss, 1979. [National Foundation-March of Dimes. *Birth Defects: Original Article Series* (Vol. 15, No. 7)].

Apgar, V. A proposal for a new method of evaluation of the newborn infant. *Current Research in Anesthesiology and Analgesia,* 1953, *32,* 260–267.

Bernbaum, J., Pereira, G. R., Watkins, J. B., & Peckham, G. J. Nonnutritive sucking during gavage feeding enhances growth and maturation in premature infants. *Pediatrics,* 1983, *71,* 41–45.

Blake, F. G. Personal communication, 1967.

Burroughs, A. K., Anderson, G. C., Patel, M. K., & Vidyasagar, D. Relation of nonnutritive sucking pressures to tcPo₂ and gestational age in preterm infants. *Perinatology–Neonatology,* 1981, *(5)*2, 54–62.

Burroughs, A. K., Asonye, U. O., Anderson-Shanklin, G. C., & Vidyasagar, D. The effect of nonnutritive sucking on transcutaneous oxygen tension in noncrying preterm neonates. *Research in Nursing and Health,* 1978, *1,* 69–75.

Desmond, M. M., Franklin, R. R., Vallbona, C., Hill, R. M., Plumb, R., Arnold, H., & Watts, J. The clinical behavior of the newly born: The term baby. *Journal of Pediatrics,* 1963, *62,* 307–325.

Desmond, M. M., Rudolph, A. J., & Phitaksphraiwan, P. The transitional care nursery: A mechanism for preventive medicine in the newborn. *Pediatric Clinics of North America,* 1966, *13,* 651–668.

Dinwiddie, R., Patel, B. D., Kumar, S. P., & Fox, W. W. The effects of crying on arterial oxygen tension in infants recovering from respiratory distress. *Critical Care Medicine,* 1979, *7,* 50–53.

Dinwiddie, R., Pitcher-Wilmott, R., Schwartz, J. G., Shaffer, T. H., & Fox, W. W. Cardiopulmonary changes in the crying neonate. *Pediatric Research,* 1979, *13,* 900–903.

Dubowitz, L., Dubowitz, V., & Goldberg, C. Clinical assessment of gestational age in the newborn infant. *Journal of Pediatrics,* 1970, *77,* 1–10.

Field, T., Ignatoff, E., Stringer, S., Brennan, J., Greenberg, R., Widmayer, S., & Anderson, G. C. Effects of nonnutritive sucking during tube feedings of ICU preterm neonates. *Pediatrics,* 1982, *70,* 381–384.

Flanagan, G. L. *The first nine months of life.* New York: Simon & Schuster, 1972. (Reprinted by Philadelphia: International Ideas, 1975.)

Hodson, W. A. Diagnosis and clinical criteria for recognition. In T. D. Moore (Ed.), *Necrotizing enterocolitis in the newborn infant.* Columbus, Ohio: Ross Laboratories, 1975.

Hooker, D. Fetal reflexes and instinctual processes. *Psychosomatic Medicine,* 1942, *4*, 199.

Huch, A., & Huch, R. Transcutaneous, noninvasive monitoring of P_{O_2}. *Hospital Practice,* 1976 *38*, 43–52.

Huch, A., Huch, R., & Lucey, J. F. (Eds.). *Continuous transcutaneous blood gas monitoring.* New York: Liss, 1979. [National Foundation-March of Dimes. *Birth Defects: Original Article Series* (Vol. 15, No. 4].

Jones, H. H. The Valsalva procedure: Its clinical importance to the physical therapist. *Journal of the American Physical Therapy Association,* 1965, *45*, 570–572.

Kessen, W., & Leutzendorff, A. M. The effect of nonnutritive sucking on movement in the human newborn. *Journal of Comparative Physiological Psychology,* 1963, *59*, 69–72.

Kessen, W., Leutzendorff, A. M., & Stoutsenberger, K. Age, food deprivation, nonnutritive sucking, and movement in the human newborn. *Journal of Comparative Physiological Psychology,* 1967, *63*, 82–86.

Kohn, C. L., Nelson, A., & Weiner, S. Gravidas' responses to realtime ultrasound fetal image. *Journal of Obstetric, Gynecologic, and Neonatal Nursing,* 1980, *9*, 77–80.

Kron, R. E., Stein, M., & Goddard, K. E. A method of measuring sucking behavior of newborn infants. *Psychosomatic Medicine,* 1963, *25*, 181–191.

Liley, A. W. Physiological observations in fetal transfusion. *Studies in physiology.* New York: Springer-Verlag, 1965.

Lind, J., Stern, L., & Wegelius, C. Human foetal and neonatal circulation. In J. Anderson (Ed.), *American Monograph in Pediatrics Series.* Springfield, Ill.: Thomas, 1964.

Look Magazine, 1969.

Mantovani, J. F., Pasternak, J. F., Mathew, O. P., Allan, W. C. Mills, M. T., Casper, J., & Volpe, J. J. Failure of daily lumbar punctures to prevent the development of hydrocephalus following intraventricular hemorrhage. *Journal of Pediatrics,* 1980, *97*, 278–281.

McKay, S. R. Second stage labor—Has tradition replaced safety? *American Journal of Nursing,* 1981, *81*, 1016–1019.

McKay, S. R. & Roberts, J. Second stage of labor: What is normal? In press.

Measel, C. P., & Anderson, G. C. Nonnutritive sucking during tube feedings: Effect upon clinical course in premature infants. *Journal of Obstetric, Gynecologic and Neonatal Nursing,* 1979, *8*, 265–272.

Moltz, H. Imprinting: Empirical basis and theoretical significance. *Psychological Bulletin,* 1960, *57*, 291–314.

Moltz, H. Imprinting: An epigenetic approach. *Psychological Review,* 1963, *70*, 123–138.

Moss, A. J., Emmanouilides, G., Adams, F. H., & Chuang, K. Response of the ductus arteriosus and pulmonary and systemic arterial pressure to changes in oxygen environment in newborn infants. *Pediatrics,* 1964, *33*, 937–944.

Nilsson, L., Furujhelm, M., Ingelman-Sundberg, A., & Wirsen, C. *A child is born* (2nd ed.). New York: Delacorte, 1976.

Nilsson, L., Ingelman-Sundberg, A., & Wirsen, C. *A child is born* (1st ed.). New York: Delacorte, 1965.

Parmelee, A. H., Jr., Kopp, C. B., & Sigman, M. Selection of developmental assessment techniques for infants at risk. *Merrill-Palmer Quarterly*, 1976, *22*, 177–199.

Sameroff, A. J. An apparatus for recording sucking and controlling feeding in the first days of life. *Psychonomic Science*, 1965, *2*, 355–356.

Volpe, J. J. Intracranial hemorrhage in the newborn: Current understanding and dilemmas. *Neurology*, 1979, *29*, 632–635.

Walsh, S. Z., Meyer, W. W., & Lind, J. *The human fetal and neonatal circulation*. Springfield, Ill: Thomas, 1974.

7

A Cross-Cultural Study of Teenage Pregnancy and Neonatal Behavior

Barry M. Lester
Cynthia T. Garcia Coll, Carol Sepkoski

The current concern with teenage pregnancy can be traced to the late 1960s and early 1970s, when it was realized that more than half of out-of-wedlock births occurred among teenagers (Osofsky, 1970). The problem of illegitimacy was redefined to emphasize adolescence, and demographic statistics began to reflect high birthrates among teenagers, especially in the number of out-of-wedlock births (Baldwin, 1976).

Some of the consequences of teenage pregnancy have been studied. The medical community regards teenage pregnancy as a medical risk for both the mother and the child; others are concerned with the social problems that

This chapter is based on a final report to the NICHD Center for Population Research, contract N01-HD-7283. We would like to express our appreciation to Doctors Norman Maldonado, Eloisa Munoz Dones, Luis A. Roman, and De Jesus and the staff at the Hospital Municipal de San Juan, Puerto Rico, and to Dr. Donald Eitzman and the staff at the Shands Teaching Hospital, University of Florida Medical School. We are grateful to the infants and mothers who participated in this study and to Maria de Los Angeles Gonzalez, Lucy Lyons, Eugene Emory, Sandy Elliot, and Kate Neff for their assistance. Portions of these data were presented at the following meetings: American Psychological Association (1979), Society for Pediatric Research (1982), and American Academy of Pediatrics (1982). Portions of these data are also published in Lester, Garcia Coll, & Sepkoski, 1982.

result from early childbearing, such as reduced educational and occupational attainment, lower income and increased welfare dependency, and marital disruption. The effects on the child in terms of personality, academic, and intellectual development beyond the effects of the background characteristics of the parents have also been studied with regard to teenage pregnancy. Reviews of the literature can be found in Baldwin and Cain (1980), Baldwin (1976), Baizerman, Sheehan, Ellison, & Schlesinger (1974), and Zackler and Brandstadt (1975). The present study examines the consequences of teenage pregnancy for the behavioral organization of the newborn infant in two cultural settings, Florida and Puerto Rico. Previous studies have suggested that the newborn of the teenage mother is at greater medical risk (e.g., Grant & Heald, 1972; Dott & Fort, 1976). This may imply that these infants are behaviorally at risk as well, that they show signs of behavioral compromise due to factors associated with early childbearing.

The notion that teenage pregnancies are associated with high rates of obstetric complications and neonatal morbidity and mortality is commonly accepted and has resulted in the classification of virtually all teenage pregnancies as being at risk (Laney, Sandler, Sherrod, & O'Connor, 1979). However, Plionis (1975) noted that although the literature is replete with studies that relate obstetrical complications of teenage pregnancies to poor fetal outcome, the assertion that teenagers are medically at risk is loosely based on disparate data from multiple sources.

Poor nutrition has also been implicated in increased rates of toxemia, prolonged labor and delivery complications, and prematurity in teenage mothers (Battaglia, Frazier, & Hellegers, 1963; Grant & Heald, 1972; Osofsky, 1970). Osofsky (1970) reported that in a group of low-income pregnant teenagers, the rate of anemia was 52 percent and that 90 percent of the sample showed evidence of nutritional inadequacy. McAnarney (1975) found complications such as toxemia, prolonged labor, and cephalopelvic disproportion to be highly associated with teenage pregnancies. Other problems include abruptio placentae, contracted pelvis, and premature labor (Battaglia, et al., 1963; Braen & Forbrush, 1975; Dott & Fort, 1976). In a study by Coates (1970), the obstetric history of young black primagravidas was compared with older mother controls. Young mothers had a higher incidence of acute toxemia, uterine dysfunction, one-day fever, and cardiovascular problems. In this group, anemia was related to fetal distress, uterine dysfunction to neonatal idiopathic hyperbilirubinemia, and asphyxia to respiratory distress. Israel and Woutersz (1963) and Marchetti and Menaker (1950) both reported a 15 percent incidence of preeclampsia in black teenagers.

By contrast, other studies have not shown increased obstetric risk in teenage mothers. In two studies of low socioeconomic status, for the infants of black teenagers receiving adequate prenatal care, the rate of toxemia was similar to that of the average population in Chicago (Zankler, Andelman, & Bauer, 1969), and in New Haven low rates of complications were reported, with a 5 percent rate of toxemia and a 10 percent rate of prematurity (Sarrel & Klerman, 1969). In a study from Nashville (Laney et al., 1979), no differences in obstetric performance or delivery outcome were found in mothers of 13–19 years receiving adequate prenatal care.

Differences in prenatal care were used to explain discrepancies among studies in teenage pregnancies and perinatal mortality by Mednick, Baker, and Sutton-Smith (1979). The authors noted that most studies report a curvilinear relation between mothers' ages and perinatal mortality, with higher mortality rates among younger and older mothers. However, in two studies, a white subsample of the American Collaborative Perinatal Project (Niswander & Gordon, 1972) and a Danish perinatal study (Zachau-Christensen & Ross, 1975), a linear relation was found, with teenage mothers in both studies showing the lowest mortality rates. Each age group in the Danish study had a higher mortality rate than the American sample, probably because the Danish study sample was drawn from a higher medical risk population than the American counterpart. The authors concluded that the lower mortality rates among the American and Danish perinatal samples were due to adequate medical care. They also suggested that previously reported higher mortality rates in teenage mothers are more likely due to social factors that result in poor medical care than to physiological factors of the mothers.

These and other studies (Dott & Fort, 1976) suggest that, given adequate prenatal care, the medical risk to mother and infant may not be appreciably greater for the teenage mother than for the population as a whole. Unfortunately, many teenagers do not receive adequate antenatal care, because it is not available or because teenage mothers are less likely to use those services that are available. Teenage mothers make fewer prenatal clinic visits and start prenatal care later in pregnancy (Dott & Fort, 1976). With less than adequate prenatal care, obstetrical complications may compromise the fetus, placing the infant as well as the mother at risk.

If teenage mothers are at greater risk for obstetrical complications, their infants may show poorer performance on neonatal behavioral measures. The association between prenatal and perinatal risk factors and neonatal behavioral compromise has been shown in a number of studies. The question of whether or not there is an additional or unique risk for the behavioral organization of the infant associated with teenage pregnancy has not been investigated.

Research on the behavior of infants of teenage mothers is just beginning. McLaughlin, Sandler, Herrod, Vietze, & O'Connor (1979) studied adolescent and older mothers from a low-income population in Nashville that had received adequate prenatal care. They found no differences between younger and older mothers on the Neonatal Behavioral Assessment Scale (Brazelton, 1973) or on scales of maternal attitudes or infant temperament. They reported tentative findings that older mothers spent more time out of contact with their babies and vocalized more to them than younger mothers. These findings were similar to those reported by Osofsky and Osofsky (1971), who found that teenage mothers were rated high on warmth and physical interaction with their infant, but low in verbal interaction. McLaughlin et al. (1979) attributed the overall lack of significant differences between infants of teenage and older mothers to the combination of selection factors for the programs in which the mothers were enrolled and the care provided by the project.

Thompson et al. (1979) used the Brazelton scale to compare the infants of 30 black teenage mothers with 30 older mother controls. The infants were selected for low risk obstetric and pediatric factors, and the families were part of an early intervention program to educate teenage mothers in infant stimulation techniques. Comparison of the 26 behavior items of the Brazelton scale showed that the teenage mother–infant group had a faster response decrement to repeated flashes of a light, but were slower in following to a ball, a human face, a human voice, and to face and voice together. Infants of teenage mothers were also less alert and cuddly, had poorer head control in pull to sit, and were less able to remove a cloth from their face. When scored on four Brazelton scale clinical dimensions, infants of teenage mothers more often received scores in the worrisome categories.

One purpose of the present study was to compare the behavioral organization of infants of teenage mothers and infants of older mothers. A second purpose was to consider the unique effects of the mother's age on neonatal behavior. We wanted to determine if the mother's age affected neonatal behavior when the effects of the maternal obstetric history were controlled. Another possibility is that maternal age may act in concert with other prenatal and perinatal factors in affecting neonatal behavior. The study of the effects of the mother's age as part of a sequence of cumulative risk factors was a third purpose. The fourth goal was to broaden our perspective on issues of teenage pregnancy through the cross-cultural approach. We wanted to see if comparable effects were found in different cultural settings and to gain some appreciation for the cultural context surrounding the pregnant teenager that would help identify the strengths and weaknesses of the support systems available to the young mother and her infant. In Puerto Rico, teenage motherhood seems to be more culturally accepted than in Florida. The teenage mother in Puerto Rico is usually married, receiving prenatal care, and is part of an extended family that provides social support. This scenario is less often the case in Florida.

METHOD

Subjects

The total sample consisted of 303 infants. Approximately half of the infants were from Florida ($n = 148$) and are referred to as the mainland sample; the other half of the infants were from Puerto Rico ($n = 155$). Infants who were being assisted by mechanical ventilation, recovering from surgery, sick, or who had congenital anomalies were excluded from the study. The infants were from low socioeconomic status families participating in state-supported programs providing prenatal and postnatal medical care. All mothers received prenatal care, although information about the number of prenatal visits was not available. Of the 303 infants, 80 were born to mothers under 18 years of age.

The 148 babies in the mainland sample were recruited from the Shands Teaching Hospital at the University of Florida Medical School and were evenly divided between males and females. Of all the infants, 38 were born to mothers below the age of 18. Most of the infants were black, with a substantially higher proportion of black infants in the younger mother group.

The sample from Puerto Rico included 155 neonates born at the Hospital Municipal of San Juan, Puerto Rico, and included 78 males and 77 females. A total of 42 of the infants were born to mothers below the age of 18.

Procedure

On the second day of life, the infants were examined with the Brazelton Neonatal Behavioral Assessment Scale (Brazelton, 1973) in a quiet, dimly lit room near the newborn nursery. Each infant was examined by a two-person team, an examiner and a scorer, who had been trained to reliability (24 of 26 items ± 1 point agreement) and who were blind to the mother's age and obstetric risk score. The 26 individual items of the Brazelton scale were summarized into seven clusters (Lester, Als, & Brazelton, 1982, see Figure 1 in Chapter 2) that have been used in other studies (Coll, Sepkoski, & Lester, 1981; Sepkoski, Coll, & Lester, 1982; Yogman, Cole, Als, & Lester, 1983). This system combines the 26 behavioral items into six behavioral clusters and uses the 16 reflexes to generate a seventh reflex cluster. To derive the six behavioral clusters, the curvilinear scale items are rescored as linear. The cluster score is the mean of the rescored items used to define the cluster. Each cluster is qualitative, with higher scores indicating "better" performance. The six behavioral clusters are habituation, the response decrement to the repeated presentation of a light, rattle, bell, and pinprick; orientation, the infant's response to animate and inanimate stimuli and his or her overall alertness; the motor cluster, integrated motor acts and overall muscle tonus; range of state, an assessment of the rapidity, peak, and lability of state changes; regulation of state, the infant's efforts to modulate his or her own state control; and autonomic stability, signs of physiological stress seen as tremors, startles, and changes in skin color. The seventh or reflex cluster is the total number of deviant reflex scores, so that higher scores indicate a greater number of deviant reflexes, hence "worse" performance.

Following the administration of the Brazelton scale, the medical records of the mother and infant were coded. Each infant was assigned an obstetrical complications score based on the system developed by Prechtl (1968). In this system, an obstetric complication refers to any prenatal or perinatal factor or group of factors that increases the risk of fetal mortality. The presence of several obstetric complications is assumed to pose a greater risk to the fetus than any single factor. Prechtl defined 42 variables, shown in Table 7-1, that were used as the criteria of optimal obstetric conditions, subdivided into maternal, parturitional, and fetal factors. For each infant a count was made of the number of conditions that did not meet the criteria

Table 7-1

Criteria of Optimal Obstetric Conditions

Maternal Factors	
Maternal age primipara	18–30 years
Maternal age multipara	20–30 years
Marital state	Married
Parity	1–6
Abortions in history	0–2
Pelvis	No disproportion
Luetic infection	Absent
Rh antagonism	Absent
Blood group incompatibility	Absent
Nutritional state	Well nourished
Hemoglobin level	70 or more
Bleedings during pregnancy	Absent
Infections during pregnancy	Absent
X Rays of abdomen during pregnancy	No
Toxemia	Absent or mild
Blood pressure	Not exceeding 90/135
Albuminuria and edema	Absent
Hyperemesis	Absent
Psychological stress	Absent
Prolonged unwanted sterility (2 years)	Absent
Maternal chronic diseases	Absent

Parturition

Twins or multiple birth	No
Delivery	Spontaneous
Duration 1st stage	6–24 hours
Duration 2nd stage	10 min–2 hours
Contractions	Moderate or strong
Drugs given to mother	O_2, local anesthetic
Amniotic fluid	Clear
Membranes broken	Not longer than 6 hours

Foetal Factors

Intrauterine position	Vertex
Gestational age	38–41 weeks
Fetal presentation	Vertex
Cardiac regularity	Regular
Fetal heart rate (2nd stage)	100–160 bpm
Cord around the neck	No or loose
Cord prolapse	No
Knot in the cord	No
Placental infarction	No or small
Onset respiration	Within first minute
Treatment, resuscitation	No
Drugs given	Nil
Body temperature	Normal
Birth weight	2500–4900 g

Reprinted with permission from Prechtl, H. F. R., Neurological findings in newborn infants after pre- and paranatal complications. In J. Jonxis, H. Visser, & J. Troelstra (Eds.), *Aspects of prematurity and dysmaturity*. Leiden: Stenfert Kroese, 1968.

for optimality. This count was the obstetric complications score. For our study, the lower cutoff of the maternal age variable was not included in the obstetric complications score.

In the present study, the ponderal index (PI) was also computed for each infant (Miller & Hassanein, 1971). The PI is a weight-for-length ratio (birth weight in grams × 100/birth length in cm³) used in the assessment of fetal malnutrition. A low PI indicates thinness, and a high value obesity. Previous studies have found effects on Brazelton scale scores and infant cry features in term underweight-for-length infants (Lester, 1979; Zeskind & Lester, 1981) and that the PI has additive effects in the presence of other perinatal factors (Lester et al., 1982).

A 5-point obstetrical medication rating scale was also scored. The medication scale ratings were no medication, analgesia only, and local, regional, or general anesthesia.

RESULTS

Medical Factors

The biomedical characteristics of the mainland and Puerto Rican groups are presented in Table 7-2. Analysis of variance (teenage or older mothers from the mainland or Puerto Rico) showed that the mean gestational age was slightly higher in the Puerto Rican infants [$F(1,286) = 7.47$, $p < .007$]. In the Puerto Rican sample 1-min Apgar scores were slightly lower [$F(1,283) = 4.33, p < .04$]. On the obstetric complications score, the mean number of total nonoptimal obstetric conditions was greater in infants of teenage mothers [$F(1,295) = 13.02, p < .002$] and in mainland infants [$F(1,295) = 17.77, p < .003$]. These differences were due to the greater number of nonoptimal obstetric conditions in the teenage mainland group, as indicated by the culture $\times$ mother's age interaction [$F(1,295) = 8.83, p < .001$]. When the total number of nonoptimal conditions was divided into its component maternal, parturitional, and fetal factors, the results show that the difference in total nonoptimal scores was due to a greater number of maternal and fetal nonoptimal factors in the teenage mainland group. A greater number of maternal nonoptimal factors was found on the mainland [$F(1,296) = 52.28, p < .001$] and teenage [$F(1,296) = 60.63, p < .001$] groups, with the significant culture $\times$ mother's age interaction showing more maternal nonoptimal factors in infants of mainland teenage mothers [$F(296) = 38.08, p < .001$]. The mean number of parturitional nonoptimal conditions was higher in Puerto Rican than in mainland infants [$F(1,295) = 11.63, p < .001$]. The mean number of fetal nonoptimal factors was greater in the mainland sample [$F(1,296) = 6.3, p < .01$], with the interaction showing that this was due to the greater number of fetal factors in the mainland teenage group [$F(1,296) = 3.97, p < .05$].

Although the majority of infants of teenage mothers were firstborn (74%, $n = 26$ on the mainland; 76%, $n = 32$ in Puerto Rico), there were 9 second-born infants of teenage mothers in Puerto Rico, and 7 on the mainland. Each teenage group had one infant who was third-born of a teenage mother. In the older mother groups, birth order ranged from first (33%, $n = 35$) to eighth in the Mainland sample and from first (4%, $n = 46$) to seventh in Puerto Rico. Most of the mainland teenage mothers were single (67%, $n = 24$). However, in Puerto Rico only 7 percent ($n = 3$) of the teenage mothers were single. Among older mothers, 27 percent ($n = 23$) were single in the mainland sample, as compared to 3 percent ($n = 3$) in Puerto Rico. On the ponderal index, the Puerto Rican infants were lower [$F(1,285) = 14.70, p = .001$]. These differences were not due to weight or length differences, since neither birth weight nor birth length showed significant main effects on interactions. No group differences were found on the 5-point obstetric medication rating scale.

Table 7-2
Biomedical Characteristics of the Sample

	Mainland				Puerto Rico			
	Teenage Mothers		Older Mothers		Teenage Mothers		Older Mothers	
Obstetric Factor	Mean	SD	Mean	SD	Mean	SD	Mean	SD
Birth weight (g)	3041.3	597.15	3233.67	802.19	3025.95	413.00	2922.5	590.26
Birth order	1.3	0.68	2.4	2.1	1.26	0.497	2.1	1.36
Gestational age (weeks)	38.6	2.23	38.77	2.4	39.79	1.4	39.19	2.25
Obstetric medication	2.29	0.93	2.3	1.1	2.195	0.72	2.3	0.88
Chest circumference (cm)	33.3	1.86	32.78	3.03	32.8	1.78	32.04	3.14
Length (cm)	50.18	2.97	50.87	3.73	51.22	2.7	50.35	3.16
Head circumference (cm)	33.87	1.76	34.16	2.17	33.39	1.4	33.94	2.2
Number of nonoptimal obstetric conditions								
Total	5.05	1.5	3.1	1.81	3.1	1.89	3.47	2.15
Maternal	2.84	0.89	1.15	0.97	1.2	0.81	1.02	0.94
Parturitional	1.11	0.98	1.04	0.92	1.38	1.06	1.66	1.06
Fetal	1.11	0.83	0.86	1.03	0.5	0.9	0.79	1.1
Ponderal index	2.39	0.25	2.4	0.298	2.55	0.23	2.26	0.31
Apgar (1)	7.5	1.87	7.86	1.95	7.32	0.986	7.15	1.35

(continued)

Table 7-2 (continued)

| Obstetric Factor | Mainland | | | | Puerto Rico | | | |
| | Teenage Mothers | | Older Mothers | | Teenage Mothers | | Older Mothers | |
	Mean	SD	Mean	SD	Mean	SD	Mean	SD
Apgar (5)	8.39	1.36	8.66	1.1	8.54	0.7	8.36	1.04
Parity	0.25	0.5	1.5	1.57	0.26	0.497	1.1	1.3
Gravida	1.28	0.51	2.59	1.6	1.36	0.69	2.3	1.47
Duration of labor (min)	705.7	478.2	629.1	354.6	481.7	285.4	482.2	396.3

Reprinted with permission from Lester, B. M., Garcia Coll, C. T. & Sepkoski, C. Teenage pregnancy and neonatal behavior effects in Puerto Rico and Florida. *Journal of Youth and Adolescence*, 1982, *11*, 385–402.

Behavioral Effects

Two types of analyses were performed to study the relation between mother's age and neonatal behavior. The first was a series of univariate analysis-of-variance comparisons by age and obstetric complications within cultural groups for the Brazelton scale cluster scores. Where significant effects were found on the cluster scores, further comparisons were made for the individual items that defined the cluster. The second type of analysis was multiple regression to study the additive effects of mother's age with other prenatal and perinatal factors in predicting the Brazelton scale cluster scores.

For the univariate comparisons, infants of adolescent mothers were each matched with infants of older mothers within each cultural group for birth weight, gestational age, the number of nonoptimal obstetric conditions, sex, and race. Infants of older and teenage mothers were then divided into high and low obstetric complications groups, based on a median split of the number of nonoptimal conditions. This represented 0–2 and 2–5 nonoptimal conditions for the Puerto Rican and mainland low complications groups, respectively. Tables 7-3 and 7-4 show the means and standard deviations of the 26 Brazelton scale items for the high and low complications groups for teenage and older mothers in Puerto Rico and the mainland. A 2 (age of mother) × 2 (high or low complications) analysis of variance on the Brazelton scale cluster scores was performed for the Puerto Rican and mainland sample. For the Puerto Rican infants two significant effects were found. Infants with low complications scored higher on regulation of state [$F(1,80) = 5.88, p < .02$], and a significant interaction showed that for the low complications group, infants of teenage mothers had a wider range of state than infants of older mothers [$F(1,80) = 4.83, p < .03$]. The single item effects from the items that defined the clusters showed that infants with fewer complications showed a better ability to mold to the examiner's cuddling maneuvers [$F(1,80) = 9.33, p < .004$] and were easier to console when crying [$F(1,33) = 18.76, p < .01$] than infants with more complications. For the low complications group, infants of teenage mothers spent more time in higher states of arousal [$F(1,80) = 13.76, p < .004$], built up faster to a crying state [$F(1,80) = 7.31, p < .009$], and changed state more often [$F(1,80) = 19.05, p < .04$] than infants of older mothers. The analysis of the cluster scores for the mainland sample showed no significant main effects of interactions.

The purpose of the multiple regression analysis was to study the additive effects of maternal age and prenatal and perinatal factors in relation to neonatal behavior. Nine biomedical variables were selected as predictors in a series of stepwise multiple regressions in which the seven Brazelton scale cluster scores served as outcome variables. The predictor variables were the age of the mother, the ponderal index, gestational age, marital status, the

Table 7-3

Means and Standard Deviations of Brazelton Scale Behavioral Items for Puerto Rico

Behavioral Items	Teenage Mothers				Older Mothers			
	Low Complications		High Complications		Low Complications		High Complications	
	Mean	SD	Mean	SD	Mean	SD	Mean	SD
Habituation Cluster								
Light	4.68	0.75	4.60	1.00	4.72	1.13	4.21	0.54
Rattle	4.77	1.75	4.38	1.32	4.48	1.29	4.00	1.10
Bell	4.10	0.78	3.90	1.18	4.24	1.41	3.95	0.76
Pinprick	3.65	2.10	3.05	2.16	2.71	1.85	3.10	2.04
Orientation Cluster								
Inanimate visual	6.10	2.10	5.74	2.10	7.10	1.37	6.29	2.33
Inanimate auditory	6.71	1.42	6.48	1.97	7.00	1.10	7.24	1.30
Animate visual	6.58	1.61	5.84	1.83	6.85	0.93	6.10	2.10
Animate auditory	6.86	1.32	6.52	1.44	6.62	1.02	6.91	0.83
Animate visual and auditory	6.70	1.34	6.63	1.57	6.85	0.93	6.60	1.53
Alertness	5.95	1.28	5.76	1.95	6.10	1.34	6.24	1.48
Motor Cluster								
General tonus	6.38	1.02	5.57	1.50	6.29	1.10	5.86	1.20
Motor Maturity	3.91	1.14	3.71	1.10	3.57	0.93	3.57	1.29
Pull to sit	4.43	1.57	4.00	2.03	4.29	1.00	4.24	1.58
Defensive movements	6.24	1.45	6.48	1.47	6.38	1.47	6.52	0.98

Range of State Cluster								
Rapidity of buildup	4.43	2.23	2.81	2.06	2.52	2.04	3.29	1.71
Peak of excitement	5.86	1.11	5.29	1.38	4.76	1.14	5.81	1.21
Irritability	4.62	1.39	4.48	2.13	3.43	1.66	4.38	2.22
Lability of state	5.24	2.21	4.29	2.13	3.43	1.66	4.38	2.22
Regulation of State Cluster								
Cuddliness	5.19	1.03	4.48	1.12	5.14	1.01	4.52	0.87
Consolability	7.71	0.61	6.00	2.36	8.00	0.00	6.56	2.13
Self-quieting	6.42	1.39	5.22	2.79	5.38	2.36	5.29	2.26
Hand to mouth	5.76	2.32	5.29	2.79	5.38	2.36	5.29	2.26
Autonomic Stability Cluster								
Tremulousness	6.33	1.96	5.43	2.36	5.29	2.41	4.24	2.93
Startle	3.62	2.20	3.62	2.22	2.91	1.41	3.29	1.85
Lability of skin color	5.76	1.55	4.76	1.95	5.71	1.82	5.62	1.77

Reprinted with permission from Lester, B. M., Garcia Coll, C. T. & Sepkoski, C. Teenage pregnancy and neonatal behavior effects in Puerto Rico and Florida. *Journal of Youth and Adolescence*, 1982, *11*, 385–402.

Table 7-4

Means and Standard Deviations of Brazelton Scale Items for the Mainland

Behavioral Items	Teenage Mothers				Older Mothers			
	Low Complications		High Complications		Low Complications		High Complications	
	Mean	SD	Mean	SD	Mean	SD	Mean	SD
Habituation Cluster								
Light	5.90	1.40	4.90	2.97	6.27	1.70	5.90	2.20
Rattle	6.30	1.70	5.50	2.90	6.70	2.30	5.50	2.20
Bell	5.90	3.10	4.46	2.38	7.10	1.40	5.30	1.89
Pinprick	3.70	1.99	3.50	2.20	4.07	1.67	3.58	2.15
Orientation Cluster								
Inanimate visual	5.80	2.56	4.89	2.40	3.75	1.90	4.40	2.26
Inanimate auditory	5.89	1.97	5.10	1.50	5.67	1.50	4.89	1.88
Animate visual	5.70	2.54	5.70	2.50	5.00	2.20	4.90	2.50
Animate auditory	5.90	1.80	5.80	1.80	6.40	1.40	5.67	1.80
Animate visual and auditory	6.10	2.46	5.05	2.97	5.25	2.40	4.16	2.10
Alertness	5.65	2.20	5.79	2.30	5.25	2.40	4.16	2.10
Motor Cluster								
General tonus	5.95	1.30	5.80	1.70	5.80	1.60	5.89	1.05
Motor Maturity	4.15	0.88	3.90	1.98	4.00	1.67	3.28	1.10
Pull to sit	5.85	2.40	5.00	2.93	5.65	2.46	4.90	2.00
Defensive movements	5.90	2.10	5.50	2.60	6.25	2.27	5.89	2.30

Range of State Cluster								
Rapidity of buildup	5.16	1.68	5.60	2.10	4.26	1.79	5.20	1.77
Peak of excitement	6.10	1.36	5.80	1.30	6.70	1.50	6.70	1.30
Irritability	4.40	2.28	5.25	1.90	4.10	1.90	5.16	1.89
Lability of state	4.25	2.40	4.40	2.10	4.80	2.00	4.90	2.40
Regulation of State Cluster								
Cuddliness	5.60	2.17	5.30	1.95	5.70	1.89	5.40	1.68
Consolability	6.10	1.40	6.00	2.10	5.26	1.87	5.18	2.30
Self-quieting	5.10	2.90	6.35	2.50	5.30	2.50	5.39	2.60
Hand to mouth	6.00	2.60	4.90	2.75	5.30	2.00	5.26	1.97
Autonomic Stability Cluster								
Tremulousness	5.60	2.10	5.80	2.89	6.80	1.98	5.70	3.26
Startle	5.35	2.30	5.37	2.20	5.25	2.00	4.95	2.50
Lability of skin color	3.45	1.50	4.26	1.80	4.85	2.37	4.50	1.87

Reprinted with permission from Lester, B. M., Garcia Coll, C. T. & Sepkoski, C. Teenage pregnancy and neonatal behavior effects in Puerto Rico and Florida. *Journal of Youth and Adolescence*, 1982, *11*, 385–402.

drug score, the 1-min Apgar score, and the number of maternal, parturitional, and fetal nonoptimal conditions. We report the combination of biomedical variables that explained the greatest amount of significant variation in neonatal behavior. In all of the regressions that follow for both mainland and Puerto Rican infants, none of the bivariate correlations between maternal age and the Brazelton scale cluster scores were significant.

For the Puerto Rican infants, the multiple regression of the habituation cluster indicated higher scores related to older, married mothers with lower medication scores and infants of a greater gestational age, higher ponderal index, and fewer fetal nonoptimal conditions [$r = .42$, $F(6,139) = 4.95$, $p < .001$]. Higher scores on the orientation cluster were related to fewer parturitional nonoptimal conditions and greater gestational age [$r = .36$, $F(3,145) = 7.33$, $p < .001$]. On the motor cluster, higher scores were related to a greater gestational age, a higher Apgar score, and a higher ponderal index [$r = .49$, $F(3,145) = 15.28$, $p < .001$]. Effects on the range of state cluster were not significant. For regulation of state, higher scores were found for older mothers with infants of greater gestational age and fewer nonoptimal conditions [$r = .28$, $F(3,145) = 4.04$, $p < .009$]. Higher scores on autonomic regulation were related to the combination of fewer fetal nonoptimal conditions, greater gestational age, and higher ponderal index [$r = .34$, $F(4,112) = 6.22$, $p < .001$]. On the reflex cluster, a smaller number of deviant reflexes was related to fewer maternal nonoptimal conditions, fewer fetal nonoptimal conditions, and a higher ponderal index [$r = .33$, $F(3,145) = 6.06$, $p < .001$].

For the mainland sample, the regression of the habituation cluster showed higher scores related to fewer maternal and parturitional nonoptimal conditions, a higher ponderal index, a greater gestational age, and higher Apgar scores [$r = .46$, $F(5,99) = 5.3$, $p < .001$]. The orientation cluster was not significantly related to the predictor variables. On the motor cluster, higher scores were found for older mothers with a lower drug score and a higher infant ponderal index [$r = .28$, $F(3,113) = 3.25$, $p < .03$]. Higher scores on range of state were associated with the combined effects of older mothers with lower drug scores and greater infant gestational age [$r = .44$, $FF(3,113) = 9.32$, $p < .001$]. On the regulation of state cluster, higher scores were related to older mothers, lower drug scores, and higher Apgar scores [$r = .29$, $F(3,113) = 3.5$, $p < .02$]. For autonomic regulation, higher scores were found from the combined effects of older mothers with lower drug scores, fewer parturitional nonoptimal conditions, and a higher infant ponderal index [$r = .32$, $F(4,112) = 3.12$, $p < .02$]. A greater num ber of deviant reflexes was due to lower Apgar scores and more parturitional and fetal nonoptimal conditions [$r = .35$, $F(3,102) = 4.78$, $p < .004$].

Comparisons with Other Samples

The mean Brazelton scale scores in Tables 7-3 and 7-4 are within the range of what is considered to be normal levels of performance. Table 7-5 shows the means and standard deviations of the Brazelton scale items for 54 infants on days 1 and 3 (Tronick, Wise, Als, Adamson, Scanlon, & Brazelton, 1976). These infants were from white middle class families in Boston and were highly selected on optimal obstetric and neurological criteria; that is, they are very low risk infants. We can compare the mean scores of days 1 and 3 from the Boston sample with the mean scores of the two teenage and older mother groups by considering scores that differ by more than one scale point. Horowitz, Ashton, Culp, Gaddis, Levin, and Reichmann (1977) have used these criteria justified by the interobserver reliability criteria of the Brazelton scale in which a one-point discrepancy between two scores on an item is considered an agreement.

Using this approach to compare the infants from the present study with the Boston sample, we find that for the mainland teenage sample, 2 of the 26 items differed by more than one point. The teenage mainland infants had lower scores on the response decrement to a bell, and on orientation to face and voice. The infants of older mainland mothers differed from the Boston babies on seven items, scoring lower on orientation to bell, face, and face and voice and alertness and consolability, and higher on rapidity of buildup and tremors. The Puerto Rico–Boston comparisons show that infants of teenage mothers scored lower than the Boston babies on five items: habituation to light, rattle, and bell, pull to sit, and cuddliness. Infants of older mothers scored lower than Boston babies on habituation to light, rattle, bell, and pinprick, pull to sit, cuddliness, rapidity of buildup, and startle. They scored higher on orientation to ball, bell, and voice and on lability of skin color.

A sample more comparable to the present study was reported by Osofsky and O'Connell (1977). They studied 328 newborn, randomly selected from the Temple University Hospital in Philadelphia. The subjects were nonwhite, from lower socioeconomic status families, with the mothers' ages ranging from 13 to 41. Unfortunately, no information concerning the obstetric histories of these infants was provided. Using the greater than one point scale difference criteria, the infants of teenage mothers from the mainland scored higher on habituation to light, bell, and pinprick and lower on motor maturity and hand-to-mouth scores than the Philadelphia infants. For the Puerto Rican sample, the infants of teenage mothers scored higher than the Philadelphian babies on habituation to light, orientation to rattle and ball, and consolability. The infants of older mothers in Puerto Rico

Table 7-5

Means and Standard Deviations of Brazelton Scale Behavioral Items

Behavioral Items	Day 1		Day 3	
	M	SD	M	SD
Habituation Cluster				
Light	6.3	1.6	7.1	1.5
Rattle	6.7	2.1	6.8	1.8
Bell	6.9	2.1	7.1	1.8
Pinprick	4.4	1.5	4.2	1.2
Orientation Cluster				
Inanimate visual	5.6	1.4	5.4	1.5
Inanimate auditory	5.5	1.1	5.8	0.8
Animate visual	6.3	1.2	6.5	1.1
Animate auditory	5.5	1.3	5.8	1.9
Animate visual and auditory	6.6	1.1	6.9	0.9
Alertness	4.9	2.3	5.5	1.9
Motor Cluster				
General tonus	5.3	0.9	5.4	1.0
Motor maturity	4.2	0.6	4.7	0.9
Pull to sit	5.6	1.2	5.8	1.3
Defensive movements	4.9	2.4	6.9	1.3
Activity level	3.9	0.8	4.6	0.9
Range of State Cluster				
Rapidity of buildup	3.5	2.2	3.6	1.8
Peak of excitement	5.4	1.3	5.8	1.3
Irritability	4.1	1.5	4.0	1.5
Lability of state	2.7	1.2	2.8	1.1
Regulation of State Cluster				
Cuddliness	5.6	1.0	5.8	1.2
Consolability	6.4	1.7	6.2	1.4
Self-quieting	5.2	1.6	5.1	1.5
Hand to mouth	4.9	2.2	6.0	1.8
Autonomic Stability Cluster				
Tremulousness	5.0	1.7	4.4	1.8
Startle	4.5	1.8	4.3	1.6
Lability of skin color	4.4	1.4	4.1	1.2

Reprinted with permission from Tronick, E., Wise, S., Als, H., Adamson, L., Scanlon, J., & Brazelton, T. B. Regional obstetric anesthesia and newborn behavior: Effect over the first ten days of life. *Pediatrics*, 1976, *58*, 94–100.

show higher scores on habituation to light, orientation to rattle and ball, and consolability, and lower scores on motor maturity, peak of excitement, rapidity of buildup, and hand-to-mouth facility than the Philadelphian infants.

DISCUSSION

The results of the comparisons of the Brazelton scale cluster scores suggest that the effects of maternal age on neonatal behavior may vary as a function of the number of obstetric complications and cultural group. In the Puerto Rican group, the effects of obstetric complications appeared to depress neonatal behavior along behavioral dimensions related to the infant's state organization. Infants with fewer complications were more responsive to being cuddled on the examiner's shoulder and horizontally in the arm when not crying, and when crying, required less intervention to stop them from crying. The effects of mother's age was also seen along state-related dimensions of behavior in these infants. The significant age × complications interactions revealed that with fewer complications, infants of teenage mothers spent more time in higher states of arousal, reached a crying state earlier in the exam, and changed state more often than infants of older mothers. With fewer complications, mother's age seems to be inversely related to the Puerto Rican infant's level of arousal.

There was no effects of mother's age or obstetric complications in the mainland sample. Since the number of obstetric complications was higher in the mainland than in the Puerto Rican sample, one possibility is that the number of complications in the mainland low complications group was too high to detect behavioral differences when these infants were compared with the higher complications group. Moreover, we might speculate that the effects of maternal age are subtle and masked by the presence of too many obstetric complications, as in the mainland sample. In Puerto Rico, with fewer complications, the effects of maternal age were visible along state-related dimensions. Infants of teenage mothers showed higher and more labile levels of arousal than infants of older mothers.

The results of the multivariate analysis showed that the obstetric and perinatal risk variables accounted for 8–24 percent of the variation of Brazelton scale cluster scores in Puerto Rico, and for 8–21 percent on the mainland. Factors indicative of greater biological risk were associated with poorer performance on the Brazelton scale cluster scores. Mother's age was entered in two of the six significant regressions in Puerto Rico and in four of the six significant regressions in the mainland sample. However, the bivariate correlations showed that mother's age did not make a significant, unique contribution to neonatal behavior in either culture. These findings may suggest that maternal age acts in concert with other variables in affecting neonatal behavior. It may be that the presence of maternal age serves to potentiate the effects of other risk factors; that is, maternal age may act in combination with other factors as a synergistic effect on neonatal behavior. The synergistic effect of maternal age may be correlated with cultural differences, as suggested by the differential impact of maternal age in Florida and Puerto Rico.

The differences reported in this study are within the range of what are considered to be normal levels of performance. As with the data reported by McLaughlin et al. (1979), most of the mean scores for the 26 Brazelton scale items represent behavior within the range of normal variations. This was also indicated by the comparison with the Boston and Philadelphia samples. In that analysis, infants of teenage mothers did not differ substantially from those of older mothers when compared to the low risk Boston or higher risk Philadelphia samples. Overall, the mainland and Puerto Rican infants did differ from both the Boston and Philadelphia samples. In fact, they seemed to be between the Boston and Philadelphia samples in terms of level of performance, which makes sense in view of the likely higher risk status of the Philadelphia babies and known low risk of the Boston babies. Interestingly, the two teenage mother groups in our study showed fewer differences from the other extreme—that is, from the Boston or Philadelphia babies—than their older mother counterparts. There were 18 total differences between the two teenage groups and the Boston and Philadelphia groups, while the older mother groups differed from the Boston and Philadelphia samples on 35 occasions. In other words, by contrast, the differences we saw among infants of teenage mothers are real but not dramatic.

Nevertheless, the purpose of this analysis is to underscore the point that while younger maternal age may indeed have some unique effects on neonatal behavior, these effects are subtle and indicate that the infants may be organized slightly differently. Moreover, the patterns of these organizational differences are likely to vary across cultural settings. This may imply that the behavior of infants of teenage mothers depends upon the meaning of those behaviors for the immediate care-giving environment and the larger cultural context.

In general, the findings from this study are in agreement with previous investigations in showing that newborns of teenage mothers display a relatively normal range of neonatal behavior. Within this range, however, there is some indication that the organization of the infant's state behavior may be affected by a younger maternal age. We might hypothesize that the later impact of teenage childbearing on infant development may be an interaction between the effects of the infant's state behavior and how the mother responds to the infant. Studies of mother–infant interaction suggest that adolescent mothers differ in the amount of time spent with the infant and the amount of verbal interaction (McLaughlin et al., 1979; Osofsky & Osofsky, 1971). Moreover, the infant may have a greater impact on a younger mother owing to a lesser familiarity with children and less realistic developmental expectation and childrearing practices (De Lissovoy, 1973; Field, Windmayer, Stringer, & Ignatoff, 1980).

We became convinced from this study of the importance of the socio-cultural context in order to understand the effects of teenage pregnancy. The impact of teenage pregnancy was stronger in Florida than in Puerto Rico. Even though both samples were from the lower socioeconomic levels, in Puerto Rico most of the teenage mothers were married and almost half of them were part of an extended family. This probably represents a very different social context for an adolescent mother and her infant than the unmarried status of the Florida sample and that associated with most teenage childbearing in the United States (Baldwin, 1976). In Puerto Rico, within these socioeconomic groups early marriage and childbearing seem to be accepted as part of normal adolescent growth and development. This might affect compliance to prenatal care visits, nutrition, and stress experienced by the mother during pregnancy and would in turn affect the association of maternal age with an additive adverse effect on newborn behavior. Our results point out the need to consider not only the reproductive and obstetric history of the mother, but also the larger family, support systems, and socioeconomic environment in which the teenage mother and her infant will negotiate their relationship.

REFERENCES

Baizerman, M., Sheehan, C., Ellison, D. L., & Schlesinger, E. R. A critique of the research literature concerning pregnancy adolescents, 1960–1970. *Journal of Youth and Adolescence*, 1974, *3*, 61–75.

Baldwin, W. H. Adolescent pregnancy and childbearing—Growing concerns for Americans. *Population Bulletin*, 1976, *31*, 1–33.

Baldwin, W. H., & Cain, V. S. The children of teenage parents. *Family Planning Perspectives*, 1980, *12*, 34–43.

Battaglia, F. C., Frazier, T. M., & Hellegers, A. E. Obstetric and pediatric complications of juvenile pregnancy. *Pediatrics*, 1963, *32*, 902–908.

Braen, B. B., & Forbush, J. B. School-age parenthood—A national overview. *Journal of School Health*, 1975, *45*, 257.

Brazelton, T. B. *Neonatal Behavioral Assessment Scale*. London: Spastics International, 1973.

Coates, J. B. Obstetrics in the very young adolescent. *American Journal of Obstetrics and Gynecology*, 1970, *108*, 68–72.

Coll, C., Sepkoski, C., & Lester, B. M. Cultural and biomedical correlates of neonatal behavior. *Developmental Psychobiology*, 1981, *14*, 147–154.

De Lissovoy, V. Child care by adolescent parents. *Children Today*, 1973, *35*, 22–25.

Dott, A. B., & Fort, A. T. Medical and social factors affecting early teenage pregnancy. *American Journal of Obstetrics and Gynecology*, 1976, *125*, 532–536.

Field, T. M., Windmayer, S. M., Stringer, S., & Ignatoff, E. Teenage, lower-class, black mothers and their pre-term infants: An intervention and developmental follow-up. *Child Development*, 1980, *51*, 426–436.

Grant, J. A., & Heald, F. P. Complications of adolescent pregnancy: Survey of the literature on fetal outcome in adolescence. *Clinical Pediatrics*, 1972, *11*, 567–570.

Horowitz, F. D., Ashton, J., Culp, R., Gaddis, E., Levin, S., & Reichmann, B. The effects of obstetrical medication on the behavior of Israeli newborn infants and some comparisons with Uruguayan and American infants. *Child Development*, 1977, *48*, 1607.

Israel, L., & Woutersz, T. B. Teenage obstetrics: A comparative study. *American Journal of Obstetrics and Gynecology*, 1963, *85*, 659–668.

Laney, M., Sandler, H., Sherrod, K., & O'Connor, S. *Biologic risks in adolescent mothers and their infants.* Unpublished manuscript, 1979.

Lester, B. M. A synergistic process approach to the study of prenatal malnutrition. *International Journal of Behavioral Development*, 1979, *2*, 377–393.

Lester, B. M., Als, H., & Brazelton, T. B. Regional obstetric anesthesia and newborn behavior: A reanalysis toward synergistic effects. *Child Development*, 1982, *53*, 687–692.

Lester, B. M., Garcia Coll, C. T., & Sepkoski, C. Teenage pregnancy and neonatal behavior effects in Puerto Rico and Florida. *Journal of Youth and Adolescence*, 1982, *11*, 385–402.

Marchetti, A. A., & Menaker, J. S. Pregnancy and the adolescent. *American Journal of Obstetrics and Gynecology*, 1950, *59*, 1013–1021.

McAnarney, E. Adolescent pregnancy. *Clinical Pediatrics*, 1975, *14*, 19–22.

McLaughlin, F. J., Sandler, H. M., Herrod, K., Vietze, P. M., & O'Connor, S. Social–psychological characteristics of adolescent mothers and behavioral characteristics of their firstborn infants. *Journal of Population*, 1979, *2*, 69–73.

Mednick, B. R., Baker, R. L., & Sutton-Smith, B. Teenage pregnancy and perinatal mortality. *Journal of Youth and Adolescence*, 1979, *8*, 343–357.

Miller, H. C., & Hassanein, K. Diagnosis of impaired fetal growth in newborn infants. *Pediatrics*, 1971, *43*, 511–515.

Niswander, K. R., & Gordon, M. *The women and their pregnancies.* Philadelphia: Saunders, 1972.

Osofsky, H. Nutritional status of low income pregnant teenagers. *Journal of Reproductive Medicine*, 1970, *5*, 18–24.

Osofsky, J. D., & O'Connel, E. J. Patterning of newborn behavior in an urban population. *Child Development*, 1977, *48*, 532.

Osofsky, H. R., & Osofsky, J. D. Adolescents as mothers: Results of a program for low income pregnant teenagers with some emphasis upon infant development. In S. Chess & A. Thomas (Eds.), *Annual progress in child psychiatry and child development.* New York: Brunner/Mazel, 1971.

Plionis, B. Adolescent pregnancy: A review of the literature. *Social Work*, 1975, *20*, 302–307.

Prechtl, H. F. R. Neurological findings in newborn infants after pre- and paranatal complications. In J. Jonxis, H. Visser, & J. Troelstra (Eds.), *Aspects of prematurity and dysmaturity*. Leyden: Stenfert Kroese, 1968.

Sarrel, P., & Klerman, L. The young unwed mother. *American Journal of Obstetrics and Gynecology*, 1969, *105*, 575–578.

Sepkoski, C., Coll, C. G., & Lester, B. M. Cumulative effects of obstetric risk variables on newborn behavior. *Infant Behavior and Development*, 1982.

Thompson, R. J., Jr., Cappleman, M. W., & Zeitschel, K. A. Neonatal behavior of infants of adolescent mothers. *Developmental Medicine and Child Neurology*, 1979, *21*, 474–482.

Tronick, E., Wise, S., Als, H., Adamson, L., Scanlon, J., & Brazelton, T. B. Regional obstetric anesthesia and newborn behavior: Effect over the first ten days of life. *Pediatrics*, 1976, *58*, 94–100.

Yogman, M., Cole, P., Als, H., & Lester, B. M. Behavior of newborns of diabetic mothers. *Infant Behavior and Development*, 1983.

Zachau-Christiansen, B., & Ross, E. M. *Babies: Human development during the first year*. London: Wiley, 1975.

Zanckler, J. Andelman, S., & Bauer, F. The young adolescent as an obstetric risk. *American Journal of Obstetrics and Gynecology*, 1969, *103*, 305–312.

Zanckler, J., & Brandstadt, W. (Eds) *The teenage pregnant girls*. Springfield, Ill. Thomas, 1975.

Zeskind, P. S., & Lester, B. M. Analysis of cry features in newborns with differential fetal growth. *Child Development*, 1981, *52*, 207–212.

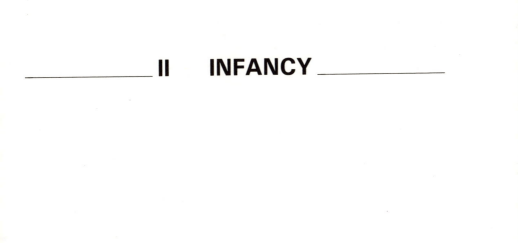

II INFANCY

8

Preterm and Full-Term Infants' Visual Responses to Mothers' and Strangers' Faces

Wendy S. Masi, Keith G. Scott

Little is known about the social development of preterm as compared to normal infants, although some literature suggests that they have deficits which may lead to patterns of interaction that are not optimal for development (Field, 1977; Field, Dempsey, & Shuman, 1979). More information is needed before optimal programs of intervention and stimulation can be devised (Als, Lester, & Brazelton, 1979).

The present study asks three questions concerning the preterm infant's early responses to social stimuli. The first question involves the ability of the preterm infant to recognize his or her primary care giver's face and voice. Normal full-term infants as young as 2 weeks of age can discriminate the animate faces of their mother and a stranger (Carpenter, 1974). Using the duration of visual fixation as a dependent measure, Carpenter found evidence that full-term females looked longer at their mother's face than that of a stranger. Preterm infants, because of their physiological immaturity and long period of separation from the mother may show a delay in this area. When the amount of experience which full-term and preterm infants have with their mother is equated, do preterm infants also show recognition of their mother?

The second question involves the patterns of visual fixation. Visual fixation of the care giver's face is one of the earliest social responses in an infant's repertoire, and it is an important component of early social interac-

The authors wish to acknowledge the support of the Mailman Foundation in conducting this research.

tion (Stern, 1974). There is evidence that preterm infants show deficits in this area. Field (1977) found that at 3½ months preterm infants looked less or averted their gaze more than full-term infants when exposed to their mother's animate face. Do preterm infants during the first 2 months of life show shorter fixations of their mother's face than do full-term infants during this same period?

The third question concerns the effects of development. Do infants' visual fixations of animate faces change over 1 month of development? That is, do the durations of visual fixations of faces by preterm and full-term infants increase with age? In order to answer these three questions, the visual fixations of mothers' and strangers' animate faces were compared for full-term and preterm infants.

METHOD

Subjects

This study involved 14 white preterm infants (8 females and 6 males) and 16 white full-term infants (8 males and 8 females) and their mothers. All preterm infants had birth weights of 1000–2000 g ($\overline{X}$ = 1700 g), gestational ages of 28–36 weeks ($\overline{X}$ = 33), and were hospitalized from 2 to 7 weeks ($\overline{X}$ = 4 weeks). Full-term infants were healthy and born to mothers who had no complications of pregnancy or delivery. Mothers of the infants ranged from 19 to 33 years of age (mean maternal age for preterm infants, 25 years; mean maternal age for full-term infants, 27 years). Here 8 of the preterm infants and 7 of the term infants were firstborn, 6 of the preterm and 9 of the term infants were later born.

At both testing sessions preterm infants were older in terms of chronological age (8 and 12 weeks versus 4 and 8 weeks for the term infants), but they were significantly younger in terms of conceptional age.

Procedure

Preterm infants were tested after they had been home for 3–4 weeks. Full-term infants were tested at 3–4 weeks of age. The second testing session for both groups occurred 4 weeks later. Thus the amount of time the infant had spent with the mother was equivalent for both groups.

The procedure was modeled after that used by Carpenter (1974). When the infant was calm and alert, he or she was placed in an infant seat and put into an observation chamber. This chamber was a three-sided partial enclosure with a trapdoor on the top through which the mother or stranger could talk to the infant. On the inside of the door there were blinking lights to maintain the infant's attention when neither the mother's nor the stranger's face was present. The infant's visual behavior was recorded by a video camera placed at the end of the periscope which projected from an opening directly below the mother's or stranger's face. This equipment was set up in a vehicle which was driven to the infant's home.

Each infant was given eight, 30-sec interaction trials of face presentations, four of the mother's face and four of the stranger's face. For some infants the mother's face was presented first and for others the stranger's face was first. The instructions to the mother and the stranger were to open the trapdoor, look at the infant, and begin talking in an attempt to elicit the infant's attention. A prepared script was used, modeled on that of Carpenter. This script consisted of repetitions of the following series of phrases: "Hello baby, how are you today? Are you a good baby? You are a good baby. You're a very good baby." Timing of the 30-sec trial was not begun until the infant oriented to the mother's or stranger's face. There was a 15-sec interval between trials during which the infant was exposed to the blinking lights. Procedures for both session 1 and session 2 were identical.

The infants' video tapes were coded through the use of a Datamyte electronic event recorder (Scott and Masi, 1977). The duration of visual fixation on the mother's or stranger's face and latencies to first fixations were recorded. Interrater reliability was determined by randomly sampling the data for two subjects within each group at each session (for a total of 16 sessions). These infants' video tapes were coded independently by two observers, and the resulting data for the duration of direct fixation on the mother and stranger were correlated. Reliability averaged .88.

RESULTS

The data for the durations of the visual fixations were analyzed by a birth condition (2) × sex (2) × stimulus condition (2) × session (2) analysis of variance with repeated measures on two factors. The repeated factors were the stimulus condition and session. For this and other analyses, mean scores across trials rather than individual trial scores were used.

The analyses showed that three of the four main effects, birth condition [$F(1,26) = 7.46$], session [$F(1, 26) = 36.35$], and social stimulus [$F(1,26) = 14.05$], were significant at the .01 level or less. There were no effects of sex and no significant interaction effects. These results, presented in Figure 8-1, indicated that full-term infants at both sessions looked more at both the mother and the stranger than did the preterm infants. All infants at both sessions looked more at their mother's than a stranger's face, and the amount of looking time for both full-term and preterm infants increased with age.

The data for latency to first fixation were analyzed with the same four-

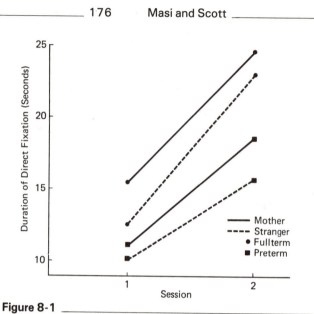

Figure 8-1

Duration of direct fixation on mother and stranger for preterm and full-term infants.

factor analysis-of-variance design used in the first analysis. The results indicated that three of the four main effects, birth condition [$F(1, 26) = 6.47$], session [$F(1, 26) = 4.28$], and stimulus condition [$F(1, 26) = 10.44$] were significant at the .05 level or less. There were no significant effects of sex and no significant interactions. These data are presented in Figure 8-2. Preterm infants were slower to orient to the stimuli than were full-term infants, both full-term and preterm infants oriented faster at the second session than the first, and infants oriented faster to the stranger than to the mother. This last result may be a testing artifact. The person interacting with the infant was responsible for judging when the infant first looked at their face. The research assistant had more experience at making this judgment than the mothers, who may have waited until they were absolutely sure their infants were looking before signaling that the trial should begin.

Another question of interest concerned the effect of conceptional age upon visual behavior. Figure 8-3 presents the data for the analysis on the duration of direct fixation on the mother's and stranger's faces. These data are presented in terms of the conceptional ages of the infants rather than by session, as it was in Figure 8-1. Figure 8-3 illustrates the increase in duration of visual fixation on both the mother and the stranger for preterm and full-term infants which occurred with increasing conceptional age.

The variable controlled in this study was time home with the mother. Because of the differences in hospitalization time and gestational age at birth, preterm infants at both ages tested were slightly younger in concep-

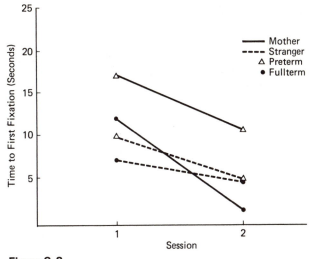

Figure 8-2 _____
Latency to first fixation on mother and stranger for preterm and full-term infants.

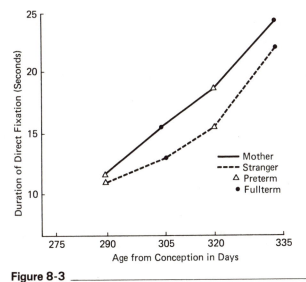

Figure 8-3 _____
Duration of direct fixation on mother and stranger by conceptional age.

tional age than full-term infants, and they were older in terms of postnatal age. A subsample of the preterm group ($n = 6$) was selected such that the conceptional age of the preterm infants at the second session equalled that of full-term infants at the first session. A comparison between the visual fixation scores of this group of preterm infants at session 2 and the full-term infants at session 1 represents a correction for prematurity. To determine if significant differences existed between these two groups, a two-way birth condition × stimulus condition analysis of variance was performed. The results indicated that while there was still a significant effect for stimulus condition [$F(1, 20) = 7.41, p < .01$], there was no longer a significant birth condition effect. Thus it appears that when we compared groups at equivalent conceptional ages, the preterm infants' visual fixations approximated those of the term infant.

DISCUSSION

The results of this study suggest that (1) both preterm and full-term infants after 3–4 weeks of experience looked more at their mother's animate face than at a stranger's, (2) preterm infants looked at their mother's and a stranger's face for shorter periods and were slower in orienting toward those faces than were full-term infants, and (3) the duration of fixations of faces by both the full-term and preterm groups increased over 1 month of development.

The demonstration that both groups of infants at both ages discriminated their mother's and a stranger's face replicates and extends Carpenter's 1974 work. Her sample consisted of female full-term infants. This sample consisted of both male and female, full-term and preterm infants. It thus appears that Carpenter's results do generalize to other samples. This suggests that even at very young ages both preterm and full-term infants can differentially respond to their primary care giver. Previous investigations suggested that infants could not recognize their mother until at least 3 months of age (Ambrose, 1961, pp. 179–196; Gewirtz, 1965). This study suggests that when the time of visual fixation is used as the dependent measure, evidence of discrimination of faces can be found much earlier.

The results confirmed the hypothesis that preterm infants are visually less responsive to social stimuli than full-term infants during the early months of life. We also noted that the preterm infants were more "difficult" to test than full-term infants. They required more time for testing, they were more fussy, and it was more difficult to elicit their attention. When questioned about their preterm infants' temperaments, mothers tended to describe them as fussy, impatient, and demanding more often than did mothers of full-term infants. Thus it appears that during this early period of developing mother–infant interactions, preterm infants do not exhibit the same visual responses as full-term infants. This may result in patterns of interaction that are less optimal.

Recently Field (1979) advanced the position that preterm infants' lesser attention to social stimuli may relate to their less developed arousal modulation and information-processing abilities. The preterm infant may require more time turned away from an interaction to process the information perceived and modulate the arousal experienced during the previous looking period. This suggests that care must be taken to provide adequate and appropriate stimulation without bombarding the infant with more stimulation than can be handled. Matching stimulation to the infant's behavior might optimize interactions with preterm infants.

REFERENCES _____

Als, H., Lester, B., & Brazelton, T. B. Dynamics of the premature infant: A theoretical perspective. In T. M. Field, A. M. Sostek, S. Goldberg, & H. H. Shuman (Eds.), *Infants born at risk*. New York: Spectrum, 1979.

Ambrose, J. A. The development of the smiling response in early infancy. In B. N. Foss (Ed.), *Determinants of infant behavior*. New York: Wiley, 1961.

Carpenter, G. Mother's face and the newborn. *New Scientist*, 1974, *21*, 742–745.

Field, T. Effects of early separation, interactive deficits, and experimental manipulations on infant–mother face-to-face interaction. *Child Development*, 1977, *48*, 763–771.

Field, T. Visual and cardiac responses to animate and inanimate faces by young term and preterm infants. *Child Development*, 1979, *2*, 179–184.

Field, T., Dempsey, J., & Shuman, H. H. Developmental assessments of infants having respiratory distress syndrome. In T. M. Field, A. M. Sostek, M. S. Goldberg, & H. H. Shuman (Eds.), *Infants born at risk*. New York: Spectrum, 1979.

Gewirtz, J. L. The course of infant smiling in four child-rearing environments in Israel. In B. M. Foss (Ed.), *Determinants of infants behavior*. London: Methuen, 1965.

Scott, K. G., & Masi, W. Use of the Datamyte in analyzing duration of infant visual behaviors. *Behavior Research Methods and Instrument*, 1977, *9*, 429–433.

Stern, D. N. Mother and infant play: The dyadic interaction involving facial, vocal, and gaze behaviors. In M. Lewis & L. Rosenblum (Eds.), *The effect of the infant on its caregiver*. New York: Wiley, 1974.

9

Responsiveness to Relational Information as a Measure of Cognitive Functioning in Nonsuspect Infants

Albert J. Caron
Rose F. Caron, Penny Glass

It is generally conceded that continuing attempts to identify infants at risk for childhood intellective disability have fallen short of the mark. Whether based on perinatal indicators or test performance, infant assessments have uniformly failed to predict future cognitive handicaps to any practical extent (Parmelee & Haber, 1973; McCall, 1976, 1979b). Although plausible explanations for this unfortunate state of affairs have been sought in the nature of intellectual development—its discontinuity or nonlinearity—it may well be that the breakdown of past predictive efforts owes less to nature than to the misplaced emphasis of our measures.

Consider first the case of perinatally defined risk. Certain complications such as prematurity and intrauterine growth retardation have indeed been implicated as preconditions of subsequent dysfunction (Kopp & Parmelee, 1979). The fact is, however, that since only 10 percent of babies are born premature or in need of intensive care, the bulk of learning impaired children (some 80 percent) have had seemingly normal, full-term birth histories (Scott, 1978; Scott & Masi, 1979). Given, too, that at least 70 percent of newborns with questionable obstetric signs emerge symptom free in childhood, it is apparent that classifications of risk restricted to infants

The preparation of this chapter was supported in part by grants from the March of Dimes–Birth Defects Foundation and W. T. Grant Foundation. We are indebted to Sue Antell and Rose Myers for their extensive contribution to the research and to Julie Hofheimer and Susan Poisson for their help in follow-up testing.

with obvious perinatal complications inevitably bypass the majority of cases who are actually in jeopardy.

While these considerations would seem to argue for greater reliance on behavioral assessment to identify vulnerable infants, psychometric efforts also appear to have been misdirected. It is now well established that standard infant tests do not predict intellective deficiency at acceptable levels of validity in either normal or high risk populations (McCall, 1979a, 1979b; Kopp & McCall, 1980). For some this finding has undermined belief in the continuity between infant and childhood intelligence and in the utility of forecasting cognitive status from infant assessments (McCall, Hogarty, & Hurlburt, 1972). For others, however, it has reinforced a conviction that the simple sensorimotor skills typically emphasized in conventional infant tests bear little relation to later cognitive functioning (Caron & Caron, 1981; Fagan & Singer, 1982; Rose, 1981, Zelazo, 1979). It has been pointed out, for example, that some infants with severe neuromotor impairment (e.g. thalidomide, cerebral palsy, and spina bifida babies) grow to maturity with intact intellect and learning competence, while others with normal motor development exhibit subsequent cognitive deficits (Zelazo, 1979). By implication, then, discontinuity may reside in the measurement of intellect rather than in its ontogeny.

Investigators subscribing to this latter view are therefore seeking to develop infant tests that tap processes more closely aligned with those underlying mature intellectual performance. In so doing, they have drawn on sophisticated laboratory research which indicates that young infants actively process information (i.e., discriminate, remember, and classify input) even before the appearance of gross motor skills. The initial forays of this group have been promising. Fagan and Fantz and their colleagues, for example, have shown that measures of recognition memory (visual preference for novel stimuli when paired with previously familiarized stimuli) not only differentiate groups of infants expected to differ in later intelligence (Fantz & Nevis, 1967; Miranda & Fantz, 1974; Fagan & Singer, 1982), but also predict variations in childhood IQ at respectable levels of validity (Fagan & McGrath, 1981). Likewise, Rose and her associates have found that cross-modal perception (visual preference for novel forms paired with forms previously familiarized tactually) is significantly more advanced in full-term than in preterm infants, even when the ages of preterm infants are corrected for early birth (Rose, Gottfried, & Bridger, 1978, 1979).

The research to be described in the balance of this chapter derives from a similar rationale. Unlike the preceding studies, however, it deals not with recognitive capacities per se, but with the infant's ability to detect and abstract a particular aspect of environmental information, namely, its configural or relational characteristics (Caron & Caron, 1981). It is assumed that the ability to interrelate elements of experience is an essential ingredient of intellect and therefore that competence in processing relational information may provide an early index of future functioning. At issue in what follows is whether differences in this capacity have concurrent or predictive implications for infants who would not typically be considered suspect, that is, full-term infants with relatively mild obstetric complications. A population at such low risk should provide a stringent test of the validity of our cognitive measures. Before presenting the research, theoretical and empirical background relevant to relational information processing is reviewed.

PROCESSING OF RELATIONAL INFORMATION AND COGNITION _____

Theoretical Perspectives _____

The environment is rich in relational information. Examples include the configural arrangements between objects deployed in space, qualitative patterns such as sameness and difference, and the temporal, functional, causal, and actional relations holding between entities in dynamic contexts (e.g., melodies, rhythms, linguistic syntax, object affordances, role relations, mechanical and social causality, etc.). Such wholistic stimulus properties, the traditional province of Gestalt psychology, have received renewed emphasis in contemporary cognitive theory, where they are seen to play a central role in the organization and functioning of adult intellect. Permanent knowledge, for example, is currently thought to have a thematic structure involving networks of object concepts bound by spatial, temporal, and causal relations (Mandler, 1979). These relational units are believed to provide essential frameworks for interpreting otherwise incomprehensible perceptual and linguistic input, and to form the basis for inferential reasoning (Bransford & McCarrell, 1974; Miller & Johnson-Laird, 1976; Schank & Abelson, 1977). As Bransford and McCarrell have observed, nothing is ever understood in isolation and things become meaningful only when we fit them into broader frames that reveal their relation to other things, their functions, actions, origins, etc. Indeed, Bransford and his colleagues have found that the propensity to impose relations on unrelated bits of information is a major factor distinguishing superior from inferior grade school students (Bransford, Stein, Shelton, & Owings, 1980).

That relational information processing appears early in life and figures prominently in perceptual/cognitive development is implicit in recent perceptual and psycholinguistic speculation. Thus James Gibson (1950, 1966, 1979) holds that the visual system is attuned from birth not to static images projected on the retina, but to the higher order, invariant relational information contained in patterns and sequences of retinal images. Elaborating on this theme, Eleanor Gibson (1969) regards the course of perceptual development as the progressive differentiation of the invariant structure of objects and the invariant relations between entities in event contexts. Similarly, current psycholinguistic analysis suggests a possible link between the processing of relational information and early language development. It has been pointed out, for instance, that the young child's ability to understand the meaning of words presupposes a preverbal capacity to form object concepts, which depends in turn on the ability to perceive structural and functional equivalences between dissimilar things (McNamara, 1972). By the same token, the ability to comprehend sentences is said to rest on a prelinguistic disposition to form relational concepts, specifically such concepts as agency of an action, recipient, possession, location, and so forth, all of which are prevalent in the rudimentary speech of children (Brown, 1973; Bloom, 1970; Schlesinger, 1971).

Infant Studies

Beyond theory, there is now considerable evidence that attests to the young infant's responsiveness to relational information (see Caron & Caron, 1981, 1982, for detailed reviews). Generally speaking, between 2 and 5 months of age infants can discriminate stationary visual patterns consisting of different arrangements of the same simple elements and can also abstract invariant configurations across stimuli whose elements differ in shape, color, or density (Caron & Caron, 1981; Cornell, 1975; Fagan, 1977; Milewski, 1979; Shwartz & Day, 1979; Vurpillot, Ruel, & Castrec, 1977). By 5 months of age, they can recognize structures composed of dissimilar elements, most notably the configuration of the human face (Caron, Caron, Caldwell, & Weiss, 1973), and beyond 5 months, they become increasingly sensitive to such abstract facial patterns as gender (Cornell, 1974; Fagan, 1976) and emotional expression (Caron, Caron, & Myers, 1982), as well as to the structural characteristics of unique faces (Cohen & Strauss, 1979; Fagan, 1976).

Prior to 5 months, furthermore, they can distinguish the complex patternings of dynamic events such as the rigid versus deforming motions of objects (Gibson, Owsley, & Johnston, 1978; Walker, Owsley, & Gibson, 1977) and are able to "match" visual and auditory patterns specifying the same event (e.g., vocalizations and their synchronized lip movements; see Spelke, 1976, 1978, 1979; Spelke & Cortelyou, 1981). Within the auditory modality per se, they can detect the melodic and rhythmic aspects of tones and speech (Chang & Trehub, 1977; Horowitz, 1974), and even as neonates can differentiate the vocalizations of their own mothers from those of a strange female (DeCasper & Fifer, 1980). Finally, as to higher order event relations, 3-month-olds apparently can comprehend certain aspects of mechanical causality (Borton, 1979), and by 10 months can distinguish it from social causality (Carlson-Luden, 1979).

Overall, these findings provide ample support for the thesis that young infants are capable of detecting relational information and at relatively abstract levels. The question of immediate concern, of course, is whether individual differences in this regard have any diagnostic value for concurrent or future intellective functioning. In the following section, we turn to the evidence bearing on concurrent validity, first as revealed in comparisons of "normal" and "risk" infants and then in a recent study of our own comparing "optimal" and "nonoptimal" infants. Subsequently, we will examine the predictive power of relational measures in samples of full-term infants.

INFANT RELATIONAL MEASURES: CONCURRENT VALIDITY

Normal–Risk Comparisons

Indirect evidence for a link between the processing of relational information in infancy and later intellective level may be found in the previously mentioned studies by Fagan, Fantz, Rose, and their co-workers. Although these investigators properly interpreted their findings in terms of differential mnemonic and discriminative capacities, the material so discriminated was often configural in content. For example, in the Miranda and Fantz (1974) experiment, normal and Down's syndrome infants were compared on the ability to distinguish stimuli varying solely in the arrangement of simple, geometric elements. Whereas normal infants could differentiate these targets at 24 weeks of age, Down's infants showed no recognition of differences at 36 weeks (the highest age examined). Likewise, the ability to discriminate two different faces—also, in the main, a configural problem—appeared at 24 weeks for normals, but not until 36 weeks for Down's infants. In a subsequent study using a test battery composed of many similar problems (Fagan & Singer, 1982), the overall performance of normal infants was superior to that of a number of high risk samples, particularly infants with diabetic mothers, those suffering from growth retardation, and those with potential central nervous system damage (seizures, ventricular hemorrhaging, etc.). Finally, Rose et al. 1978, 1979) reported that preterm infants at 12 months after expected date of birth were deficient relative to comparably aged, full-term infants in the visual recognition of object shapes following tactual exposure. The ability to integrate temporally distributed inputs into a spatial gestalt would appear to be an essential requirement for success on this task.

In our own research (Caron & Caron, 1981), we sought to obtain more direct evidence for the hypothesis that vulnerability to cognitive deficit would manifest itself early in life as a difficulty in abstracting relational information. The performance of preterm and full-term infants at equivalent conceptional ages was compared on the four problems shown in Figure 9-1 (administered, respectively, at 12, 18, 21, and 24 weeks postnatal

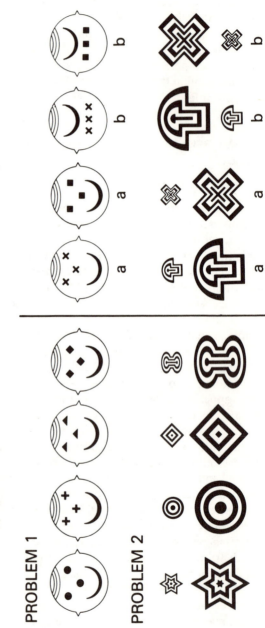

HABITUATION

TEST

PROBLEM 1

PROBLEM 2

a a b b

186

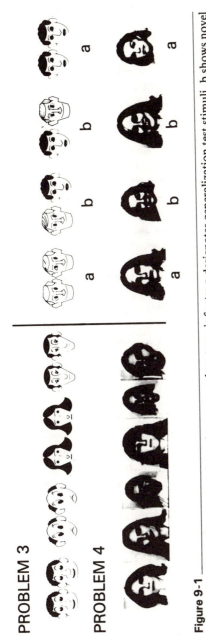

Figure 9-1
Four relational problems administered to term and preterm infants; a designates generalization test stimuli, b shows novel test configurations.

187

age). As illustrated, the procedure involved visual habituation of infants to a series of stimuli representing multiple instances of the same configural concept. In an immediately following test phase, the subjects were shown four novel stimuli: two representing new instances of the familiarized configuration (i.e., new elements in the original arrangement) and two depicting a new configuration (i.e., the same new elements in a novel configuration). The ability of infants to abstract the invariant configural information is inferred from (1) generalization of habituation (absence of response recovery) to the new instances of the familiar configuration and (2) discrimination of the novel configuration (i.e., stronger recovery to the novel relative to the familiar test patterns). This response pattern—generalization or nonrecovery to element change in conjunction with recovery to configural change—constitutes the operational definition of relational concept formation. By contrast, recovery to element change alone (i.e., in the absence of further recovery to configural change) implies that only the component features have been processed during the habituation phase. Nonrecovery to both element change and configural change, on the other hand, would mean that neither property has been encoded during familiarization (assuming that the infant had not become generally fatigued or otherwise disinterested in the situation).

On all four problems the full-term infants yielded significantly greater recovery to the configural change than to the element change stimuli, whereas the preterm infants failed to do so in any instance. The differences between groups were significant on each problem. On three of the four tasks, full-term infants generalized (showed no recovery) to the element change stimuli, while the preterm infants recovered to element change in every case. On the four problems combined, 40 percent of term infants yielded a clear-cut conceptual response pattern and an additional 31 percent recovered significantly to configural change while also recovering to component change. By contrast, the respective figures for preterm infants were 20 and 16 percent. Conversely, 37 percent of the preterm subjects responded to element change alone, as opposed to 19 percent of the full-term subjects. In sum, while the preterm and full-term infants had each processed aspects of the habituation stimuli, the preterm infants focused primarily on the elements, and the full-term infants primarily on the relations between elements.

Optimal–Nonoptimal Comparisons

Encouraged by the magnitude and consistency of these differences, we decided to put the sensitivity of our tasks to a more stringent test, specifically, to determine whether performance might reveal subtle effects associated with perinatal events within groups of full-term infants. To this end, we took a different approach to the problem of classifying infant status, an approach similar in many respects to that advocated by Prechtl (1981). Generally, perinatal studies tend to define "risk" (in terms of various maternal, fetal, and infant indices) and to categorize the remaining cases as "normal." However, given that many unrecognizably hazardous birth events may be omitted from risk inventories and that there is often no clear consensus on those items to be included (or on their cutoff points or weightings), a group of infants classified as normal, healthy, full-term could harbor a substantial number of cases who are compromised by seemingly innocuous perinatal conditions. Needless to say, this would attenuate group differences in a comparison with "risk" infants. Consequently, it seemed preferable to approach the problem from the other end of the continuum—to define "optimal" and classify all other infants as "nonoptimal." As Prechtl (1981) observed, optimality in infancy has a much higher predictive value for later normality than does any abnormal indicator for later abnormality. Indeed, focusing on the optimal provides a more homogeneous base line from which to assess the effects of less patently traumatic obstetric factors.

Subjects

We had already collected relational abstraction measures on a large number of full-term babies in connection with both our preterm study and other ongoing experiments. Since it was our practice to include all but obvious risk cases in our full-term samples, we essentially had data from a demographically homogeneous population of infants (typically firstborn of white college-educated parents) who were not otherwise classified as preterm or high risk and who had been exposed to a variety of perinatal conditions. Within the limits of information provided by the mother, we assigned infants retrospectively to optimal or nonoptimal categories according to stringent criteria. Specifically, infants were regarded as optimal if they met the following conditions:

1. They were a singleton birth.
2. They had undergone an estimated gestational period of 40 weeks ± 10 days.
3. Their birth weight was appropriate for their gestational age.
4. They had Apgar scores of 8 and 9 or better at 1 and 5 min, respectively.
5. Pregnancy involved no drugs, including fertility drugs, no metabolic disturbance or bleeding, no threat of prematurity, and so on.
6. Labor was of normal duration (3–20 hours), with no induction.
7. Their delivery was vaginal, with vertex presentation, occiput anterior; no (or low) forceps were used; local or regional anesthesia was administered; or cesarean section was performed without trial labor and without general anesthesia.

8. Postnatally, they were healthy, thriving infants having had no major physical anomalies or neurological signs, no metabolic disturbance requiring treatment or prolonged observation, no stay in intensive care as newborn, and no illness requiring hospitalization.

Full-term infants who failed to meet any of these criteria were classified as nonoptimal. There were 54 optimal infants (27 male, 27 female) and 100 nonoptimal infants (61 male, 39 female) who had all previously participated in at least one of four tasks administered at 12, 18, 21, and 24 weeks of age, respectively. The sessions of 8 nonoptimal infants who had been tested on more than one task were treated as independent data,* yielding an overall total of 110 nonoptimal sessions (65 male, 45 female). The two samples were highly similar in socioeconomic status as reflected in the mean maternal educational level (optimal, 15.4 years; nonoptimal, 15.5 years). The disproportionate number of males in the nonoptimal group is not discrepant with the distributions usually found in nonoptimal children.

Tasks

Three of the four tasks ("face configuration," "above–below," and "neutral–happy" face expressions) were the same as those used in the preterm study. The "same–different" problem, which had been the least discriminating in that study, was replaced by a second face expression task—"happy–surprise"—which had subsequently been found to yield strong term–preterm differences at 21–24 weeks (see Fig. 9-2).

Procedures

The infants were brought to the laboratory by one or both parents, who remained with them throughout the procedure. The baby (in a reclining infant seat) was placed in a three-sided chamber whose front wall had a 7 × 7-inch window at 13 inches distance on which stimuli were rear projected. Fixation was scored by the standard corneal reflection technique (Fantz, 1956) from a television monitor, each trial terminating when the infant looked away from the target for at least 0.5 sec. The habituation stimuli were presented in sequence (i.e., S_1, S_2, S_3, S_4, S_1, S_2, . . . until a specified habituation criterion was met—defined *relatively* as a 50 percent decrement from initial looking levels (based on blocks of three trials), or *absolutely* as a decline to 8 sec of viewing or less on three trials (to ensure that subjects whose initial looking was brief would not undergo prolonged habituation). To provide a check on the infant's terminal level of alertness, each session began and ended with the presentation of the same attractive art slide. Ses-

---

*Since there were no performance differences as a function of multiple testing, we felt justified in including these data.

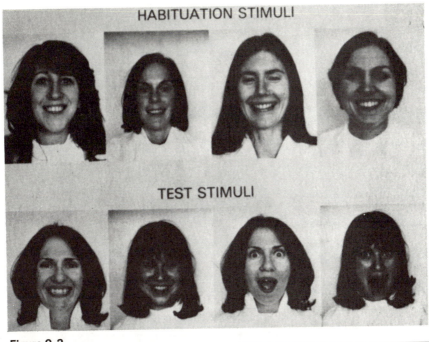

Figure 9-2
Happy–surprise face expression problem administered in the optimality study.

sions were excluded as data if they failed to meet minimum criteria of overall looking during habituation (15 sec) and during test (10 sec).

Results

Two test scores were of central interest: a *generalization* or *element
discrimination* score, calculated as total fixation of the two familiar test
configurations (F) relative to the last two habituations trials (H), or
$F/F+H$, and a *configural discrimination score*, calculated as total fixation
of the two novel test configurations (N) relative to the two familiar test configurations (F), or $N/N+F$. A chance value of 50 percent or less on either
measure would imply nondiscrimination, and a value significantly in excess
of 50 percent would imply discrimination. Again, a conceptual test pattern
would consist of scores of 50 percent or less on element discrimination, and
scores of greater than 50 percent on configural discrimination.

As shown in Figure 9-3, the mean scores of the optimal infants approximated the ideal conceptual pattern on each task. Specifically, the optimal
subjects were nonresponsive (yielded chance or lower scores) to element
change, but were highly responsive to configural change. Nonoptimal infants, by contrast, recovered almost exclusively to element change on each

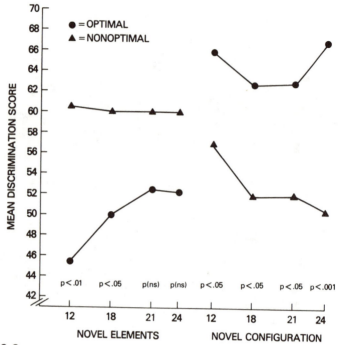

Figure 9-3

Configural discrimination scores of optimal and nonoptimal infants across four age (task) levels.

problem. As indicated, six of the eight group comparisons were statistically significant.

The nonparametric data perhaps best reveal the extent of the difference between the two groups. Using a criterion for recovery of 55.6 percent or greater (the percentage representing a significant deviation from chance based on all cases combined), we were able to classify the performance of each infant according to one of four possible categories of discrimination/nondiscrimination:

1. Recovery to configuration only (the ideal pattern)
2. Recovery to both elements and configuration
3. Recovery to elements only
4. Recovery to neither

The resulting distribution for all tasks combined (Fig. 9-4) differed markedly between the optimal and nonoptimal subjects (chi square = 22.51, $p < .001$). While the two groups did not diverge in their response to novelty per se (categories A, B, and C combined), the optimal group, as expected, was more likely to discriminate the novel configuration than the

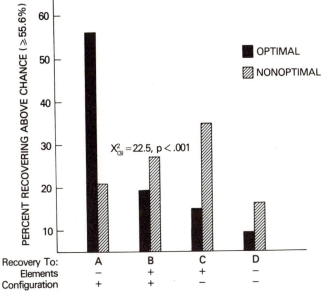

Figure 9-4
Distribution of optimal and nonoptimal infants across four recovery categories. A, recovery to configural change; B, recovery to both configural and element change; C, recovery to element change; D, recovery to neither configural nor element change.

nonoptimal group (categories A and B combined, 76 versus 48%) and less likely to discriminate the novel elements (categories B and C combined, 33 versus 63%). More importantly, the optimal group was more likely than the nonoptimal group to discriminate the novel configuration alone, that is, to respond in a manner reflecting concept acquisition (category A, 57 versus 21%).

In order to determine whether these differences might be attributable to any particular subgroup of nonoptimal infants, the responses of two subclasses that were represented in sufficient numbers to form distinct groups were separately examined. These included infants who had 1 min Apgar scores of 6 or less ($n = 16$) and those who had an estimated gestational age of 42 weeks or more ($n = 31$). Because there were too few low-Apgar cases for direct comparison with the optimal group, the low-Apgar subgroup was eliminated from the nonoptimal sample, and the remaining infants compared with the optimal sample. The resulting optimal–nonoptimal comparison was minimally changed (chi square$_3$ = 20.46, $p <$ .001), suggesting that the difference between the optimal and nonoptimal groups was robust and not due simply to the deviant performance of a few less healthy infants. Similarly, when the post-term subgroup was directly compared with the optimal infants, the difference remained significant (chi square$_3$ = 9.95, p < .01). Since this category included many infants normally not considered at risk, it appears that performance on our tasks was sensitive to subtle perinatal complications.

Finally, to determine whether our obtained effects might be sex linked, optimal–nonoptimal comparisons were conducted separately for males and females. The distributions of optimal and nonoptimal infants were significantly discrepant within each sex group (chi square$_3$ = 9.11 and p < .01 for males, chi square$_3$ = 7.45 and p < .01 for females), indicating that our results were not primarily a function of the overrepresentation of males in the nonoptimal sample.

Habituation Data

A further question may be raised as to whether the nonoptimal infants might have been generally less efficient than the optimal infants in processing information. We therefore compared the two groups in terms of (1) the number of trials to reach criterion during habituation and (2) the total accumulated fixation time during habituation. There were no significant between-groups differences for either of these variables on any of the tasks. Although processing differences have been reported between risk and nonrisk samples (e.g., Rose, 1980), it appears that the present effects were due less to differences in efficiency of processing than to differences in the *content* of processing: optimal infants primarily encoded configurations, and nonoptimal infants, elements.

The preceding findings suggest that measures of relational information processing obtained in infancy are sensitive to obstetric complications associated with full-term birth. It remains to be determined, however, whether these performance differences represent transient effects or differences in functioning having long-term consequences. We turn now to the evidence bearing on this issue, beginning first with published work to date and concluding with ongoing research in our laboratory.

INFANT RELATIONAL MEASURES: PREDICTIVE VALIDITY

Previous Studies

Indirect evidence for the predictive validity of infant relational measures may be gleaned from recent reports by Fagan and his colleagues. Specifically, Fagan and McGrath (1981) administered vocabulary tests to children at 4 and 7 years who had previously been tested between 5 and 7 months on pairings of novel and familiar element arrangements and face photographs. The obtained correlations between infant novelty preference and childhood verbal IQ of .37 at 4 years and .57 at 7 years were each significant and were apparently unrelated to socioeconomic status as measured by parental education level. In a further investigation (Fagan, 1981), a correlation of .36 was found between novelty preference scores for faces at 7 months and 3-year vocabulary scores. The magnitude of these relations is not particularly robust, but, as Fagan has observed, given the relatively low reliability of the infant measures and the restricted range of intelligence scores (90–130), the obtained coefficients very likely underestimate predictive validity.

Preliminary Study in Our Laboratory _____

In view of these findings, we were moved to inquire whether our own relational measures might yield comparable correlations with childhood performance. For a variety of reasons, however, we were not particularly sanguine about the possibility of obtaining definitive data. For one thing, most of our subjects had received one or at most two relational tasks in infancy, an insufficient number to ensure adequate levels of reliability. In addition, the majority of cases had barely reached their second birthday, which restricted our choice of outcome measure and meant that younger children would be assessed differently from older ones. Moreover, the child tests employed (the Bayley Mental Development Scale and the Stanford-Binet Intelligence Scale) yield global performance measures that may be affected by factors unrelated to those tapped by our infant tests. Finally, our sample was markedly homogeneous with respect to social class, thus reducing the potential range of intellective variations and hence the magnitude of outcome correlations. Despite these reservations, we felt that the resulting information might at least tell us whether we were moving in the right direction and, if sizable correlations were to occur regardless of the above limitations, it would reflect dramatically on the predictive power of our tasks.

Subjects _____

Thus far 64 of our infant subjects (32 boys and 32 girls) have been given either the Bayley Mental Development Scale or the Stanford-Binet Intelligence Scale (form L-M) between 2 and 3½ years of age. All were full-term infants, 31 of whom (12 boys, 19 girls) had been classified optimal, and 33 (20 boys, 13 girls) nonoptimal. Only infants who had been tested on one or both of our face expression problems—"happy-surprise" and "neutral-happy" (administered between 21 and 24 weeks)—were selected for follow-up. These tasks were used as a predictive base because they were administered to many more infants than the "schematic face" and "above-below" problems (thus yielding better normative data and a larger subject pool) and because they were presented at 5-6 months, when infant performance is likely to be more stable. The scores of subjects who had been tested on both problems ($n = 15$) were averaged for present purposes. Testers were unaware of the children's infant data.

Results

The means and standard deviations of the infant and childhood test scores and the relevant parental data are summarized for the optimality and sex subgroups in Table 9-1. Turning first to the optimality groups, we find that, contrary to expectation, there were no overall differences between the optimal and nonoptimal subjects on the childhood tests. The optimal children did score somewhat higher on the Binet Scale than the nonoptimal children, but neither this difference nor that for the combined Bayley and Binet scores were significant. This finding may be due in part to the fact that there were also no differences between the two groups on our infant measures. As can be seen, the nonoptimal subjects recovered as strongly to novel expressions as the optimal subjects, indicating that this subgroup was not entirely representative of our nonoptimal infant population (who, it will be recalled, yielded chance, 50% recovery to facial expressions; see Fig. 9-3). While this sampling bias is unfortunate, it should be emphasized that it could have no bearing on the extent of correlation between our infant and childhood measures (each of which showed considerable variability) and in fact may have served to eliminate the possible confounding effect of optimality on childhood performance. Finally, it should be noted that there were no differences in parental age or education between the optimal and nonoptimal subjects, underscoring again the homogeneous socioeconomic status of the sample. Given the overall high level of parental education, the above-average intellective mean of the children is understandable.

Examination of the gender breakdowns in Table 9-1 reveals that the childhood quotients of females tended to be somewhat higher than those of the males (particularly on the Bayley Scale) but here too the differences were not significant. There were also no sex differences on the infant measures, which again was unexpected, since proportionately more girls than boys had been rated optimal. Apparently, the strong recovery to expressions of the nonoptimal sample was confined primarily to males ($\overline{X} = 60.2\%$ for nonoptimal boys; $\overline{X} = 54.6\%$ for nonoptimal girls). Nevertheless, the range of both recovery scores within each sex group was considerable (about 25–85%) and approximately half the children of each gender recovered significantly to expressions and half to persons. Lastly, the parents of boys and girls too were comparable in age and education.

The correlations between our infant and childhood scores are shown in Table 9-2. As can be seen in the first row of the table, the coefficients for all subjects combined were exceedingly modest. The correlation of .24 between recovery to expressions and childhood performance was marginally signifi-

Table 9-1

Mean Performances on Infant and Childhood Tests (Bayley Mental Development Scale and Binet IQ) and Mean Parental Data of the Optimality and Sex Subgroups

	Optimal Subjects	Nonoptimal Subjects	Girls	Boys	All Subjects
Bayley					
Mean	111.9	112.6	115.2	108.3	112.3
SD	22.9	13.3	7.9	25.6	17.9
Range	58–150	84–133	104–130	58–150	58–150
n	15	18	19	14	33
Binet					
Mean	119.4	110.9	115.9	114.6	115.2
SD	20.0	14.9	23.4	13.5	18.0
Range	80–159	88–151	80–151	100–159	80–159
n	16	15	13	18	31
Bayley and Binet					
Mean	115.8	111.9	115.5	111.8	113.7
SD	21.5	13.8	17.2	19.8	18.1
n	31	33	32	32	64
Percentage recovery to expressions					
Mean	59.2†	58.0†	55.5†	61.6†	58.6†
SD	14.7	18.2	16.4	16.2	16.5
Percentage recovery to persons					
Mean	54.0	56.7*	55.7*	55.1*	55.4*
SD	15.1	11.1*	13.5*	13.0*	13.3*

(continued)

Table 9-1 (continued)

	Optimal Subjects	Nonoptimal Subjects	Girls	Boys	All Subjects
Trials to criterion					
Mean	9.3	8.5	8.1	9.7	8.9
SD	6.6	3.9	3.6	6.7	5.4
Mother's ed					
Mean	15.7	15.7	15.8	16.0	15.9
SD	2.0	2.0	2.2	1.8	2.0
Father's ed					
Mean	17.0	16.7	16.5	17.0	16.8
SD	1.9	2.3	2.0	2.3	2.1
Mother's age					
Mean	30.3	30.1	29.2	30.9	30.1
SD	4.3	4.2	3.6	4.6	4.3
Father's age					
Mean	32.1	31.6	31.4	32.0	31.7
SD	5.0	5.1	6.1	4.6	5.3

$*p < .05.$
$†p < .01.$

Table 9-2 _____

Correlations Between Three Infant Test Measures and Childhood Intellective Scores for Optimality, Sex, and Childhood Test Subgroups

	Percentage Recovery to Expressions	Percentage Recovery to Persons	Trials to Criterion
All subjects (n = 64)	.24*	−.06	.19
Nonoptimal (n = 33)	.33*	−.03	.14
Optimal (n = 31)	.19	−.06	.20
Girls (n = 32)	.53‡	−.39†	−.11
Boys (n = 32)	.06	.18	.35†
Binet (n = 31)	.42‡	−.29	.23
Bayley (n = 33)	−.02	.20	.10
Girls–Binet (n = 13)	.68‡	−.57†	−.09
Girls–Bayley (n = 19)	.30	−.06	−.19
Boys–Binet (n = 18)	.20	.03	.51†
Boys–Bayley (n = 14)	−.20	.37	.25
Nonoptimal–girls (n = 13)	.67‡	−.41	−.08
Optimal–girls (n = 19)	.44*	−.40*	−.14
Nonoptimal–Binet (n = 15)	.62‡	−.51†	.11
Optimal–Binet (n = 16)	.23	−.16	.30

*p < .05, one tail.
†p < .025.
‡p < .01.

cant ($p < .05$, one tail), but hardly represented an improvement over the median correlation of .23 between standard infant tests and 3-year IQ (McCall et al., 1972). To determine whether these values might differ between our various subgroups (optimal versus nonoptimal subjects, girls versus boys, Binet versus Bayley tests), separate coefficients were computed for each of these categories.

As shown in the next six rows of Table 9-2, the pattern of correlations was markedly discrepant for girls and boys and for the Binet and Bayley tests, but was roughly comparable for optimal and nonoptimal children. Specifically, whereas for girls recovery to expressions and recovery to persons were both correlated significantly and in opposite directions with the combined IQ and Bayley MDI scores (.53 for expressions, $-.39$ for persons), for boys these coefficients were negligible. On the other hand, trials to criterion were correlated significantly with later performance for boys, but not for girls (.35 versus $-.11$, respectively). The difference between the three pairs of male and female coefficients were significant or near significant ($p < .05$, $p < .025$, and $p < .075$. respectively).

A somewhat similar pattern of differences emerged for the Binet and Bayley tests, with the Binet coefficients being generally stronger. Thus recovery to expressions had a .42 correlation with Binet IQ, and recovery to persons a $-.29$ correlation ($p < .10$), whereas in the Bayley matrix neither of these coefficients approached significance. Trials to criterion failed to be significantly correlated with either scale when considered independently of gender. The differences between the Binet and Bayley recovery coefficients were not quite significant ($p < .075$ in each case).

As might be expected in view of the preceding discussion, the most clear-cut infancy–childhood correlations occurred for girls tested with the Binet IQ (eighth row of Table 9-2), where coefficients of .68 ($p < .01$) and $-.57$ ($p < .025$) were obtained for recovery to expressions and recovery to persons, respectively. The trials to criterion correlation previously found for males was also strongest for those males tested with the Binet ($r = .51$, $p < .025$). By contrast, the Bayley correlations were nonsignificant for both sexes. Examination of the sex × optimality and test × optimality subgroups (last four rows of Table 9-2) revealed that in general the female and Binet correlations tended to be better articulated for nonoptimal subjects. Unfortunately, there were not enough cases to obtain meaningful correlations for the three-way (sex × test × optimality) breakdowns.

In addition to the infancy–childhood test correlations, matrices of intercorrelations were computed involving the Binet and Bayley scores, the three infant test measures, the parental data, and one additional variable, birth order, which had previously been found to be negatively correlated with verbal IQ in a sample comparable to our own (Fagan, 1981). (Unfortunately, only 10 of our 64 subjects—4 girls and 6 boys—were later born, which would seriously attenuate correlations involving this variable). Three aspects of these data merit comment. First, recovery to expressions and recovery to persons were correlated negatively with each other for both girls and boys (overall $r = -.48$, $p < .001$), thus suggesting that both scores reflect a single dimension having to do with the ability to categorize face expressions. Given our obtained pattern of IQ correlations for these two variables (positive for recovery to expressions, negative for recovery to persons), it would appear, then, that the ability to classify face expressions at 5–6 months (i.e., to generalize to new persons in a familiar expression and to detect novel expressions) is predictive of Binet IQ at 3 years, particularly for girls. By contrast, the trials to criterion measure was not correlated with either recovery to expressions or recovery to persons (overall $r = -.05$ and $r = .21$, respectively). Hence the obtained correlation for boys between this variable and childhood IQ likely reflects the influence of a factor unrelated to the capacity to detect expressive invariants.

The second point to be noted in this context is that none of the parental variables were correlated with either the Bayley, Binet, or infancy scores, a finding that is no doubt due again to the homogeneously high socioeconomic level of the sample.

Finally, although birth order was modestly correlated with overall childhood performance ($r = -.24$, $p < .05$), the relation was stronger for the Bayley ($r = -.34$, $p < .05$) than for the Binet ($r = -.09$). It also tended to be correlated more strongly with childhood scores for boys ($r = -.32$, $p < .05$) than for girls ($r = -.12$), but given the small number of later born children, these differences are hardly definitive. Since birth order also related negatively to trials to criterion for boys ($r = -.30$, $p < .05$), no added predictability to childhood performance could be derived from this variable over and above that from the trials measure alone.

Summary and General Comment

The major findings of our preliminary study are threefold. First, the ability to form face expression concepts at 5–6 months was found to be predictive of Binet IQ at 3 years, but not of Bayley MDI at 2 years. Second, the predictive power of this infant capacity proved to be considerably stronger for girls than for boys. Finally, a second infant variable, degree of attentiveness to habituation stimuli, was positively associated with childhood performance for boys but not for girls. Consider each of these results in turn.

The overall correlation of .42 between recovery to novel expressions and Binet IQ represents a significant advance over the median correlation of .23 previously obtained between conventional tests of infant sensorimotor development and IQ at 3 years. It also compares favorably with the correlations of .36 and .41 reported by Fagan (1981) and by Fagan and McGrath

(1981), respectively, between recognition memory scores at 5–7 months and verbal intelligence at 3 years. The extent of correlation is particularly encouraging, if one further takes into account the limited number of test items employed and the homogeneous nature of the sample, both of which would tend to attenuate infant test reliability and hence predictive validity. Fagan and Singer (1982), on the basis of their own data, have estimated the reliability of infant tests based on 1.5 items (as in our situation) at a value of only .24. If this estimate approximates that of our measures and if one also assumes a reliability of .90 for the Stanford-Binet, then the maximum validity coefficient that could have been expected in this study is .47 (the square root of the joint reliabilities), a value not much greater than our obtained coefficient of .42. Thus the magnitude of our correlation lies pretty much at the limit of validity allowed by the underlying test reliabilities. If the aforementioned sources of attenuation could be substantially reduced, it is conceivable that our validity coefficient would show appreciable gain. Although improved reliability does not ensure greater validity, there is presently no good reason to refrain from pursuing this objective.

The failure of the Bayley test to yield significant correlations with our infant measures is perhaps not too surprising, given that the Bayley Scale includes fewer conceptual–relational items than the Binet. On the other hand, Lewis and Brooks-Gunn (1981) recently obtained correlations of .52 and .40 between recovery to novel colors and forms at 3 months and 24-month Bayley performance. If the Bayley MDI can be assumed to measure discriminative ability more than conceptual ability, this inconsistency is perhaps explainable. Indeed, the relatively modest correlation of .53 between the 24-month Bayley mental scale and the Stanford-Binet (McCall, 1976) indicates that the two tests harbor more distinctive than shared variance. Nevertheless, the discrepancy between the two studies remains to be resolved.

As to the obtained gender differences, two points invite consideration. First, there is other evidence that infant tests predict later IQ better for girls than boys (Goffeney, Henderson, & Butler, 1971; McCall et al., 1972). McCall et al. (1972), for example, found that correlations between Gesell scores at 6, 12, 18, and 24 months and Stanford-Binet IQ at 3½, 6, and 10 years were uniformly higher for girls than boys. Likewise, in Fagan's research, where male and female correlations were not significantly different, the coefficients nevertheless tended to be larger for girls than for boys—.40 versus .31 at 4 years and .62 versus .49 at 7 years, respectively (Fagan & McGrath, 1981). It would appear, then, that our sex differences are not exceptional, although one is hard pressed to account for them.

One possible explanation derives from a recent study of our own (Caron, Caron, & Myers, 1982), where infants of three ages (4, 5½, and 7 months) were given the "happy–surprise" problem. While overall performance improved with age, at each age more girls than boys yielded a conceptual test pattern (nonrecovery to person change, recovery to expression change), with 4-month girls performing as well as 5½-month boys, and 5½-month girls nearly as well as 7-month boys. Boys in the main tended to respond either to person change alone or to both person and expression changes. It was suggested that girls may become attuned at a younger age than boys to expressive configurations, and that boys of 4–6 months may be more responsive to specific facial features. As we have seen, however, our present sample included as many boys as girls who responded conceptually at test. Is it perhaps possible that these scores mean different things for boys and girls? Specifically, could it be that younger boys who yielded a conceptual test pattern had abstracted only specific facial features (e.g., toothy versus open mouths), whereas girls who produced this pattern abstracted a configural gestalt (happy versus surprise expressions)? If there is any merit to this speculation, then predictability for boys should improve if tested at 7–8 months rather than at 5–6 months. Unfortunately, we presently do not have enough cases to test this prediction, but the previously cited data of McCall et al. (1972) do in fact suggest that correlations to later IQ occur earlier for girls than boys. For the moment, it is unclear whether this or some other factor underlies our sex differences, or whether we are dealing simply with random sampling fluctuations.

The second point to be made in this context pertains to our last finding, that prolonged attentiveness to stimuli during habituation was related to superior childhood performance for boys. In a recent study, Kopp and Vaughn (1982) reported somewhat comparable data, namely, "sustained attention" to objects at 8 months improved predictability to 24-month Bayley scores for males but not for females. Interestingly, their sample was highly variable with respect to socioeconomic status and ethnicity, the primary predictors of 2-year performance, and only when these factors were controlled did the contribution of sustained attention to the MDI emerge for males. In our own sample, on the other hand, where variation due to these sources was negligible, the attentional relation was manifested in the simple correlation. Be that as it may, this sex difference is also something of an enigma, particularly since infant boys have been found to habituate faster than girls (Tighe & Powlison, 1978).

GENERAL CONCLUSIONS

The preceding findings lend support to a number of interrelated propositions advanced in the beginning of this chapter. First, they tend to confirm the general thesis that prediction of later intellective functioning is likely to be better for infant tests that involve processes related to those underlying mature cognitive performance. In addition, they suggest, together with Fagan's predictive data, that there is individual stability in early intellectual growth. Finally, the results are consistent with the specific assumption that the ability of infants to detect invariant configural–relational properties of stimuli is continuous with conceptual–relational capacities in childhood.

The possibility that intellectual development involves a continuum of processing skills prompts consideration of the formal relation between early and later skills. In particular, do the same basic abilities underlie infant and childhood cognition or are these abilities somehow transformed or supplemented by other skills during development? As we have seen, Fagan and Singer (1982) opt for an identity relation between early and later processing. As they put it, "to predict later intelligence, the task is to sample behaviors during infancy which are similar in kind or which tap the same processes as behaviors known to be related to later intelligence" (p. 12). Thus they see no essential differences between the processes underlying early recognition memory tasks and those involved in later tests of intelligence. This is a straightforward continuity position and is shared by others on the contemporary developmental scene, albeit for different processes. The Gibsons (E. Gibson, 1969; J. Gibson, 1979), for example, believe that perceptual mechanisms promoting information pick-up are central to cognition and function from birth without major transformation. By contrast, Piagetian theory posits a fundamental change in the character of representational thought from infancy to childhood. Unlike the child, the sensorimotor infant is held to be preconceptual, presymbolic, and premnemonic. Still another conception of continuity, intermediate between these positions, is a building-block or hierarchic model in which later abilities are taken to result from the incorporation, integration, and refinement of earlier skills. Thus, the processes underlying our infant relational tasks may be viewed as rudiments of more complex functions such as analogic and inferential reasoning where higher-order relational information (relations between relations) predominate, not only at the perceptual level but also symbolically. Such a model would leave room for maturational and/or environmental contributions to intellectual growth and for both discontinuity and continuity in development. Needless to say, there is as yet no compelling evidence for any of these developmental positions, although the predictive research reviewed in the present chapter as well as recent studies of infant and childhood memory (see Mandler, 1983), would appear to rule out a radical Piagetian or epigenic formulation.

Assuming there is continuity in development, a question remains as to the specific abilities that persist from infancy to childhood. The Gibsons, as noted, stress a perceptual capacity. Critical invariant information is thought to be directly extracted from the environment through mulitiple perceptual channels. In this scheme, internal representational structures, memory, and processes that transform input are presumed to play minimal roles at all ages. On the other hand, Fagan and Singer (1982) view their recognition memory tasks as involving not only perception and discrimination, but also a registration–storage mechanism that mediates comparison of later with earlier input. Our own view would combine elements of both these positions. It emphasizes both detection and encoding, specifically encoding of invariant relational information. It differs from Gibsonian theory, in that it posits an encoding process, and from Fagan and Singer's approach, in that it stresses the encoding of a particular kind of environmental attribute (relational). While there is as yet no basis for choosing between these alternatives, it would appear from our own research that encoding per se is not the critical predictor of later IQ but rather encoding of invariant relational information. It will be recalled that our infants were required to ignore one aspect of the stimuli—their variable elemental properties (e.g., eye color, nose width, etc.)—and to focus instead on their invariant configural properties (e.g., smiling expressions). As we have seen, those who encoded elemental information under these circumstances (i.e., those who responded to person change alone) tended to perform poorly at 3 years, while those who encoded configural information tended to perform well. Fagan and Singer (1982) do suggest that recognition of similarity across differing contexts is one of a triumvirate of processes, together with discrimination and retention, that may be basic to intelligent functioning. What remains to be resolved is whether all, some, or none of these processes carry the major predictive weight from infancy to childhood.

Aside from these conceptual fine points, one has finally to confront the issue of whether the various findings reported above have any practical implications for infant assessment. Obviously, at this stage there is room for skepticism. McCall (1981), for example, is not overly impressed with the potential utility of infant cognitive measures as screening devices. He points out that the best single predictor of childhood IQ is parent education, socioeconomic status, or IQ (at levels of .50 or greater), and he suggests that since the correlations thus far obtained for infant recognition memory tasks do not exceed this level, there is little pragmatic benefit to be derived from these measures. It should be noted, however, that in both Fagan and McGrath's and our own studies, the samples were quite homogeneous with respect to parental education, and significant correlations between infant scores and childhood IQ were found nevertheless. Consequently, the tasks involved may have been tapping sources of variance that are independent of the factors reflected in parental education level. If this is the case, then the infant measures could be combined with the parental data to yield greater predictability than might be obtained from either alone. Moreover, parental scores cannot, in principle, be used to identify infants who will subsequently deviate from the mental levels of their parents—e.g., the developmentally delayed offspring of educated parents or the precocious children of uneducated parents—and yet these constitute target groups of major social interest. Nor can parental measures forecast specific developmental disabilities that may eventually occur in otherwise competent children. In sum, while we may still be a long way from developing robust screening instruments based on infant cognitive measures, their potential pragmatic value cannot be summarily dismissed.

REFERENCES

Bloom, L. *Language development*. Cambridge, Mass.: MIT Press, 1970.

Borton, R. W. *The perception of causality in infants*. Unpublished doctoral dissertation, University of Washington, 1979.

Bransford, J. D., & McCarrell, N. S. A sketch of a cognitive approach to comprehension. In W. B. Weimer & D. S. Palermo (Eds.), *Cognition and the symbolic processes*. Hillsdale, N.J.: Erlbaum, 1974.

Bransford, J. D., Stein, B. S., Shelton, T. S., & Owings, R. A. Cognition and adaptation: The importance of learning to learn. In J. Harvey (Ed.), *Cognition, social behavior and the environment*. Hillsdale, N.J.: Erlbaum, 1980.

Brown, R. W. *A first language: The early stages*. Cambridge, Mass.: Harvard University Press, 1973.

Carlson-Luden, V. *Causal understanding in the ten-month-old*. Unpublished doctoral dissertation, University of Colorado, 1979.

Caron, A. J., & Caron, R. F. Processing of relational information as an index of infant risk. In S. L. Friedman & M. Sigman (Eds.), *Preterm birth and psychological development*. New York: Academic, 1981.

Caron, A. J., & Caron, R. F. Cognitive development in early infancy. In T. Field, A. Huston, H. Quay, L. Troll & G. Finley (Eds.), *Review of human development*. New York: Wiley, 1982.

Caron, A., Caron, R., Caldwell, R., & Weiss, S. Infant perception of the structural properties of the face. *Developmental Psychology*, 1973, *9*, 385–399.

Caron, R. F., Caron, A. J., & Myers, R. S. Abstraction of invariant face expressions in infancy. *Child Development*, 1982, *53*, 1008–1015.

Chang, N., & Trehub, S. Auditory processing of relational information by young infants. *Journal of Experimental Child Psychology*, 1977, *24*, 324–331.

Cohen, L. B., & Strauss, M. S. Concept acquisition in the human infant. *Child Development*, 1979, *50*, 419–424.

Cornell, E. H. Infants' discrimination of photographs of faces following redundant presentations. *Journal of Experimental Child Psychology*, 1974, *18*, 98–106.

Cornell, E. H. Infant's visual attention to pattern arrangement and orientation. *Child Development*, 1975, *46*, 229–232.

DeCasper, A. J., & Fifer, W. P. Of human bonding: Newborns prefer their mothers' voices. *Science*, 1980, *208*, 1174–1176.

Fagan, J. F. Infant's recognition of invariant features of faces. *Child Development*, 1976, *47*, 627–638.

Fagan, J. F. An attention model of infant recognition. *Child Development*, 1977, *48*, 345-359.

Fagan, J. F. *Infant memory and the prediction of intelligence.* Paper presented at the Society for Research in Child Development meeting, Boston, April, 1981.

Fagan, J. F., & McGrath, S. K. Infant recognition memory and later intelligence. *Intelligence*, 1981, *5*, 121-130.

Fagan, J. F., & Singer, L. T. Infant recognition memory as a measure of intelligence. In L. P. Lipsitt (Ed.), *Advances in infancy research* (Vol. 2). Norwood, NJ: Ablex, 1982.

Fantz, R. L. A method for studying early visual development. *Perceptual and Motor Skills*, 1956, *6*, 13-15.

Fantz, R. L., & Nevis, S. The predictive value of changes in visual preference in early infancy. In J. Hellmuth (Ed.), *The exceptional infant* (Vol. 1). Seattle: Special Child Publications, 1967.

Gibson, E. J. *Principles of perceptual learning and development.* New York: Appleton, 1969.

Gibson, E. J., Owsley, C. J., & Johnston, J. Perception of invariants by five-month-olds: Differentiation of two types of motion. *Developmental Psychology*, 1978, *14*, 407-415.

Gibson, J. J. *The perception of the visual world.* Boston: Houghton Mifflin, 1950.

Gibson, J. J. *The senses considered as perceptual systems.* Boston: Houghton Mifflin, 1966.

Gibson, J. J. *The ecological approach to visual perception.* Boston: Houghton Mifflin, 1979.

Goffeney, B., Henderson, N. B., & Butler, B. V. Negro-white, male-female eight-month developmental scores compared with seven-year WISC and Bender test scores. *Child Development*, 1971, *42*, 595-604.

Horowitz, F. D. Visual attention, auditory stimulation, and language discrimination in young infants. *Monographs of the Society for Research in Child Development*, 1974, *39*, 5-6.

Kopp, C. B., & McCall, R. B. Stability and instability in mental performance among normal, at-risk, and handicapped infants and children. In P. B. Baltes & O. G. Grim, Jr. (Eds.) *Life-span development and behavior* (Vol. 4). New York: Academic, 1980.

Kopp, C. B., & Parmelee, A. H. Prenatal and perinatal influences on infant behavior. In J. D. Osofsky (Ed.), *Handbook of infant development.* New York: Wiley, 1979.

Kopp, C. B., & Vaughn, B. E. Sustained attention during exploratory manipulation as a predictor of cognitive competence in preterm infants. *Child Development*, 1982, *53*, 174-182.

Lewis, M., & Brooks-Gunn, J. Visual attention at three months as a predictor of cognitive functioning at two years of age. *Intelligence*, 1981, *5*, 131-140.

MacNamara, J. Cognitive basis of language learning in infants. *Psychological Review*, 1972, *79*, 1-13.

Mandler, J. M. Categorical and schematic organization in memory. In C. R. Puff (Ed.), *Memory organization and structure.* New York: Academic, 1979.

Mandler, J. M. Representation and retrieval in infancy. In M. Moscovitch (Ed.), *Infant Memory.* New York: Plenum, 1983.

McCall, R. B. Toward an epigenetic conception of mental development in the first three years of life. In M. Lewis (Ed.), *Origins of intelligence: Infancy and early childhood.* New York: Plenum, 1976.

McCall, R. B. Qualitative transitions in behavioral development in the first three years of life. In M. Bornstein & W. Kessen (Eds.), *Psychological development from infancy.* Hillsdale, N.J.: Erlbaum, 1979. (a)

McCall, R. B. The development of intellectual functioning in infancy and the prediction of later IQ. In J. D. Osofsky (Ed.), *Handbook of infant development.* New York: Wiley, 1979. (b)

McCall, R. B. Early predictors of later IQ: The search continues. *Intelligence*, 1981, *5*, 141–147.

McCall, R. B., Hogarty, P. S., & Hurlburt, N. Transitions in infant sensori-motor development and the prediction of childhood IQ. *American Psychologist*, 1972, *27*, 728–748.

Milewski, A. E. Visual discrimination and detection of configurational invariance in 3-month infants. *Developmental Psychology*, 1979, *15*, 357–363.

Miller, G. A., & Johnson-Laird, P. N. *Language and perception.* Cambridge, Mass.: Harvard University Press, 1976.

Miranda, S. B., & Frantz, R. L. Recognition memory in Down's syndrome and normal infants. *Child Development*, 1974, *45*, 651–660.

Parmelee, A. H., & Haber, A. Who is the "risk infant"? *Clinical Obstetrics and Gynecology*, 1973, *16*, 376–387.

Prechtl, H. F. R. Optimality: A new assessment concept. In C. C. Brown (Ed.), *Infants at risk.* Johnson & Johnson Baby Products, 1981.

Rose, S. A. Enhancing visual recognition memory in preterm infants. *Developmenal Psychology*, 1980, *16*, 85–92.

Rose, S. A. Lags in the cognitive competence of prematurely born infants. In S. L. Friedman & M. Sigman (Eds.), *Preterm birth and psychological development.* New York: Academic, 1981.

Rose, S. A., Gottfried, A. W., & Bridger, W. H. Cross-modal transfer in infants: Relationship to prematurity and socio-economic background. *Developmental Psychology*, 1978, *14*, 643–652.

Rose, S. A., Gottfried, A. W., & Bridger, W. H. Effects of haptic cues on visual recognition memory in full term and preterm infants. *Infant Behavior and Development*, 1979, *2*, 55–67.

Schank, R., & Abelson, R. *Scripts, plans, goals, and understanding.* Hillsdale, N.J.: Lawrence Erlbaum, 1977.

Schlesinger, I. M. Production of utterances and language acquisition. In D. I. Slobin (Ed.), *The ontogenesis of grammar.* New York: Academic, 1971.

Schwartz, M., & Day, R. H. Visual shape perception in early infancy. *Monographs of the Society for Research in Child Development*, 1979, *44*, 7.

Scott, K. G. The rationale and methodological considerations underlying early cognitive and behavioral assessment. In F. D. Minifie & L. L. Lloyd (Eds.), *Communicative and cognitive abilities—Early behavioral assessment.* Baltimore: University Park Press, 1978.

Scott, K. G., & Masi, W. The outcome from and utility of registers of risk. In T.

Field, A. Sostek, S. Goldberg, H. Shuman (Eds.), *Infants born at risk.* Jamaica, N.Y.: Spectrum, 1979.

Spelke, E. Infants' intermodal perception of events. *Cognitive Psychology*, 1976, *8*, 553–560.

Spelke, E. *Intermodal exploration by four-month-old infants: Perception and knowledge of auditory-visual events.* Unpublished doctoral dissertation, Cornell University, 1978.

Spelke, E. S. Perceiving bimodally specified events in infancy. *Developmental Psychology*, 1979, *15*, 626–636.

Spelke, E. S., & Cortelyou, A. Perceptual aspects of social knowing: Looking and listening in infancy. In M. E. Lamb and L. R. Sherrod (Eds.), *Infant social cognition.* Hillsdale, N.J.: Lawrence Erlbaum, 1981.

Tighe, T. J. & Powlison, L. B. Sex differences in infant habituation research: A survey and some hypotheses. *Bulletin of the Psychonomic Society*, 1978, *12*, 337–340.

Vurpillot E., Ruel, J., & Castrec, A. L'organisation perceptive chez le nourrisson: Réponse au tout ou à ses' elements. *Bulletin de Psychologie*, 1977, *327*, 396–405.

Walker, A., Owsley, C., & Gibson, E. J. *Differentiation of motions and shapes in motion by human infants.* Paper presented at the meeting of the Eastern Psychological Association, Boston, April 1977.

Zelazo, P. R. Reactivity to perceptual–cognitive events: Applications for infant assessment. In R. B. Kearsley & I. E. Sigel (Eds.), *Infants at risk.* Hillsdale, N.J.: Lawrence Erlbaum, 1979.

10

The Cognitive Development of
Failure to Thrive Infants:
Methodological Issues and New Approaches

Lynn Twarog Singer
Dennis Drotar, Joseph F. Fagan III
Linda Devost, Robin Lake

The purpose of the present chapter is to critically review prior research, particularly salient methodological issues, on the cognitive development of infants at developmental risk owing to environmentally based or organic failure to thrive (FTT). In addition, two studies are presented which advance our knowledge of this complex and important pediatric population. The first is a descriptive study of the intellectual development of a large sample of hospitalized FTT infants. The second is a controlled, prospective study which examines the relation of the early cognitive development of FTT infants to their cognitive development at age 20 months. One theme of the present review is that research on infants with problematic developmental outcome has been characterized by fragmented study which has paid little attention to basic information processing and sensory skills, areas which can provide a data base for theory development and intervention strategy (Kopp & Parmelee, 1979; Fagan & Singer, 1981). Thus the second study investigated a specific perceptual–cognitive skill, visual recognition

---

The authors wish to thank Marcy Bush, Jayne Lytle, Sue McGrath, Judy Negray, Lisa Polack, Elizabeth Shaver, and Ann Shepherd for their help with data collection and preparation.

This work was supported by Multiple Research Project Grant HD-11089 from the National Institute of Child Health and Human Development and by Grant Nos. 30274-03 and 35220-01 from the National Institute of Mental Health.

memory, and its relation to other sensorimotor skills in early and late infancy in groups of failure to thrive and normal infants.

Despite its high incidence as a pediatric referral problem among infants during the first year of life, the condition "failure to thrive" has been relatively neglected in the literature concerned with developmental risk conditions. Since infants who are failure to thrive can be identified both objectively and early in life, they form an ideal population in which to study the specific features of cognition which interact with environmental factors to predict risk for intellectual deficit later in life.

DEFINITION OF FAILURE TO THRIVE

Infants are diagnosed as failure to thrive when weight for age falls below the third percentile on standardized norms (Barbero & McKay, 1969). The growth failure may or may not be accompanied by organic dysfunction, which can include neurological, cardiac, and gastrointestinal disease, as well as an extensive number of less prevalent causes such as cystic fibrosis, congenital anomaly, fetal alcohol syndrome, and respiratory, endocrine, or skeletal disease (Shaheen, Alexander, Truskowshy, & Barbero, 1968; Hannaway, 1970). Symptomatology, chronicity, and outcome are dependent on the nature and severity of the physical illness involved.

When studied as a group, infants who fail to thrive and who also have observed organic dysfunction (such infants are commonly called organic failure to thrive) appear to do quite poorly developmentally, even in comparison to other failure to thrive infants who do not have specifiable organic impairment. Unfortunately, since the literature on organic failure to thrive infants is extremely sparse, few generalizations can be made from available data except to note that the condition appears to signal severe developmental risk.

The term *nonorganic failure to thrive* (NOFT) is commonly used to describe infants and children who fall significantly below age expectations in height and/or weight based on national growth norms, in the absence of a physical basis for growth failure.

Although the specific causes of this condition remain a subject of controversy (Kotelchuck, 1980), there is general agreement that NOFT signals risk for the developing infant (Leonard, Rhymes, & Solnit, 1966; Hufton & Oates, 1977; Fraiberg, 1980). Table 10-1 summarizes studies of the intellectual development of infants with this condition. Although the majority of studies have identified significant delays in cognitive development, estimates of severe intellectual deficits such as mental retardation are quite variable and range from 8 percent (Glaser et al., 1968) to 66 percent (Elmer & Gregg, 1969). The findings of prior studies note a higher than average in-

Table 10-1
Intellectual Development of Failure to Thrive Infants

Authors	n (Total)*	Age Range	Method	Initial Assessment	Follow-up Period (Age at Assessment)	Final Assessment
Glaser et al. (1968)	40 (50)	2 mo–5 yr	Cattell, Stanford-Binet		3 mo–5 yr (8 mo–8 yr)	8% retarded, 66% average or above 25% borderline
Elmer & Gregg (1969)	15	8–30 mo	Oppenheimer Scales		3–11 yr (3–11 yr)	66% mildly retarded, 33% normal
Leonard et al. (1966)	13	2–27 mo	Gesell	20% generalized delay	6 mo–4 yr (7 mo–8 yr)	All within average range
Whitten et al. (1969)	11 (16)	3–24 mo	Cattell	85% IQ below 80, 15% normal	1 mo (4–25 mo)	No change
Ramey et al. (1975)	9 (12)	6–16 mo	Bayley	Mean DQ 60	4 mo (10–20 mo)	Experimental mean DQ, 80; control, 73
Fitch et al. (1975, 1976)	29 (35)	4–24 mo	Bayley	Mean IQ 87, compared with matched normal control IQ of 106	6–18 mo (10 mo–3 yr)	No change
Eckels (1968)	8	3–12 mo	Composite Developmental Inventory	All delayed mental age 1–6 mo behind chronological age	4 mo (7–16 mo)	No change

n = number of subjects assessed; total = total number in study.

213

cidence of intellectual deficit. Although the available literature on NOFT infants is more extensive than that on organic FTT infants, the studies have been fraught with significant methodological problems which severely limit the validity and generalizability of their conclusions.

METHODOLOGICAL ISSUES

Sample Selection

The lack of uniform criteria with which to select infants with nonorganic failure to thrive has been a major impediment to systematic research. Nonorganic failure to thrive infants are usually hospitalized and given a variety of diagnostic tests to rule out the many organic conditions that could affect the infant's weight gain (Barbero & McKay, 1969). The demonstration of weight gain with proper nutrition in a hospital setting is, in itself, an important diagnostic test which excludes a number of physical problems that could affect weight gain. However, the exclusion of organic conditions responsible for poor weight gain does not provide positive operational criteria which objectively define the environmental factors potentially responsible for this condition (Kotelchuck, 1980). Failure to thrive infants are a complex population with considerable inter- and intrasample variations with respect to a variety of factors that may affect cognitive development. Such factors include the nature of their relationships with their parents, the degree of neglect and/or stimulation experienced in the home situation, economic level, family size, birth order, and parental intelligence. Moreover, different subgroups of NOFT infants reflect differing parent-child interaction patterns which can be identified within this population (Whitt, 1981).

Criteria for sample selection assume particular importance in view of the heterogeneity of the nonorganic failure to thrive population. The varied incidence of intellectual deficit associated with NOFT found in studies to date may be at least partially attributable to differences in sample selection from study to study. Even more important, selection criteria used in prior studies have sometimes confounded the criteria for sample selection with the response measure under question. For example, some investigators (Whitten, Pettit, & Fischoff, 1969; Ramey, Starr, Pallas, Whitten & Reed, 1975) have included the presence of developmental delay as a criterion to constitute their sample, a practice which introduces a serious sampling bias that may result in a spuriously high incidence of cognitive deficit. In addition, maternal deprivation has been used as a criterion for failure to thrive (Whitten et al., 1969). In the absence of detailed observation of the parent-child interaction in the home situation, judgments of maternal deprivation are inherently subjective. Until subgroups of failure to thrive infants can be objectively and reliably identified, use of open criteria for this condition which are not confounded with outcome measures of cognitive development is indicated. Criteria that can be objectively specified include (1) weight more than two standard deviations below the age expectations based on objective norms, (2) no organic problems which would affect growth or cognitive development based on physical diagnosis, and (3) significant weight gain in hospital (Schmitt, 1978).

Sample Size and Characteristics

With a few exceptions (Glaser, Heagarty, Bullard, & Pivchik, 1968; Fitch, Cadol, Goldson, Jackson, Swartz, & Wendel, 1975; Fitch, Cadol, Goldson, Wendal, Swartz, & Jacoson, 1976), the total sample sizes employed in studies of the cognitive development of FTT infants have been quite small, and in most instances smaller than 15. Small sample sizes are particularly troubling because of the variability of the FTT population with respect to factors such as family income level, parents' occupation, presence of life stress, and family size. Although many hospitalized infants with failure to thrive come from highly stressed impoverished backgrounds (Evans, Reinhart, & Succop, 1972), NOFT infants come from middle-class homes as well. Unfortunately, most studies have not described the demographic characteristics of their samples in sufficient descriptive detail. In addition, although some failure to thrive infants have had repeated hospitalizations for this problem, investigators have generally not reported whether the infant had prior admissions for failure to thrive, or the duration of these hospitalizations.

Samples of failure to thrive infants have also been heterogeneous with regard to age at hospitalization. Furthermore, the length of time the infant had been failing to thrive and/or experienced the effects of inconsistent stimulation and deprivation also differs widely from infant to infant. It is important to recognize that the age at intellectual testing does not necessarily correspond to the onset of the infant's poor weight gain. Many infants who are hospitalized for failure to thrive had been growing poorly for long periods of time before the hospital admission in which they are assessed (Drotar, Malone, Negray, & Dennstedt, 1981). However, it should be noted that since failure to thrive tends to be a chronic condition, age at testing may be highly correlated with the duration of the child's FTT and/or nutritional and stimulation deficits. For example, it is quite likely that very young infants may have experienced deficits in nutrition and/or stimulation for shorter periods of time than older infants.

Variability of initial assessment age within samples is also important, because the abilities tapped by traditional infant tests vary so dramatically with age that results of such assessments are not strictly comparable from age to age (McCall, Hogarty & Hurlburt, 1972). For this reason, it may be very useful to analyze data from samples which include infants with a wide age variation.

ASSESSMENT CONDITIONS

Infants who fail to thrive when hospitalized are in varying states of nutritional and/or stimulus deprivation and vary widely in social responsiveness, particularly at the time of initial testing. For this reason, in evaluating the failure to thrive infants' abilities, careful attention must be given to the effects of infant state on their responses to the test items (Drotar, Malone, & Negray, 1979a). Initially, upon hospital admission, many failure to thrive infants have a frozen, alert appearance termed radar gaze (Barbero & Shaheen, 1967), which includes a withdrawn demeanor, hesitance in social interaction, and limited exploration of objects, skills that are heavily represented in traditional infant assessment procedures such as the Bayley Scale (Bayley, 1969). The comprehensiveness of the assessment and hence the inferences that can be reasonably drawn from the intellectual test data from a single assessment are sometimes quite limited. For example, it is likely that the findings from tests given to unresponsive FTT infants reflect a performance deficit rather than a true deficiency in cognitive or information processing. For this reason, assessments given early during the hospitalization may seriously underestimate the child's potential. In addition, during their hospitalization, many infants who fail to thrive undergo a variety of tests for physical diagnosis which may further limit their responsiveness to testing. For this reason, multiple administrations of infant assessment instruments are often needed to obtain a reasonable evaluation of the infant's abilities (Drotar et al., 1979a). Given the difficulty involved in obtaining a valid sample of the FTT infant's intellectual development, it is unfortunate that investigators have not included detailed information about the conditions of assessment.

Study Design

With one exception (Fitch et al., 1976), the majority of investigations have involved single group study designs without a comparison group. However, without comparison groups, one cannot reasonably infer that the cognitive deficits found in a population of failure to thrive infants are associated with their poor weight gain versus a host of possible factors which may be highly correlated with the FTT. Failure to thrive infants are from families with a high level of social disorganization, life stress, and poverty, factors which themselves may be associated with a higher than average incidence of intellectual deficits. In support of this notion, a recent controlled study (Mitchell, Gorell & Greenberg, 1980) found that social class variables, rather than the presence of poor weight gain, accounted for the intellectual deficits found in a group of infants with poorer than average weight gain. In a similar vein, Elmer (1977) reported that the very high incidence of cognitive deficits found in a group of children who had suffered child abuse also occurred in a matched sample of nonabused children from equivalent social backgrounds and living circumstances.

Cross-sectional and/or short-term prospective designs have dominated the study of the cognitive development of FTT infants. Most investigators have assessed the cognitive development of failure to thrive children either at one point in time (Glaser et al., 1968; Elmer, Gregg, & Ellison, 1969) or after short follow-up periods of 4 months or less (Whitten et al., 1969; Ramey et al., 1975; Eckels, 1968). The brief follow-up period in studies of intellectual development and failure to thrive severely limits inferences that can be made concerning the predictive validity of the findings concerning the infant's later cognitive development. As shown in Table 10-1, studies show inconsistencies in the stability of developmental risk at follow-up. Prospective follow-up of initial assessments made during infancy is particularly important because single developmental assessments have such limited predictive validity during infancy (McCall, Hogarty, & Hurlburt, 1972), partly because of the dramatic changes in the sensorimotor abilities sampled during the first few years of life (McCall, Eichorn, & Hogarty, 1977).

Measures of Cognitive Ability

Standard infant tests have been the sole measure of intellectual development in studies of cognitive functioning of FTT infants. However, the reliance on the IQ or DQ as the only measure of intellectual abilities may obscure potentially significant patterns of cognitive strength and deficit in different areas of skill. For example, the severe environmental problems which culminate in failure to thrive may contribute to selective deficiencies in areas such as expressive language which have major implications for the child's competence. At least one investigator (Leonard et al., 1966) has commented on the "unevenness of development" in their subjects, although no study has investigated specific areas of cognitive development in infants either during or recently after their hospitalization for failure to thrive. Thus a more detailed exploration of the cognitive abilities of NOFT infants may be useful, either through the breakdown of standard infant test instruments through factor or cluster analyses (Kohen-Raz, 1967), or through a study of individual sensory processes.

Finally, the measures of cognitive functioning that have been used with FTT infants have also posed problems. Some investigators (Elmer, Gregg,

& Ellison, 1969; Eckels, 1968) have employed rarely used infant assessment procedures of questionable reliability, standardization, and predictive validity. Unfortunately, even the better standardized infant assessment instruments such as the Bayley Scale of Mental Development have questionable or no predictive validity, particularly for scores within the normal range (McCall et al., 1972). Traditional infant assessment measures are heavily dependent on items involving sensorimotor functioning, which may not correspond to the processes involved in cognitive development in later life (McCall et al., 1972). Also, it is possible that traditional measures of infant intelligence, which are so dependent on the infant's social responsiveness and/or interest in objects, may not be as suitable for the FTT population as cognitive tasks that are less dependent on infant state.

In summary, the conclusiveness of prior research concerning the impact of failure to thrive on infant cognitive development has been limited by ambiguities of definition, subject selection, assessment context, and method, as well as the use of small, heterogeneous samples and a lack of controls for relevant variables such as socioeconomic status and prematurity. The studies outlined in this chapter represent preliminary attempts to acquire a more reliable and valid data base on a condition which poses significant developmental risk for the young infant. The present studies advance our understanding by documenting intellectual development and its correlates within a large, heterogeneous sample of NOFT infants and by using perceptual–cognitive and standard sensorimotor assessments to describe and predict the later intellectual abilities of NOFT infants and comparison groups of normal infants and those with organically based failure to thrive.

STUDY I

The first study was conducted as a pilot phase, in a prospective study of home-based treatment of nonorganic failure to thrive infants (Drotar, Malone, & Negray, 1979b).

Subjects

This sample consisted of 80 infants hospitalized for evaluation of FTT at the Cleveland Metropolitan General Hospital and Rainbow Babies' and Childrens' Hospital, the major pediatric and teaching hospitals for Case Western Reserve University's School of Medicine. The sample included consecutive referrals of infants, ages 1–25 months, over a 4-year period (1976–1981) to pediatric psychology and the Infant Growth Project, a clinical research project which involved a highly visible consultation service on the pediatric infant divisions (Drotar & Malone, 1980; Drotar & Malone, in press). All infants had poor weight gain which was more than two standard deviations below age expectations based on National Center for Health Statistics (NCHS) norms (Hamil, Drizd, Johnson, Reed, Roche, & Moore, 1979) and had a diagnosis of environmentally based failure to thrive as demonstrated by (1) an absence of organic disease that could explain the growth failure as shown by physical diagnosis and detailed laboratory testing and (2) presence of significant weight gain in hospital (Schmitt, 1978).

The final sample included 35 females and 45 males from Cleveland and surrounding suburban communities, with a mean age of 8 months. The majority of the sample (71/80, 83%) were 1 year old or younger; 30 infants (45%) were 6 months old or younger. The length (median 10th percentile) and head circumference (median 10th to 25th percentile) of the sample were within age expectations based on NCHS norms (Hammil et al, 1979). Most infants (67%) were either firstborn (31%) or second born (36%). A total of 22 infants (28%) were premature (average gestational age of 35 weeks). The duration of hospitalization ranged from 4 days to 4 weeks. By definition, all children were undernourished relative to age expectations, but only a few were severely malnourished as assessed by associated symptoms, such as wasting.

Over half the families (42/80) were on welfare; 24 of the fathers were unemployed. In 12 instances, fathers were totally uninvolved in family activity. A total of 44 of the fathers (55%) were employed and the mean class ranking of their occupations was 5.5 (skilled manual according to Hollingshead, 1957); 12 mothers (15%) were working (occupational rank of 4.8, Hollingshead, 1957).

Procedure _____

Infants were tested in the hospital environment, at their crib in the case of young infants or in a testing room in the case of older infants, with the Bayley Scale of Mental Development (Bayley, 1969).

A total of 11 infants were referred too late in the hospital admission to warrant a complete assessment of their abilities in the hospital. In these cases, assessments were completed in their homes. As is characteristic of this population, infants were in varying states of nutritional impairment and responsiveness when they were first seen for assessment. Infants were not evaluated during the first few days of their hospitalization. Most had been in the hospital for at least 3 days prior to the assessment. Those infants who were not at all responsive to testing initially were seen on subsequent occasions to allow a representative assessment. The examiners were all trained and experienced with the Bayley Scale and included clinical psychologists on the hospital staff and/or research assistants with the Infant Growth Project.

Results _____

Infants' mental development indices (MDIs) followed the normal curve, but were skewed to the low average end of the distribution ($\overline{X}$ = 94.2, SD = 17.0). The MDI of the total sample using uncorrected MDIs was slightly lower ($\overline{X}$ = 90.5, SD = 20.2). The majority of scores (61%) clustered within the average range (85–115). One-fifth of the sample scored within the borderline range of functioning (70–84). Only 7.5 percent of the sample could be considered at risk owing to DQs below 70.

Pearson product–moment correlations were obtained between a number of child and family characteristics and MDI, including birth order (r = −.17), the number of siblings, (r = .08), the father's occupational rank (r = .17), and age (r = −.28). Only the correlation between age and MDI was significant (p < .01), indicating that older infants had lower MDIs.

Discussion _____

Study I indicated that the developmental scores of failure to thrive infants as measured by the Bayley Scale were approximately normally distributed, but skewed toward the low average end of the distribution. Although a greater than usual number of infants scored within the borderline range, or range of mild mental retardation, the intellectual development of this sample was surprisingly intact (at least as measured by the Bayley Scale), in contrast to other studies (Elmer & Gregg, 1969; Whitten et al., 1969; Ramey et al., 1975; Fitch et al., 1975, 1976; Eckels, 1968) which noted a much higher incidence of delayed cognitive development in such a population. The present findings are closest to those of Glaser et al. (1968) and Fitch et al. (1976). Using the Cattell Infant Intelligence Scale, Glaser et al. (1968) found that the abilities of FTT infants approximated those of the normal distribution, but were skewed to the lower end. In the study of Glaser et al., 6 percent of the sample were retarded, 66 percent had abilities within the average range or above, and 25 percent were within the borderline range, proportions comparable to the present findings. The finding of Fitch et al. (1976) of a mean DQ of 87 on the Bayley Scale is also comparable to the present findings.

Discrepancies in these versus prior findings may reflect differences in method, the most compelling of which may have to do with sample selection. The present study sample was selected using an open-ended criterion which included infants showing poor weight gain owing to environmental factors, rather than more restrictive criteria involving additional assumptions about the nature of NOFT. One would expect that the abilities of NOFT infants selected on the basis of open-ended criteria would be higher than those of a sample constituted on the basis of developmental delay or maternal deprivation. The present sample was also recruited by pediatric referral to a pediatric psychology service and a clinical research project that was highly visible on the pediatric infant division, and involved weekly rounds with pediatric staff (Drotar & Malone, 1980) and an independent chart review by project staff. These methods of case identification may have led to identification of NOFT infants at earlier ages, and with less severe cognitive deficiencies than is usually the case. The fact that the majority of the present sample were under 1 year of age and younger than the other study samples supports this notion.

The present findings suggest caution about the generalizability of findings from samples of NOFT infants gathered by traditional means, since such samples tend to be comprised of only the most impaired NOFT infants. In support of this notion, a chart review of admissions for FTT in this setting long before the beginning of this study (Drotar, Malone, Negray & Dennstedt, 1981) indicated that less than half of those infants with environmentally based failure to thrive were referred by pediatric staff for psychological consultation. Moreover, the smaller number of infants that were referred tended to be older and to have greater cognitive impairments than those infants who were subsequently referred. It is also quite likely that the sample characteristics of infants referred for consultation may vary dramatically with the pediatric population served by the hospital, as well as with the nature of psychological services provided by the hospital. The present findings are most representative of samples gathered at a large, acute care pediatric teaching hospital serving as a major referral center for a metropolitan area.

Among a variety of family and subject characteristic variables, only age at testing was significantly correlated with the level of intellectual ability. Younger infants tended to have higher abilities than older infants. This finding may be understood as a reflection of the potentially chronic nature of this condition: failure to thrive is a chronic problem. Once an infant has fallen off the growth course, he or she is likely to continue to gain weight at a less than normal rate. For this reason, as a group, older infants have been gaining weight at a less than normal rate and have suffered the effects of environmental and nutritional privation (which can accompany NOFT) for longer periods of time than younger infants. As a consequence, their abilities may have been more compromised. It should be noted that the relative homogeneity of the sample with respect to social class variables may have attenuated the correlations between other factors and developmental test scores.

The findings of this cross-sectional, descriptive study do not shed light on the factors which relate to the low average intellectual abilities of NOFT infants or whether these early patterns are associated with problematic, longer term outcome. It is very possible that similar findings could have been obtained by assessing a sample of age-matched infants from the same family and economic backgrounds of these infants. Thus the presence or absence of NOFT per se may be less important than social class and family variables in determining intellectual deficits.

STUDY II

The second study was designed to examine a number of questions which have not been addressed in prior studies of the cognitive development of failure to thrive infants.

Whether or not specific cognitive deficits might be present early in life and persist to affect later cognitive functioning is an important question, with implications for the treatment of infants with growth impairment. Intellectual retardation observed later in life may be a consequence of specific preexisting cognitive deficits which might prevent the failure to thrive infant from adaptively using aspects of the environment that promote social and emotional development. Not being able to take in or process information would be expected to interfere with an infant's responsivity and affect mother–infant interaction. One might ask whether or not the failure to thrive infant can perceive, discriminate, and remember visual–social stimuli as well as normal infants. The inability or ability to perform such tasks could be expected to have significant effects on an infant's cognitive and social development. At least one previous study has suggested a link between one aspect of early information processing, that is, visual attentiveness, and both care-taker–infant interaction and intellectual outcome (Sigman, Cohen, & Forsythe, 1981). Alternatively, subsequent intellectual problems reported later in life in children who had experienced failure to thrive during infancy may be the effect of cumulative experiences, such as frequent hospitalizations, low socioeconomic status, and social deprivation, which tend to occur with growth failure, with or without organic involvement. Failure to thrive infants experience a range of care-taking environments which have not been considered in previous studies.

Thus a prospective investigation of the concurrent cognitive functioning of infants hospitalized for organic and nonorganic failure to thrive was done within the first year of life, with follow-up assessment at 20 months of age. Groups of such infants were initially compared with normal infants on their ability to demonstrate recognition memory for visual–social stimuli, that is, face photographs and abstract designs, as well as on the basis of a standard infant development assessment, the Bayley Mental Scale of Infant Development. A breakdown of Bayley Mental Scale items into four subdomains was also employed in an attempt to delineate the relative proficiency of FTT infants on other, more specific cognitive skills.

Visual Recognition Memory _____

Infants' visual recognition memory has been widely investigated with the visual preference technique, which uses the activity of the eyes themselves to measure the infant's ability to discriminate among stimuli. By at least the third month of age, if total maturational level is considered, infants demonstrate more interest in novel than in previously exposed targets, implying recognition memory. The age at which an infant demonstrates immediate recognition memory depends on both the nature of the stimuli to be discriminated and the amount of study time given the infant (Fagan, 1975). Varying the nature of the stimuli used as targets reveals age differences in recognition memory among infants from 2 to 8 months of life. Recognition memory for social stimuli, for example, photographs of faces, has been studied extensively in infants. The normal infant, at 4 months of age, can discriminate between a rotated and an upright version of the same face photograph (Fagan, 1973). By 5-6 months of age, distinctions between categorically different faces (male versus female) can be made (Fagan, 1973), and by 7 months distinctions within some categories (male versus male) can be made (Fagan, 1976).

Infants who can be expected to differ in intellectual functioning later in life have also been shown to differ in the development of visual preferences and their ability to perform recognition memory tasks. For example, infants who develop neurological problems later in life have also differed in their visual fixations in patterns in the first weeks of life (Miranda, Hack, Fantz, Fanaroff, & Klaus, 1977). In a home-reared sample of infants of university faculty members versus institution-reared infants of women of average intelligence, preference for novel over previously exposed targets developed approximately 1 month earlier (Fantz & Nevis, 1967).

In addition, evidence has recently been presented which suggests that tests of infant visual recognition memory may be valid predictors of later intelligence (Fagan & McGrath, 1981; Lewis & Brooks-Gunn, 1981). Specifically, in the Fagan–McGrath study, significant correlations which compared favorably in magnitude to predictive validity coefficients of other more well-established tests were found between normal infants' preferential visual fixations and scores on standard vocabulary tests 4–6 years later. A complete review of the concurrent and predictive validity of infant recognition memory tests as tests of intelligence is contained in Fagan and Singer (in press).

Subjects _____

The initial sample included 39 infants from three local hospitals and well-child care clinics in Cleveland, Ohio. A diagnosis of failure to thrive had been made for 26 of the 39 infants. All 26 of the FTT infants had been hospitalized at least once between the ages of 5 and 9 months, and weighed below the third percentile for their conceptional age at testing. The absence of known organic etiology and weight gain during or shortly after hospitalization constituted the criteria in the present study for a diagnosis of nonorganic failure to thrive for 13 of the 26 infants (9 male, 4 female; 4 black, 9 white). Documented organic etiology was the criterion for a diagnosis of organic failure to thrive for the other 13 failure to thrive infants (4 male, 9 female; 7 black, 6 white). Of the 13 infants in the organic FTT group, 3 had primary neurological disease, 2 had choanal atresia, 2 had fetal alcohol syndrome, and 1 infant was failure to thrive due to methadone addiction; 1 infant had cerebral palsy and congenital heart disease, 1 had pulmonary stenosis and cyanotic heart disease, and 3 had polycystic renal disease, necrotizing enterocolitis, and Aarskoog syndrome, respectively. The remaining 13 infants tested of the total 39 were infants who were not FTT (6 male, 7 female; 4 black, 9 white). These normal control subjects had been recruited from well-child care clinics and through county birth records.

The data in Table 10-2 allow comparisons among the nonorganic failure to thrive, the organic failure to thrive, and the normal control infants at initial examinations in terms of gestational age at birth (weeks), postnatal age at test (weeks), conceptional age at test (weeks), birth weight (grams), and highest educational level attained by either parent (years of schooling completed). Means, standard deviations and ranges are listed for each characteristic. Separate analyses of variance indicated that the three groups of subjects did not differ significantly on the basis of gestational, postnatal, or conceptional age, birth weight, or on levels of parental education at initial assessment.

Table 10-3 describes the 11 infants who were available for follow-up assessment at 20 months of age (corrected for prematurity). Loss of subjects was related to moves out of state (2), death (1), and untraceability (3). Another series of analyses of variance indicated that, except for birth weight, groups were not reliably different at follow-up on the demographic and birth status variables noted previously. Based on an orthogonal comparison, the organic failure to thrive group available for follow-up was characterized by a lower birth weight compared to that of the other two comparison groups. At follow-up, a new variable was also described in an attempt to account for some of the variability in care taking consistency that had emerged in our study of both failure to thrive groups. At least half the subjects in both FTT groups had experienced one to three relatively long-term placements outside their original home. Thus the number of such placements in a different care-taking setting, for example, foster home, group home, or rehabilitation facility, was computed for each subject.

Table 10-2

Comparison of Nonorganic Failure to Thrive, Organic Failure to Thrive, and Normal Control Infants on Gestational Age (GA), Postnatal Age (PA), Conceptional Age (CA), Birth Weight (BW), and Parents' Education (P. Ed.) at Initial Test

Group		Measure				
		GA	PA	CA	BW	P. Ed.
Nonorganic failure to thrive (n = 13)	Mean	39.0	30.0	69.0	2847	11.8
	SD	1.8	7.0	7.3	592	1.9
	Range	36-40	20-44	60-84	1927-3828	8-16
Organic failure to thrive (n = 13)	Mean	37.0	30.0	67.0	2378	11.6
	SD	3.5	7.5	6.1	862	1.8
	Range	28-40	21-44	61-84	1035-4195	10-16
Normal controls (n = 13)	Mean	38.0	30	69.0	3027	11.9
	SD	1.8	10.1	6.9	694	2.3
	Range	36-40	20-44	60-84	2041-4368	7-16

Table 10-3

Comparison of Nonorganic Failure to Thrive, Organic Failure to Thrive, and Normal Control Infants on Gestational Age (GA), Chronological Age (CA),* Birth Weight (BW), Highest Educational Level of Parents (HiEd), and Number of Placements (Placements) at Follow-up

Group		Measure				
		GA	CA	BW	HiEd	Placements
Nonorganic failure to thrive (*n* = 11)	Mean	38.9	21.4	2838	12.5	1.0
	SD	1.9	3.5	680	1.4	1.3
	Range	36–40	18–27	1808–3828	11–16	0–3
Organic failure to thrive (*n* = 11)	Mean	37.0	19.8	2259	11.4	1.4
	SD	3.6	3.22	897	1.4	1.0
	Range	28–40	17–27	1035–4195	10–15	0–3
Normal controls (*n* = 11)	Mean	38.9	19.6	3091	12.5	0.0
	SD	1.9	2.11	685	1.8	0.0
	Range	36–40	18–25	2041–4368	11–16	0.0

*In months.

226

Short-term, acute care hospitalizations were not included. Normal control infants had experienced no placements outside the home and were reliably differentiated from both FTT groups, who did not differ from each other on this characteristic.

All subjects were tested by means of a portable apparatus, the details of which have been illustrated by Fagan (1970). Targets employed in the present study were chromatic and achromatic photographs of men's, women's, and babies' faces (4 babies, 4 women, and 2 men) and two abstract black and white patterns. Each face photograph measured approximately 5½ inches from crown to chin and was mounted on a 7 × 7-inch white stimulus plaque. Each abstract pattern measured approximately 6 × 6 inches and was mounted on a 7 × 7-inch white stimulus plaque.

Procedure

On initial assessment, all nonorganic FTT infants were tested in the hospital as soon as weight gain had stabilized or, if necessary, in the home within 1 week after hospital discharge. Organic FTT infants were tested in the hospital after their medical condition had stabilized. Control subjects were tested in the home. All follow-up assessments were completed in the home or at an office appointment. Tasks for recognition memory differed according to the age of the infant. They were similar to those that had elicited differential fixation in previous studies of normal 5- and 7-month-old infants (Fagan, 1973, 1976) and were also similar to tasks which differentiated groups of normal and Down's syndrome infants (Miranda & Fantz, 1974) and which were predictive of individual differences in later intelligence at 4–6 years for children in the normal to superior range of intelligence (Fagan & McGrath, 1981). All infants were also given the Bayley Mental Scale test of the Bayley Scales of Infant Development at initial testing ($\overline{X}$ = 8 months) and at follow-up at 20 months. For 15 of the 39 infants, the initial Bayley Scale was given by a separate examiner who was unaware of the results of the visual recognition testing. All follow-up testing was done by clinical psychology graduate students who were uninformed of the purpose of the study or the status of the infants.

Bayley Mental Scale items were also computed using the Kent Scoring Adaptation of the Bayley Scales of Infant Development (Reuter, Stancin, & Craig, 1981), as well as by obtaining an overall mental development index (MDI) based on Bayley's (1969) norms. The Kent Adaptation renders four separate behavioral domains, that is, cognitive, language, social, and fine motor, based on face validity of the items. The Kent Adaptation provides a developmental age equivalent for each infant for each cognitive domain when a total score of items passed for each domain is computed.

Results

Several analyses of the data were undertaken in order to address the following questions: (1) Did infants with nonorganic or organically based failure to thrive differ from normal control infants on the basis of visual recognition memory and sensorimotor tasks early in life? (2) Were there differences among groups on cognitive tasks later in life? (3) How was performance on early assessment related to performance at 18 months? (4) Did the groups show differential patterns of functioning on the basis of an item-by-item breakdown of the Bayley Mental Scale into behavioral domains? (5) Finally, which demographic and environmental variables were most highly related to outcome?

Visual Recognition Memory

To compare the three groups of infants (organic FTT, NOFT, and normal) on the basis of visual recognition memory and the Bayley standardized infant developmental measure, each infant's duration of fixation to the novel relative to the familiar targets during recognition testing was computed for each problem. The total ratio of fixation to all novel versus all familiar targets was then computed for each subject, and a percentage of novelty score assigned to each subject. Mean percentages of total fixation time devoted to novel targets during recognition testing are listed in the left column of Table 10-4 for each of the three groups. In terms of performance, recognition tasks were easily done by both the NOFT and control

Table 10-4

Mean Percentage of Fixation to Novelty Targets and Mean Bayley Mental Development Index Quotients (MDI) Achieved by Nonorganic Failure to Thrive, Organic Failure to Thrive, and Normal Control Infants at Initial Assessment

| | | Measure | |
		Percentage of Fixation Time Devoted to Novel Targets	MDI
Group			
Nonorganic failure to thrive	Mean	68.0	77.6
	SD	9.1	20.5
	Range	55–83	50–100
Organic failure to thrive	Mean	52.6	67.7
	SD	8.5	13.8
	Range	34–62	60–101
Normal controls	Mean	62.5	120.2
	SD	9.2	10.7
	Range	45–75	76–150

infants as measured by means of 68 percent [SD = 9.1, $t(12)$ = 7.2, $p <$ .001] and 62.5 percent [SD = 9.2, $t(12)$ = 4.9, $p <$ .001], respectively. Organic FTT infants, however, demonstrated only chance performance, with a mean of 52.6 percent [SD = 8.5, $t(12)$ = 1.1].

A one-way analysis of variance was used to compare the three groups of infants on the basis of novelty scores. The results indicated a reliable difference among the three groups [$F(2,36)$ = 9.87, $p <$ .005] in responsiveness to novelty. Two orthogonal comparisons were made. When nonorganic failure to thrive infants were compared with the control infants, no reliable differences emerged. A second orthogonal comparison indicated that the organic failure to thrive group was reliably different from the other infants ($F(1,36)$ = 19.88, $p <$ .001], with 87 percent of the total treatment variance accounted for by such a comparison. Thus, when assessed for visual recognition memory, infants who were FTT without organic cause did as well as normal controls, while those FTT infants with organic etiology did significantly more poorly than both the NOFT and the normal control infants. Developmentally, then, NOFT infants demonstrated visual perceptual–cognitive abilities equivalent to normal infants, while organic FTT infants, as a group, demonstrated significant deficits or delays.

Sensorimotor Abilities _____

Each infant also received a mental development index quotient (MDI) derived from his performance on the Bayley Mental Scale of Infant Development. An MDI is a standardized score which allows comparison of an individual infant with his age peers. Mean MDI quotients computed for each group are also listed in Table 10-4. Control infants did quite well on the Bayley Mental Scale, as reflected in the mean MDI for that group, 120, which is one standard deviation above the expected average of 100 for the general population. Both failure to thrive groups did quite poorly, however, with mean MDIs of 77.6 for the NOFT infants and 67.7 for the organic FTT infants.

A one-way analysis of variance revealed reliable differences among the three groups of infants on the basis of Bayley Mental Scale performance [$F(2,36)$ = 23.98, $p <$ .001]. Again, two orthogonal comparisons were made to determine where the differences among groups occurred. In the case of sensorimotor abilities, no reliable differences were found when NOFT and organic FTT groups were compared [$F(1,36)$ = 0.15]. However, high and reliable differences were found [$F(1,36)$ = 46.45, $p <$ .001] accounting for 96 percent of the total mental scale variance when normal control infants were compared to both FTT groups. Thus, when compared on the basis of sensorimotor development, organic FTT and NOFT infants did equally poorly, lagging considerably behind their nonfailure to thrive age mates in development.

At both ages, infants' Bayley Mental Scale responses were used to derive separate age equivalents for every infant on all the domains of the Kent Scoring Adaptation, that is, cognitive, language, social, and fine motor domains. Each infant's developmental age equivalent score was then converted to a ratio score based on the infant's chronological age at testing.

Follow-up Study

At follow-up (mean age, 20.6 months), data from the Bayley Mental Scale on the 11 remaining subjects in each group were entered into a $3 \times 2 \times 4$ analysis of variance with repeated measures on the last two factors, using groups, age at testing, and Bayley Scale domain scores from the Kent Adaptation as factors. A Pearson product–moment correlation was calculated between Bayley MDIs at each age and the mean score across the Kent Scale scores for each domain. Since the correlation was quite high ($r = .96$, $p < .0005$), the Kent scores were used in the interpretation of the data at follow-up. A significant main effect due to groups emerged [$F(2,30) = 21.3$, $p < .001$]. For the cases remaining at follow-up, results of the initial 8-month Bayley Scale assessment were replicated, indicating that normal control infants had more advanced sensorimotor skills than both groups of FTT infants, who, in turn, were not reliably different from each other. Since there were no main effects due to time of testing [$F(1,90) = 0.06$, NS], the sensorimotor lags in the FTT groups seen at original assessment apparently were still evident at follow-up approximately 1 year later.

An additional main effect due to Bayley subtest scales was noted [$F(3,90) = 3.92$, $p < .05$]. However, there were no interactions involving Bayley subtests and groups [$F(6,90) = 1.88$], time of test [$F(3,90) = 1.80$], or groups and time combined [$F(6,90) = 0.22$]. Thus, although some Bayley subtests were more difficult than others, they were equally difficult for all groups studied. Also, no variability in patterns of cognitive abilities dependent on diagnostic category appeared in the present data. Neither group of FTT infants was differentially disadvantaged in any one of the four skill areas tapped on the Kent Scale Adaptation of the Bayley Mental Scale.

A significant group $\times$ time interaction was found [$F(2,90) = 4.82$, $p < .025$] When results were graphed, the organic failure to thrive group appeared to be at a disadvantage on the Bayley first assessment relative to the other two groups. Comparison of the four subtest scores for the organic FTT group showed somewhat lowered scores on language and social domains ($\overline{X} = 61$), a relation that was not apparent at follow-up and which therefore might be related to state variables at initial assessment. There was virtually no change in mean Bayley scores over time for any group, with both organic FTT and normal control infants' MDIs showing only slight regression toward the mean, and with the NOFT group's follow-up score remaining almost identical to its first assessment score.

Prediction of Outcome _____

In order to address the questions of the predictive ability of the infant assessments and of the relation of demographic and social variables to outcome, several correlational and regression analyses were conducted. Table 10-5 illustrates the interrelation among several demographic, cognitive, and environmental factors for all groups combined ($n = 33$).

As might be expected, birth weight and gestational age were highly intercorrelated ($r = -.66, p < .001$). For the sample as a whole, black infants tended to have lower birth weights than white infants ($r = -.38, p < .02$). The number of placements outside the home an infant had experienced was highly and negatively related to 20-month Bayley MDI scores. Although the number of placements was the only single variable which was significantly related to outcome, birthweight and parental education were reliably associated with the number of placements an infant had experienced ($r = -.48, r = -.38$, respectively; $p < .02$). Thus lower birth weight FTT infants, who tended to be black of less-educated parents, were placed more often in foster homes or institutions and had poorer developmental outcomes at 20 months.

Demographic and social variables related somewhat differently to outcome when individual diagnostic groups were examined, as illustrated in Table 10-6. Because of the large number of correlations involved, only the $p < .005$ level of confidence was used to determine significance within each group.

Within the NOFT group, both gestational age ($r = .74, p < .005$) and the number of placements ($r = -.71, p < .005$) were highly related to the level of sensorimotor ability at 18 months. The number of placements was also reliably related to Bayley MDI at 8 months ($r = -.74, p < .005$), indicating that infants performing most poorly on sensorimotor tasks at 8 months were more likely to be placed outside the home, were more likely to experience multiple placements, and ultimately manifested more sensorimotor lags at outcome. Within the NOFT group, those infants placed outside the home also tended to be those who were premature at birth ($r = -.73, r = -.77$, respectively; $p < .005$) and of lower socioeconomic status ($r = .67$ between birth weight and parental education).

Among the organic FTT infants, a number of variables were all moderately related to outcome, including birth weight ($r = -.50$), gestational age ($r = -.43$), parental educational level ($r = .52$), and the number of placements ($r = -.43$). In this group, the number of placements and parental educational level were confounded ($r = -.71, p < .005$). How-

Table 10-5

Correlations Among Race, Birth Weight (BW), Gestational Age (GA), Parents' Education (P. Ed.), Number of Placements (No. Place), Mean Novelty Preferences (%N), and Bayley Mental Scale Scores (MDI) at 20 Months ($n = 33$)

	Race	BW	GA	P. Ed.	No. Place	%N	8-mo MDI	20-mo MDI
Race		-.38	-.24	-.26	.13	-.21	.21	-.22
BW			.81	.34	-.48	-.01	.28	.25
GA				.21	-.33	-.03	.12	.11
P. Ed.					-.38	.29	.17	.34
No. place						-.12	-.57	-.66
%N							.11	.29
8-mo MDI								.82*
20-mo MDI								

*$p < .001$.

232

Table 10-6

Correlations Among Race, Birth Weight (BW), Gestational Age (GA), Parents' Education (P. Ed.), Number of Placements (No. Place), Mean Novelty Preferences (%N), and Bayley Mental Scale Scores (MDI) at 20 Months ($n = 11$)

	Race	BW	GA	P. Ed.	No. Place	%N	8-mo MDI	20-mo MDI
Nonorganic failure to thrive								
Race		-.17	.00	-.45	-.05	.01	-.14	-.23
BW			.85†	.67	-.73*	.26	.28	.67
GA				.29	-.77*	.15	.41	.74*
P. Ed.					-.23	.06	-.13	-.21
No. place						-.14	-.74*	-.71*
%N							-.21	.25
8-mo MDI								.51
20-mo MDI								
Organic failure to thrive								
Race		-.52	-.38	.20	-.11	.25	.06	.39
BW			.78*	-.03	-.17	-.63	-.41	-.50
GA				-.08	-.03	-.53	-.52	-.43
P. Ed.					-.71*	-.07	-.16	.52
No. place						-.14	.08	-.43
%N							.54	.54
8-mo MDI								.61
20-mo MDI								

(continued)

233

Table 10-6 (continued)

	Race	BW	GA	P.Ed.	No. Place	%N	8-mo MDI	20-mo MDI
Normal controls								
Race		.05	.29	−.26		−.71*	.27	−.11
BW			.83†	.18		−.36	.18	−.14
GA				.28		−.45	.09	−.27
P. Ed.						.52	.18	.15
No. place								
%N							.06	.52
8-mo MDI								.75†
20-mo MDI								

*$p < .005$.
†$p < .001$.

234

ever, neither factor was at all related to either of the variables reflecting prematurity ($r = -.03, r = -.17, r = -.08, r = -.03$, respectively), nor were they related to Bayley MDIs at 8 months ($r = -.16, r = .08$, respectively). Thus, among a group of infants already compromised by prematurity, physical illness, malnourishment, and delayed perceptual–cognitive and sensorimotor abilities early in life, the suggestion of the cumulative and exacerbating effects of care taking disruption and socioeconomic status factors can be seen in the rising correlations between the number of placements (from $r = .08$ to $r = -.43$), parental education (from $r = -.16$ to $r = .52$), and 8- and 20-month outcome measures.

Among the normal control infants, none of the variables significantly related to outcome in the malnourished groups bore any reliable relation to the outcome of the normal infants. Only the relation between novelty score and race was significant ($r = -.71, p < .005$). However, an examination of the sample indicated that the correlation was based on only 2 black infants in the sample who did quite poorly on the novelty test. Since previous studies based on larger groups have found no relation between novelty scores and race (Fagan & Singer, in press), the relation is probably spurious.

Correlations were also examined to assess the predictive power of perceptual–cognitive and sensorimotor measures to 20-month outcome. As expected, since the Bayley Mental Scale was used as the outcome measure, performance on this sensorimotor measure during the first year of life was highly related to performance on the same measure at 20 months ($r = .82, p < .001$) for the entire sample. The correlations for the NOFT, organic FTT, and control groups between the two Bayley scores were similar ($r = .51, r = .61, r = .75$, respectively).

Except for the organic FTT group ($r = .54$), visual recognition task performance was unrelated to Bayley MDIs achieved in the first year. Correlations for the normal control and combined groups were $-.21, .06$, and $.11$, respectively. By 20 months, correlations between infant perceptual–cognitive measures and standard infant intellectual assessments for the same groups had risen to $.54, .25, .52$, and $.29$ for organic FTT, NOFT, control, and combined samples, respectively. Thus visual recognition memory performance was unrelated to skill on sensorimotor measures within the first year of life, except for the most severely compromised group of infants. By the end of the second year of life, however, visual recognition tasks bore a substantially increasing relation to later performance on the standard infant assessment for all groups of infants.

Two subsidiary analyses were undertaken to investigate issues which arose during the first analysis of the data. The first question which surfaced was concerned with the fact that by time of follow-up, a large proportion of infants in both failure to thrive groups had experienced some placement outside the home. This variable, considered to be a gross measure of changes in care takers, had been uncontrolled for when the normal comparison group was recruited. Since both individual correlations and a multiple-regression analysis had indicated that the number of placements related to 20-month outcome, the normal control infants were not comparable to the other two groups of infants on this measure. Thus, within the two FTT groups, the mean MDIs of those infants who had been reared at home were compared to the mean MDIs of those infants who had been moved out of the home, as well as to the scores of the control infants. FTT infants who were home reared, whether organic or NOFT, attained Bayley MDIs in the low average range at 20 months (mean MDI, 87.5), whereas infants placed outside the home achieved scores which would place them at risk for continued developmental delay (mean MDI, 68.8).

A final subsidiary analysis was done in order to understand the nature of the finding that all groups displayed little variability in cognitive skills on the basis of the Bayley Scale domains derived from the Kent Scoring Adaptation. One explanation for this finding might lie in the construction of the Kent Scale rather than in an absence of any differential functioning between groups on discrete cognitive skills. When intercorrelations among Kent scale domains were computed, almost all scales were so highly related to one another that little evidence of the scale's ability to measure independent skills was apparent.

In summary, the second study compared groups of NOFT, organic FTT, and normal control infants on the basis of visual recognition memory and a standard sensorimotor assessment, the Bayley Mental Scale of Infant Development, with follow-up at 20 months of age. Within the first year of life, all FTT infants showed delayed sensorimotor development in comparison to normal control infants, but only organic FTT infants demonstrated impairment on a visual recognition memory task. At 20-month follow-up, significant lags in sensorimotor development were still evident for both FTT groups. At both early and later assessments, no evidence for differential abilities in specific cognitive skills within any group, based on the Kent Scoring Adaptation of the Bayley Mental Scale, were found. However, the lack of differences may be an artifact of poor validity of the Kent Scale.

Of the demographic and environmental variables related to outcome for all infants, a care taking variable, that is, the number of placements, was the only one found to be reliable. This factor was in turn highly associated with variables of race and prematurity. Within the NOFT group, only care taking consistency and prematurity were reliably related to 20-month outcome, while placements outside the home were related to lower Bayley performance at first test, prematurity, and lower socioeconomic status. For organic FTT infants, care taking consistency was related to socioeconomic status and to outcome, but not to prematurity or sensorimotor deficits early in life. Organic FTT infants were, however, of overall lower birth weight than the other two groups. For control infants, no variable was reliably related to outcome. Prediction to 20-month outcome was greatest with first-year Bayley scores, the number of placements outside the home, and visual recognition memory performance.

Discussion _____

The second study corroborates the impression of previous investigators that early in life, NOFT infants show delayed sensorimotor development relative to their peers, even when variations in age, race, prematurity, and socioeconomic status are controlled (Elmer, Gregg, & Ellison, 1969; Ramey et al., 1975; Fitch et al., 1975). Based on the present study, such lags are still present well into the second year of life. The present study differs from the first study of this chapter in the high percentage of subjects who were placed outside their homes for care taking. The importance of considering such care taking variables which had not previously been examined in the study of NOFT infants is underscored, since those NOFT infants who were home reared achieved MDIs within the average range at 20 months. The development of home-reared NOFT infants was similar to that achieved by the NOFT infants in the first study.

Thus the discrepancies among findings of previous studies with regard to the cognitive functioning of NOFT infants may be the result of gross disruption of care-taking environments within the population, rather than the result of socioeconomic or prematurity variables per se, since the NOFT and control groups were matched on the latter variables. The recruitment of appropriate control groups for NOFT infants is problematic, however. In the present study, there appeared to be a strong self-selection bias operating in the control infants of lower socioeconomic status, since more lower socioeconomic status parents refused to participate in the study than agreed to enter the study as controls. One possibility might be that those parents who refused to participate were more socially isolated (Elmer, Gregg, & Ellison, 1969). The relatively high Bayley scores of the control infants is not an unusual finding and may be the result of shifting norms on that test, or a ceiling effect in the normal group (Field, Dempsey, & Schuman, 1981).

Nonorganic FTT infants demonstrated a visual recognition memory equivalent to that of normal control infants, illustrating at least one information-processing skill which differentiates them from organic FTT infants. This finding suggests that developmental delay in NOFT infants may be related to a confluence of environmental factors rather than impaired central nervous system functioning. Using a conceptually similar perceptual–cognitive task on older NOFT children, Kearsely (1979) and his associates reported case studies of NOFT children from 18 to 30 months of age who demonstrated a normal level of cognitive development based on a perceptual–cognitive task, but who showed delayed development on the basis of the Bayley Scales. Since, with intervention, those NOFT children studied achieved a normal level of intellectual competence, their sensori-motor delays were attributed to environmental rather than intrinsic factors. Thus the heavy reliance of the Bayley test on sensorimotor and productive language functioning may result in lower scores in very young children and be misleading as an estimate of intellectual potential. Perceptual–cognitive measures, such as the visual recognition task, may be less susceptible to motivational factors and be more representative of the types of information-processing tasks characteristic of later cognitive functioning.

On the basis of the visual recognition task, organic FTT infants would be considered to be at higher risk for neurological problems and intellectual delay that nonorganic FTT or normal infants, supporting the data of previous investigators (Riley, Landiworth, Kaplan, & Collip, 1968; Ambuel & Harris, 1963). Since organic FTT infants in the present study tended to be of lower gestational age at birth, prematurity may be an additional factor contributing to their lowered Bayley scores at outcome.

Perhaps the most interesting implication of the present results for future research is the fact that both the Bayley sensorimotor scales and the visual recognition tests agree that infants who are failing to thrive secondary to organic disease show major continuing lags in development. Future studies of the early and later cognitive functioning of organic failure to thrive infants will need to focus on those factors associated with a diagnosis of organic failure to thrive which may be responsible for the severe cognitive deficits observed in such infants. It is unclear, for example, whether the delay in perceptual–cognitive development is due to the specific disease associated with the growth failure, the malnourishment, the interaction of physical illness with malnourishment, or the lower socioeconomic status and deprivation frequently associated with certain physical problems. The present study attempted to control for degree of malnourishment in the failure to thrive groups, since all infants were under the third percentile in weight for age. However, the degree of malnourishment in organic failure to thrive infants may still be greater or less than that of the nonorganic infants (i.e., infants may be under the first percentile rather than the third), may be more pervasive (i.e., affecting length and head circumference as well as weight), or may be more chronic. In fact, the latter condition is suggested by an examination of the weight gains made during hospitalization by the two failure to thrive groups in the present study. Organic failure to thrive infants tended to gain less weight over a longer period of time than nonorganic failure to thrive infants.

The fact that any group of organic failure to thrive infants is comprised of a heterogeneous population with diverse etiologies and outcomes also makes generalization from the present data difficult. Some organic diagnoses per se (i.e., not accompanied by a diagnosis of failure to thrive), such as primary central nervous system dysfunction, fetal alcohol syndrome, and drug addiction, are generally thought to be prognostic of later delayed or impaired intellectual status (Streissguth, 1977; Streissguth, Herman, & Smith, 1978). Other diagnoses, such as cyanotic heart disease and cystic fibrosis, have not been found to be associated with poorer later intellectual development (Rasof, Linde, & Dunn, 1967; Lloyd-Still, Hurwitz, & Wolff, 1974).

However, not all infants with organic diseases fail to thrive, and whether or not malnourishment in conjunction with organic disease poses additional risk for later intellectual delay, as is suggested by the present data, is unknown. Virtually no studies have compared organic failure to thrive infants with a specific disease to their nonfailure to thrive counterparts. When a group of middle-class children with cystic fibrosis who had been severely malnourished in the first year of life were compared 7-10 years later with a similar group of cystic fibrosis children who had not been malnourished, no differences were found in intellectual development on the basis of the Wechsler Intellectual Scale for Children or the Wide Range Achievement Test (Ellis & Hill, 1975). Thus future work will need to examine the effect of malnourishment within specific physical illnesses.

REFERENCES _____

Ambuel, J., & Harris, B. Failure to thrive: A study of failure to grow in height and weight. *Ohio State Medical Journal* 1963, *XX*, 998-1000.

Barbero, G, & McKay, N. Failure to thrive. In W. E. Nelson (Ed.), *Textbook of pediatrics*. Philadelphia: Saunders, 1969.

Barbero, G. J., & Shaheen, E. Environmental failure to thrive: A clinical view. *Journal of Pediatrics*, 1967, *71*, 639-644.

Bayley, N. *The Bayley Scales of Infant Development manual*. New York: Psychological Corporation, 1969.

Drotar, D., & Malone, C. A. The developmental case conference as a method of teaching pediatricians about child development on inpatient service. *Clinical Pediatrics*, 1980, *19*, 261-262.

Drotar, D., Malone, C. A. Psychological consultation on a pediatric infant division. *Journal of Pediatric Psychology*, 1982, *7*, 23-32.

Drotar, D., Malone, C. A., & Negray, J. Intellectual assessment of young children with environmentally based failure to thrive. *Child Abuse and Neglect*, 1979, *3*, 927-935. (a)

Drotar, D., Malone, C. A., & Negray, J. Psychosocial intervention with the families of failure to thrive infants. *Child Abuse and Neglect*, 1979, *3*, 927-935. (b)

Drotar, D., Malone, C. A., & Negray, J. Environmentally based failure to thrive and childrens' intellectual development. *Journal of Clinical Child Psychology*, 1980, *9*, 236–240.

Drotar, D., Malone, C. A., Negray, J., & Dennstedt, M. Psychosocial assessment and care for infants hospitalized with non-organic failure to thrive. *Journal of Clinical Child Psychology*, 1981, *10*, 63–66.

Eckels, J. Home follow-up of mothers of failure to thrive children using planned nursing interviews. *ANA Clinical Sessions*, 1968, 12–24.

Ellis, C., & Hill, D. Growth, intelligence and school performance in children with cystic fibrosis who have had an episode of malnutrition during infancy. *Journal of Pediatrics*, 1975, *87*, 565–568.

Elmer, E. The follow-up study of traumatized children. *Pediatrics*, 1977, *59*, 273–279.

Elmer, E., Gregg, G. S., & Ellison, P. Late results of the "failure to thrive" syndrome. *Clinical Pediatrics*, 1969, *8*, 584–589.

Evans, S. L., Reinhart, J. B., & Succop, R. A. Failure to thrive. A study of 45 children and their families. *Journal of the American Academy of Child Psychiatry*, 1972, *11*, 440–459.

Fagan, J. F. Memory in the infant. *Journal of Experimental Child Psychology*, 1970, *9*, 217–226.

Fagan, J. F. Infants' delayed recognition memory and forgetting. *Journal of Experimental Child Psychology*, 1973, *16*, 424–450.

Fagan, J. F. Infant recognition memory as a present and future index of cognitive abilities. In N. Ellis (Ed.), *Aberrant development in infancy: Human and animal studies*. New York: Wiley, 1975.

Fagan, J. F. Infants' recognition of invariant features of faces. *Child Development*, 1976, *47*, 627–638.

Fagan, J. F., & McGrath, S. K. Infant recognition memory and later intelligence. *Intelligence*, 1981, *5*, 121–130.

Fagan, J. F., & Singer, L. T. Intervention during infancy: General considerations. In S. Friedman & M. Sigman (Eds.), *Preterm birth and psychological development*. New York: Academic, 1981.

Fagan, J. F., & Singer, L. T. Infant recognition memory as a measure of intelligence. In L. Lipsitt (Ed.), *Advances in infancy research* (Vol. 2). Hillsdale, N.J.: Ablex, in press.

Fantz, R., & Nevis, S. Pattern preferences and perceptual cognitive development in early infancy. *Merrill-Palmer Quarterly*, 1967, *13*, 77–108.

Field, T. M., Dempsey, J., & Shuman, H. Developmental follow-up of pre- and post-term infants. In S. Friedman & M. Sigman (Eds.), *Preterm birth and psychological development*. New York, Academic, 1981.

Fitch, M. J., Cadol, R. V., Goldson, E. J., Jackson, E. K., Swartz, D. F., & Wendel, T. P. *Prospective study in child abuse: The child study program*. Unpublished manuscript, Denver Department of Health and Hospitals, 1975.

Fitch, M. J., Cadol, R. V., Goldson, E., Wendal, T., Swartz, D., & Jacoson, E. Cognitive development of abused and failure to thrive children. *Pediatric Psychology*, 1976, *1*, 32–37.

Fraiberg, S. *Clinical studies in infant mental health*. New York: Basic Books, 1980.

Glaser, H., Heagarty, M. C., Bullard, D. M., & Pivchik, E. C. Physical and psychological development of children with early failure to thrive. *Journal of Pediatrics*, 1968, *73*, 690-698.

Hammil, P. V., Drizd, T. A., Johnson, C. L., Reed, R. B., Roche, A. F., & Moore, W. M. Physical growth: National Center for Health Statistics percentages. *American Journal of Clinical Nutrition*, 1979, *32*, 607-629.

Hannaway, P. Failure to thrive: A study of 100 infants and children. *Clinical Pediatrics*, 1970, *9*, 96-99.

Hollingshead, A. B. *Two-factor index of social position*. Unpublished manuscript, 1957.

Hufton, I. W., & Oates, R. K. Nonorganic failure to thrive: A long-term follow-up. *Pediatrics*, 1977, *59*, 73-79.

Kearsley, R. Iatrogenic retardation: A syndrome of learned incompetence. In R. Kearsley & I Siegel (Eds.), *Infants at risk: Assessment of cognitive functioning*. Hillsdale, N.J.: Lawrence Erlbaum, 1979.

Kohen-Raz, R. Scalogram analysis of developmental sequence of infant behavior as measured in the Bayley Scale. *Genetic Psychology Monographs*, 1967, *76*, 3-21.

Kopp, C. B., & Parmelee, A. H. Prenatal and perinatal influences on infant behavior. In J. Osofsky (Ed.), *Handbook of infant development*. New York: Wiley, 1979.

Kotelchuck, M. Nonorganic failure to thrive: The status of interactional and environmental etiologic theories. In B. W. Camp (Ed.), *Advances in behavioral pediatrics* (Vol. 1). Greenwich, Conn.: Jai Press, 1980.

Leonard, M. F., Rhymes, J. P., & Solnit, A. J. Failure to thrive in infants: A family problem. *American Journal of Diseases of Children*, 1966, *3*, 600-612.

Lloyd-Still, J., Hurwitz, I., Wolff, P., & Schwachmann, H. Intellectual development after severe malnourishment in infancy. *Pediatrics*, 1974, *54*, 306-309.

McCall, R. B., Eichorn, D. H., & Hogarty, P. S. Transitions in early mental development. *Monographs of the Society for Research in Child Development*, 1977, *42*, 3.

McCall, R. B., Hogarty, P. S., & Hurlburt, N. Transitions in infant sensorimotor development and the prediction of childhood IQ. *American Psychologist*, 1972, *27*, 728-748.

Miranda, S., & Fantz, R. Recognition memory in Downs syndrome and normal infants. *Child Development*, 1974, *45*, 651-660.

Miranda, S., Hack, M., Fantz, R., Fanaroff, A., & Klaus, M. Neonatal pattern vision: A predictor of future mental performance? *Journal of Pediatrics*, 1977, *4*, 642-647.

Mitchell, W. G., Gorell, R. W., & Greenberg, R. A. Failure to thrive: A study in a primary care setting: Epidemiology and follow up. *Pediatrics*, 1980, *65*, 971-977.

Ramey, C. T., Starr, R. H., Pallas, J., Whitten, C. F., & Reed, V. Nutrition, response contingent stimulation and the maternal deprivation syndrome: Results of an early intervention program. *Merrill-Palmer Quarterly*, 1975, *21*, 45-55.

Rasoff, B., Linde, J., & Dunn, O. Intellectual development in children with congenital heart disease. *Child Development*, 1967, *38*, 1043-1047.

Reuter, J., Stancin, T., & Craig, P. *Kent Scoring Adaptation of the Bayley Scales of Infant Development*. Unpublished manuscript, First Chance Project, Kent State University, 1981.

Riley, R., Landiworth, J., Kaplan, S., & Collip, R. Failure to thrive: An analysis of 83 cases. *California Medicine*, 1968, *108*, 32–38.

Schmitt, B. (Ed.). *The child protection team handbook*. Garland, TX: STM Press, 1978.

Shaheen, E., Alexander, D., Truskowsky, M., & Barbero, G. Failure to thrive: A retrospective profile. *Clinical Pediatrics*, 1968, *7*, 255–261.

Sigman, M., Cohen, S., & Forsythe, A. The relation of early infant measures to later development. In S. Friedman & M. Sigman (Eds.), *Preterm birth and psychological development*. New York: Academic, 1981.

Streissguth, A. P. Maternal drinking and the outcome of pregnancy. *American Journal of Orthopsychiatry*, 1977, *47*, 422–426.

Streissguth, A. P., Herman, C., & Smith, D. Intelligence, behavior and dysmorphogenesis in the fetal alcohol syndrome: A report on 20 patients. *Journal of Pediatrics*, 1978, *92*, 363–366.

Whitt, K. Personal communication, January 1981.

Whitten, C., Pettit, M., & Fischoff, J. Evidence that growth failure from maternal deprivation is secondary to undereating. *Journal of the American Medical Association*, 1969, *209*, 1675–1680.

Yarrow, L. T., Rubinstein, J. L., & Peterson, F. A. *Infant and environment: Early cognitive and motivational development*. New York: Wiley, 1975.

11

Bronchopulmonary Dysplasia: Its Relation to Two-Year Developmental Functioning in the Very Low Birth Weight Infant

Edward Goldson

One of the results of the advances in the delivery of neonatal intensive care has been the increasing numbers of very small infants who survive the newborn period (Koops, 1980; Stewart, 1977, 1981; Yu, 1979). Furthermore, with the increasing survival of the very low birth weight infant, there have been significant numbers of children with bronchopulmonary dysplasia (BPD) (Wung, 1979; Tooley, 1979; Northway, 1979). Most, if not all, of these infants have difficult and complicated perinatal courses, yet are able to be discharged home in relatively stable condition. However, one of the questions we all have about these infants concerns their long-term developmental outcome. There have been a number of recent reports in the literature suggesting that there is a decrease in the mortality and morbidity among infants with very low birth weights (Hack, 1979). It has also been suggested that the long-term outcome for the low birth weight population with and without BPD is now much improved (Kumar, 1980; Markestad, 1981). On the other hand, several studies have noted an increase in the incidence of sudden infant death (Werthhammer, 1982) and a higher incidence of severe neurological and developmental abnormalities among children with BPD (Rothberg, 1981; Vohr, 1982). This discussion will address some of the long-term follow-up issues for the low birth weight infant with and without severe BPD.

Appreciation is extended to C. A. Wells, R.P.T., and C. A. Sullivan, O.T.R., for the neuromotor assessments, to Dennis Luckey, M.S., for statistical evaluation, and to Ms. Chere Lyles for secretarial assistance.

PATIENTS AND METHODS

A total of 17 children with birth weights of less than 1101 were evaluated at 2 years chronological age. All of the children were born between 1976 and 1979 and were transported to The Children's Hospital Neonatal Intensive Care Unit. For the purposes of this study, the children were divided into two groups: one with severe lung disease at the time of discharge from the nursery, and the second with mild or no lung disease at the time of discharge. Birth measures appear in Tables 11-1. None of the children had clinical evidence of intracranial hemorrhage (ICH) or retrolental fibroplasia.

The diagnosis of severe BPD was made on the basis of the radiographic findings on the chest X ray using Northway's classification (Northway, 1967). The radiographs used were taken at the time the infants had reached term or were discharged from the nursery. Severe disease was defined as being present when alveolar septae were thickened, cystic changes were evident, and there was unequal aeration with hyperexpansion of the lungs.

All of the children were seen as part of the Newborn Follow-up Program at The Children's Hospital. At 2 years chronological age the Bayley Scales of Infant Development (Bayley, 1969) were administered to the children by a developmental pediatrician. When infants scored below 50 on the Bayley Scales, a developmental index was derived for the mental and motor scales by using the following formula:

$$\text{Developmental index (DI)} = \frac{\text{mental (motor) age}}{\text{chronological age}}$$

This was required in three cases on the motor scale (see Tables 11-1 and 11-2). The derived DI was then included with the other developmental quotients for statistical analysis. During the Bayley assessment, a neuromotor assessment was also made by an occupational and physical therapist who rated the children as being normal or as having pathological or suspicious neuromotor findings. The children were classified as being pathological if they exhibited at least two of the following findings: abnormal eye movements, asymmetric movements, obligatory asymmetric reflex behavior, sustained clonus, increased deep tendon reflexes, and marked hypo- or hypertonicity. The children rated as suspicious had at least one pathological finding and problems with sensory integration, visual motor difficulties, or oral–motor and language problems, as well as unsustained clonus, mild asymmetries, and mild hypo- or hypertonicity. Children were rated as normal if they had none of the preceding findings. At the time of the evaluation, none of the children were oxygen dependent and none showed any evidence of cor pulmonale.

Table 11-1

Characteristics of Infants with and Without Severe Lung Disease

Birth Weight (Grams)	Gestational Age (Weeks)	Bayley Scale MDI/PDI*	Neurodevelopmental Assessment
	Infants with Severe Lung Disease		
650	26	76/37	Path†
709	26	57/66	Path
760	26	68/68	Path
790	26	92/101	Susp‡
820	26	77/78	Path
900	27	79/89	Susp
1000	31	71/64	Path
1080	30	76/43	Path
1100	30	80/81	Path
868§	27§	75/70§	
	Infants Without Severe Lung Disease		
630	27	90/92	Susp
860	27	90/76	Susp
1000	28	85/83	Susp
1040	30	140/93	Susp
1060	32	93/96	Susp
1070	28	108/97	Susp
1090	29	79/46	Path
1100	31	101/87	Susp
981§	29§	98/83§	

*MDI, mental developmental index; PDI, psychomotor developmental index.
†Path = pathological.
‡Susp = suspicious.
§Mean values.

RESULTS

The data for each subject are presented in Table 11-1. Only 1 child without severe lung disease had a mental score below 84, while only 1 of the severely ill group had a mental score above 84. On the motor scale, 2 of the healthier children had scores below 84, while 7 of the sicker children had scores below that level. The mean mental scores for the children with and without severe lung disease were 75 and 98, respectively, and the mean motor scores were 70 and 83, respectively. A Mann–Whitney test revealed a statistically significant difference on the mental scale scores ($p < .005$). Thus children with severe lung disease appeared to do worse on developmental testing, particularly on the mental scale, than did the

Table 11-2

Developmental Status of Infants with and Without Severe Lung Disease
Matched by Birth Weight and Gestational Age

Birth Weight (Grams)	Gestational Age (Weeks)	Bayley Scale MDI/PDI*	Neuromotor Assessment
Patients with Severe Lung Disease			
650	26	76/32	Path†
820	26	77/78	Path
1000	31	71/64	Path
1080	30	76/43	Path
1100	30	80/81	Path
930 §	29 §	76/63 §	
Patients Without Severe Lung Disease			
630	27	90/92	Susp‡
860	27	90/76	Susp
1000	28	85/83	Susp
1070	28	108/97	Susp
1100	31	101/87	Susp
932 §	28 §	95/87 §	

*MDI, mental developmental index; PDI, psychomotor developmental index.
†Path = pathological.
‡Susp = suspicious.
§Mean value.

healthier children. Furthermore, as can be seen from the data, the sicker children had a higher incidence of pathological findings on the neuromotor assessment than did the healthier children.

It should be noted that although these groups did not statistically differ in birth weight, there still was a difference in mean birth weights, which could bias the findings described above. Therefore the groups were matched on the basis of birth weight and gestational age, making the groups comparable but necessitating the exclusion of several subjects who could not be matched. The birth measures and developmental follow-up data for the matched groups are presented in Table 11-2. The only difference between the two groups is the presence of or lack of severe BPD at the time of discharge from the nursery.

When the developmental scores and the results of the neuromotor assessment are examined (see Table 11-2), one can see that there are considerable differences in the two groups which are similar to the differences noted for the unmatched groups. The children with severe disease all had developmental quotients below 84 and pathological neuromotor findings. In contrast, among the children with mild or no lung disease, none had a mental developmental index of less than 84 and only 2 had psychomotor developmental indices below 84. Furthermore, none of the children had pathological findings, but all of them had suspicious findings. On the mental scale, the mean score for the severely ill children was 76, and that for the healthier children was 95. A Wilcoxon paired signed rank test revealed statistically significant differences between the groups on the Bayley Mental Scores ($p = .03$). On the motor scale, the sicker children had a mean score of 63, while the healthier children had a mean score of 87, a difference which approached significance ($p = .06$).

DISCUSSION

There has been considerable interest in the pediatric community as to the outcome of the very low birth weight infant. There has also been concern that perhaps the increased survival of the low birth weight infant has entailed increasing numbers of children with significant handicapping conditions (Paneth, 1981). There is no question that there are many factors which influence the developmental outcome for this population of babies. These babies all have very immature lungs and most of them required assisted ventilation. Many, if not all, sustain some degree of oxygen toxicity and barotrauma and some degree of asphyxia. Many are hyperbilirubinemic and have electrolyte and glucose imbalances. Furthermore, these babies also frequently have increased nutritional needs (Weinstein, 1981) with some difficulty in fulfilling these needs, so that they may experience a degree of malnutrition at the time the brain is undergoing significant growth and development (Dobbing, 1973). Among the most significant neonatal complications, aside from prematurity itself, is the occurrence of ICH and the development of BPD. The occurrence of ICH with or without hydrocephalus has been associated with developmental delays and neurological deficits (Chaplin, 1980; Krishnamoorthy, Shannon, DeLong, Todres, & Davis, 1979). It is for this reason that along with birth weight and gestational age, ICH and hydrocephalus were also controlled. At the time these children were hospitalized computerized axial tomographic scans of the head were not being routinely done on all infants with very low birth weight cared for in The Children's Hospital. But the few infants on whom this study was done during their hospital stay did not have evidence of ICH or hydrocephalus. This was also the case when these children were seen at 2 years of age. Also, no child was oxygen dependent at the time of his or her evaluation, and none had rentrolental fibroplasia.

In this study the independent variable was the presence of severe BPD at the time of discharge from the nursery. Markestad and Fitzhardinge (1981) have suggested that the developmental outcome is not related to the presence of BPD but, rather, to the child's perinatal and neonatal experiences. However, it should be noted that the severity of BPD is related to the degree of prematurity and neonatal difficulties. Finally, the authors gave the overall impression that these children as a group were doing quite well and were generally free from neurological or developmental deficits. This study suggests a somewhat different picture. The data suggest that those children with severe BPD at the time of discharge from the nursery did significantly worse on achieving developmental milestones on the mental portion of the Bayley Scales, approached significance in being delayed on motor milestones, and had an increased incidence of neuromotor pathology compared to those children with mild or no lung disease at the time of discharge.

Those children with no disease or only mild lung disease who were matched for birth weight and gestational age did better on achieving mental and motor milestones than the sicker children. However, even in the face of normal developmental functioning as reflected in the Bayley scores, all of these children had suspicious neuromotor findings. This is, of course, disturbing and suggests that none of these low birth weight infants were completely normal at 2 years of age. The significance of these suspicious neuromotor findings is still somewhat unclear, but there is evidence in the recent literature to suggest that this is a group of children who will later emerge with learning difficulties and require special educational support (Hertzig, 1981).

It would seem, based on the data reported in this chapter, that several issues need to be addressed. First, one must bear in mind that children with bronchopulmonary disease are not a homogeneous group. There are differences between those children who have severe lung disease and those who do not have severe lung disease at the time they are discharged from the nursery. Physicians should be aware of these differences and counsel parents accordingly. Second, children with severe lung disease are at very high risk for developmental and neuromotor problems at 2 years of age. Moreover, it must be acknowledged that even less ill children with very low birth weight are also at risk for these problems. Consequently, active monitoring of both groups should be instituted at discharge as a means toward the early identification of problems that may emerge. Finally, the physician assuming the primary outpatient care for the "graduates" of intensive care nurseries must be careful not to ignore or minimize the impact of prematurity and severe BPD as it relates to growth and development. The emergence of these problems among the survivors of neonatal intensive care is something that must be addressed. If we remain committed to saving these very small and sick babies, we must also be committed to their long-term support. We must be realistic with parents, while not being totally negative. Parents should not be deluded into thinking that their very tiny baby with significant lung disease is always going to be the perfect infant so cherished in our society. On the other hand, we must be careful not to paint such a bleak picture that parents feel hopeless about their infant. Instead, a realistic picture of the infant's capacities, identifying both strengths and weakness, must be presented, and then support and counseling on an ongoing basis must be provided.

REFERENCES

Bayley, N. *Bayley Scales of Infant Development.* New York: Psychological Corporation, 1969.

Chaplin, E. R., Goldstein, G. W., Myerberg, D. Z., Hunt, J. V., & Tooley, W. H. Posthemorrhagic hydrocephalus in the preterm infant. *Pediatrics*, 1980, *65*, 901-909.

Dobbing, J., & Sand, J. The quantitative growth and development of the human brain. *Archives of Disease in Childhood*, 1973, *48*, 757-767.

Hack, M., & Fanaroff, A. The low birth weight infant: Evaluation of a changing outlook. *New England Journal of Medicine*, 1979, *301*, 1162-1165.

Hertzig, M. E. Neurological "soft" signs in low birthweight children. *Developmental Medicine and Child Neurology*, 1981, *23*, 778-791.

Koops, B. L., & Harmon, R. J. Studies on long-term outcome in newborns with birthweights under 1500 grams. *Advances in Behavioral Pediatrics*, 1980, *1*, 1-28.

Krishnamoorthy, K. S., Shannon, D. C., DeLong, G. R., Todres, I. D., & Davis, K. R. Neurologic sequelae of neonatal ventricular hemorrhage. *Pediatrics*, 1979, *64*, 233-237.

Kumar, S. P., Anda, E. K., Sacks, L. M., Ting, R. Y., & Delivoria-Papadopoulos, M. Follow-up studies of very low birthweight infants (1250 grams or less) born and treated within a perinatal center. *Pediatrics*, 1980, *66*, 438-444.

Markestad, R., & Fitzhardinge, P. M. Growth and development in children recovering from bronchopulmonary dysplasia. *Journal of Pediatrics*, 1981, *98*, 587-602.

Northway, W. H. Observations of bronchopulmonary dysplasia. *Journal of Pediatrics*, 1979, *95*, 815-818.

Northway, W. H., Rosan, R. C., & Dorter, D. Y. Pulmonary disease following respirator care of hyaline membrane disease. *New England Journal of Medicine*, 1967, *276*, 357-368.

Paneth, N., Kiely, J. L., Stein, Z., & Susser, M. Cerebral palsy and newborn care III: Estimated prevalence rates of cerebral palsy under differing rates of mortality and impairment of low-birthweight infants. *Developmental Medicine and Child Neurology*, 1981, *23*, 801-817.

Rothberg, A. D., Maisels, M. J., Bagnato, S., Murphy, J., Gifford, K., McKinley, K., Palmer, E. A., & Vannuci, R. C. Outcome for survivors of mechanical ventilation weighing less than 1250 grams at birth. *Journal of Pediatrics*, 1981, *96*, 106-111.

Stewart, A. L., Reynolds, E. O. R., & Lipscomb, A. P. Outcome for infants of very low birthweight: Survey of world literature. *Lancet*, 1981, *1*, 1038-1041.

Stewart, A. L., Turcan, D. M., Rawlings, G., & Reynolds, E. O. R. Prognosis for infants weighing 1000 grams or less at birth. *Archives of Disease in Childhood*, 1977, *52*, 97–104.

Tooley, W. H. Epidemiology of bronchopulmonary dysplasia. *Journal of Pediatrics*, 1979, *95*, 851–855.

Vohr, B. R., Bell, E. F., & Oh, W. Infants with bronchopulmonary dysplasia: Growth pattern and neurologic and developmental outcome. *American Journal of Diseases of Children*, 1982, *136*, 443–447.

Weinstein, M. R., & Oh, W. Oxygen consumption in infants with bronchopulmonary dysplasis. *Journal of Pediatrics*, 1981, *99*, 958–961.

Werthammer, J., Brown, E. R., Neff, R. K., & Taeusch, H. W. Sudden infant death syndrome in infants with bronchopulmonary dysplasia. *Pediatrics*, 1982, *69*, 301–304.

Wung, J. T., Koons, A. H., Driscoll, J. M., & James, L. S. Changing incidence of bronchopulmonary dysplasia. *Journal of Pediatrics*, 1979, *95*, 845–847.

Yu, V. Y. H., & Hollingsworth, E. Improving prognosis for infants weighing 1000 grams or less at birth. *Archives of Disease in Childhood*, 1979, *55*, 422–426.

12

Attention and Exploratory Behavior in Infants with Down's Syndrome

Peter M. Vietze
Mary McCarthy, Susan McQuiston
Robert MacTurk, Leon J. Yarrow

Until recently, it was thought that infants with Down's syndrome showed little developmental delay in the first year of life when compared with infants thought to be normal. Despite the fact that children with Down's syndrome generally achieve average IQ scores of about 50, there was little evidence of delay in their early test performance. One of the problems in this research was that the studies were cross-sectional. More recent studies (e.g., Carr, 1975; Dicks-Mireaux, 1972) suggest that clear declines in developmental progress appear in infancy, as early as 10 months. It is of some interest to note that these studies, as well as many before them, relied on standardized tests of development which provide only summary measures of developmental status. There is little or no indication of which psychological or behavioral process is instrumental in accounting for the developmental decline observed. Do infants with Down's syndrome have problems attending to stimuli? Do they lack some processing abilities or are they merely slower to develop or slower in processing information? During the past 20 years, we have learned to appreciate the abilities of normal infants and have developed sophisticated research methodologies to study their behavior. More recently, these developments have been applied to the study of delayed infants, both to learn more about the particular processes and to provide information which might be applied to intervention efforts.

Robert Fantz, and his colleagues Simon Miranda and Joseph Fagan

251

have conducted several studies of visual perception and memory in Down's syndrome infants. In one study, Miranda and Fantz (1973) compared 20 Down's syndrome infants with 20 normal infants when both groups were about 8 months of age. They found that the Down's syndrome infants spent more time than the normal infants looking at the 13 pairs of visual stimuli. Furthermore, the Down's syndrome infants showed differential looking for only 3 of the 13 pairs, whereas the normal infants showed differential attention in 11 of the pairs of stimuli. The results indicated that the Down's syndrome infants had pattern perception, though they did not show differential attention to the more complex stimuli.

In the earliest experiments by this group (Miranda, 1970; Fagan, 1971), it was found that both Down's syndrome and normal infants showed selective attention for novel versus familiar stimuli. The authors concluded that no inferences regarding cognitive ability could be drawn from these results, since the task may have been too simple for the Down's syndrome infants at 5 months. They pointed out, however, that the Down's syndrome infants took twice as long as the normal infants to "learn" the familiar stimuli, suggesting longer processing times for the Down's syndrome infants. In order to explicate these findings further, Miranda and Fantz (1974) conducted a study in which 3-, 5-, and 8-month-old normal and Down's syndrome infants were given recognition memory tasks varying in difficulty and with shorter familiarization times than in the previous studies. Normal infants were able to show recognition memory (as indexed by differential looking at the novel stimulus) at younger ages than were the Down's syndrome infants. In addition, this pattern was more evident for the difficult problems than for the easier ones. The results also showed that varying length of familiarization and recall time did not yield any differences between the normal and Down's syndrome subjects. The authors suggested that it is not possible to make inferences about any individual process, be it perception, memory, or selective attention from these data, ascribing, rather, the results to more global differences in cognitive processing ability.

In a more recent paper, Miranda (1976) reviewed the earlier studies and suggested that since Down's syndrome can be identified at birth or soon after, the utility of the various experimental techniques for identifying infants with defects in cognitive processing ability might not be great. He reasoned that there is no advantage in knowing that infants who are sure to be retarded also may show delays in basic cognitive processes. We take issue with that line of reasoning. First of all, given the wide variability in developmental status displayed by Down's syndrome infants, it would be useful to differentiate among these infants in functional rather than descriptive terms. Secondly, emphasis should be placed on similarities rather than differences between Down's syndrome and other groups. In short, we believe attention should be focused on individual differences in Down's syndrome infants. Such focus would greatly enhance future intervention efforts, allowing for prescription according to individual needs. Unfortunately, Miranda, Fantz, and Fagan did not attempt to examine individual performance results for the various processes they were studying. At this point it might be useful to continue to examine infants with Down's syndrome on a variety of tasks in order to develop a more complete profile of their processing abilities.

In order to do this, we sought to study more diverse responses than merely visual fixation. From an investigation of exploratory behavior in infancy, we developed procedures for studying how infants approached a variety of problems in which they could apply both visual and manual behaviors in order to achieve some outcome.

The theoretical bases for our research were drawn from Piaget's (1952) contention that intellectual development originates in the infant's exploration of the environment, R. W. White's (1959) notion that infants possess a motivation to engage in effective interaction with the environment (effectance), and Hunt's (1965) theory of intrinsic motivation. The studies of McCall and his associates (McCall, Applebaum, & Hogarty, 1973; McCall, Eichorn, & Hogarty, 1977) suggested that there are predictable transformations in the development of infant abilities which originate in exploratory behavior and predict later cognitive functioning. In normal infants, exploratory behavior on a variety of problems predicted concurrent and subsequent developmental status during the sensorimotor period (Yarrow, Morgan, Jennings, Harmon, & Gaiter, 1982; Yarrow, McQuiston, Mac-Turk, McCarthy, Klein, & Vietze, 1983). In the present chapter, we report the results of a similar investigation with Down's syndrome infants.

The present study sought to examine the performance of infants with Down's syndrome using procedures developed with normal infants. These procedures allowed the infants to spend relatively long periods of time exploring toys and objects which had been grouped according to three types of tasks: in *Effect Production tasks*, the infant can produce a visual or an auditory effect by operating a manipulandum; the *Sensorimotor Skills tasks* involve containers from which objects or pieces can be removed; and *Problem-Solving tasks* involve situations in which an object can be obtained by overcoming a barrier of some kind. Each of these types of tasks calls for different solutions to simple problems and relies on different cognitive skills. Several levels of exploratory behaviors may be utilized to achieve a solution to the problem, but lower level behaviors, such as banging and mouthing, may also be used with the materials. Studies with normal infants (Yarrow et al., 1983) support a developmental sequence which orders the types of tasks as follows: Effect Production, Sensorimotor Skills, and Problem Solving. We sought to discover whether the sequence was the same for infants with Down's syndrome.

In contrast to the studies of Fantz and his colleagues, discussed previously, in the present study the infants could interact physically with the stimulus materials or they could merely look at them. It was expected that the Down's syndrome infants would resemble normal infants by interacting with the three types of tasks in accordance with their increasing complexity. Thus for the Effect Production tasks we expected the most manipulation and the least visual attention; for the Sensorimotor Skills tasks we expected an intermediate amount of visual attention and manipulation; and for the Problem-Solving tasks we expected the most visual attention and the least manual interaction. Thus visual attention was hypothesized as a marker for lack of cognitive engagement. Furthermore, we expected these relations to change as we observed older infants. We expected visual attention to decrease and exploratory behavior to increase as the infants got older.

METHOD

Sample

The sample consisted of 32 infants with Down's syndrome. All of the infants were pure trisomy 21 with no mosaic cells, as determined by karyotype analysis of a sufficient number of cells. Table 12-1 describes the sample by gender, birth order, and age. There were 7 infants tested at 6 months chronological age, with 12 at 8 months, and 13 at 12 months. Subjects were given the Bayley Scales of Infant Development each time they were seen. The Bayley Scales were administered by one of the authors (R. M.) in a laboratory playroom with the mother present. The mean raw scores are also given in Table 12-1. Eight of the 8-month olds were also tested at 12 months.

All infants were referred by two local pediatricians. Criteria for exclusion were limited to neurological defects. Infants with minor cardiac problems were included. All the infants were living at home at the time of the study. Parents were given a small financial emolument to cover any expenses incurred for participating in the study.

Procedures

A total of 12 tasks, designed for 6-month-old normal infants, were presented to the infants on two different days following administration of the Bayley Scales earlier the same week. The tasks were grouped according to the three types of tasks mentioned earlier: Effect Production, Sensorimotor Skills, and Problem Solving. Half the tasks in each type were presented on each of the two days in an order which assured that no two tasks from the same group followed one another. Although each type con-

Table 12-1

Description of Sample

	Group		
	6 Months	8 Months	12 Months
n	7	12	13
Percentage of males (%)	42	43	43
Mean birth order	2.9	2.5	2.4
Mean Bayley mental development raw score	52.9	67.4	81.5
Mean Bayley motor development raw score	23.4	28.1	33.8
Mean maternal age (yr)	34.6	32.9	31.3
Mean paternal age (yr)	34.3	34.7	32.9
Mean level of maternal education (yr)	14.6	13.9	14.5
Mean level of paternal education (yr)	15.6	15.4	15.8

tained some aspects of the other two types, each task was chosen to be mainly characteristic of the type it represented. Thus all tasks might be construed to produce visual or auditory effects as a result of the infant's action although the Effect Production tasks emphasized this aspect. Table 12-2 lists the 12 tasks and their descriptions.

The infants were administered the tasks in a laboratory playroom. For each session, the infant sat on the mother's lap facing a table. The examiner sat across from the infant and presented each task one at a time. Prior to administration of the tasks, two experimental warm-up items were given, each consisting of an object handed to the infant by the examiner. All sessions were video-taped through a one-way screen. Each task was administered in a standard fashion by one of two female examiners. Each time the examiner first demonstrated the task and then allowed the infant to explore the materials for 3 min. The examiner provided no words of encouragement or reinforcement other than demonstrating the item and saying, "Can you do it?" After the initial presentation, the examiner sat quietly while the child attempted the task. Further details on the method used to present the tasks are reported elsewhere (Vietze, Pasnak, Tremblay, McCarthy, Klein, & Yarrow, 1981).

Following the sessions, the video tapes were coded using an electronic digital recording device (Datamyte, 900, Electro-General Corporation, Minnetonka, Minnesota). This allowed the duration and sequence of behaviors to be analyzed. Table 12-3 gives the coding scheme used to score the sessions. The raw data were the number of seconds the infant engaged in each behavior. The task for the coder was to indicate any change in behavior. As can be seen, the codes are arranged hierarchically, from visual attention alone, to simple exploration and complex exploration, then task-

Table 12-2

Tasks for Assessing Exploratory Behavior at 6 Months

Type of Task	Task Name	Description
Effect production	Activator	An apparatus consisting of two small balls on strings which, when pulled, causes a lever to hit a bell or hollow cylinder. It is hung on a boom stand in front of the infant.
	Chime ball	A transparent spherical toy containing small toy animals which move and make noise when the ball is hit or rolled.
	Baby bubble	A transparent spherical toy containing a butterfly and small colorful balls which spin about when the bubble is hit or pushed.
	Activity center	A rectangular board containing dials and levers which, when manipulated, produce sounds and color.
Practicing sensorimotor skills	Three men in a tub	A yellow plastic bucket containing three toy men which can be removed from the holes in which they are placed.
	Objects in a tub	A red plastic bucket containing a variety of small plastic toys which can be removed.
	Peg board	A yellow plastic board containing six removable pegs.
	Eggs in a carton	A blue plastic carton containing 12 white plastic eggs which can be removed.
Problem solving	Toy behind barrier	A lion squeeze toy is placed behind a clear plastic rectangular barrier. The child can obtain the toy by reaching.
	Animal on a string	A brightly colored plastic animal on wheels, attached to a string, is placed such that the string is within reach of the child and the toy is out of reach. The child can obtain the toy by pulling the string.

256

| Toy on a pad | A squeeze toy is placed out of reach of the child, on a blanket. The child can obtain the toy by pulling the blanket. |
| Object permanence | One tan and one white cloth are used to cover small plastic toys in a series of steps adapted from the Uzgiris–Hunt object permanence assessment procedures. |

related behaviors, and, finally, goal-directed and success behaviors. The latter result in a solution or successful completion of the task goal. In addition, the observer codes any of the social behaviors indicated, as well as any behavior which is neither relevant to the task nor any of the other behaviors being coded. In this way, all of the time may be accounted for. Interrater reliability was assessed by having two observers independently code video tapes of 30 sessions from the earlier studies with normal children. Pearson product–moment correlations for the behaviors coded ranged from .53 to .94, with a mean of .80. In order to obtain a manageable number of behaviors, the codes were collapsed prior to analysis. Thus there were five dependent measures formed:

1. Visual attention alone
2. Exploratory behavior
3. Task- and goal-directed behavior (mastery behavior)
4. Off-task behavior
5. Social behavior

For each of these measures, the percentage of the 3-min session in which the infant engaged in the behavior represented the dependent variable. These variables were tabulated for each task and then summarized according to the three task groups, with the average percentage of time computed by task type. Finally, an average score for all the tasks was computed for each dependent variable.

Data Analysis

For the three types of tasks as well as for performance on all the tasks, one-way analyses of variance were performed with age as the independent variable with each of the measures. Analyses of simple effects were carried out when the main effect of age was significant. In addition, Pearson product–moment correlations were computed between the measures of exploratory behavior at each age and the raw scores for the Bayley mental and motor development scales.

Table 12-3

Laboratory Mastery Codes

Level	Code	Behavior	Measures
0	00	Only look at apparatus	Visual attention
1	11	Only touch apparatus	
	12	Only mouth apparatus	
	13	Only passively hold apparatus	
2	21	Manipulate	
	22	Examine	
	23	Bang	
	24	Shake	Exploration
	25	Hit or bat	
	26	Drop object	
	27	Reject object	
	28	Offer, give	
3	31	Task-related behavior (relating two objects)	
	33	Grasping or holding	
	34	Reach for apparatus	
4	41	Goal-directed maneuver (correct)	Task-related, goal-directed behavior (mastery)
	42	Resets problem or task	
5	51	Effect produced	
	52	Problem solved	
	53	Motor task accomplished	
8	81	Looks at examiner	
	82	Vocalizes to examiner	
	85	Looks at mirror	
	86	Looks at mother	Social behavior
	87	Vocalizes to mother	
	88	Leans back on mother	
	80	End social behavior	
9	95	Engaged with nontask object	Off-task behavior
	99	Other	

RESULTS

The results will be presented in two parts. First, the results taken across all 12 tasks will be presented. This will allow an understanding of how the infants distributed their time in exploring the materials, regardless of the type of task. Subsequently, the results for each of these types of tasks will be presented.

Figure 12-1 shows the results based on all 12 tasks. As can be seen,

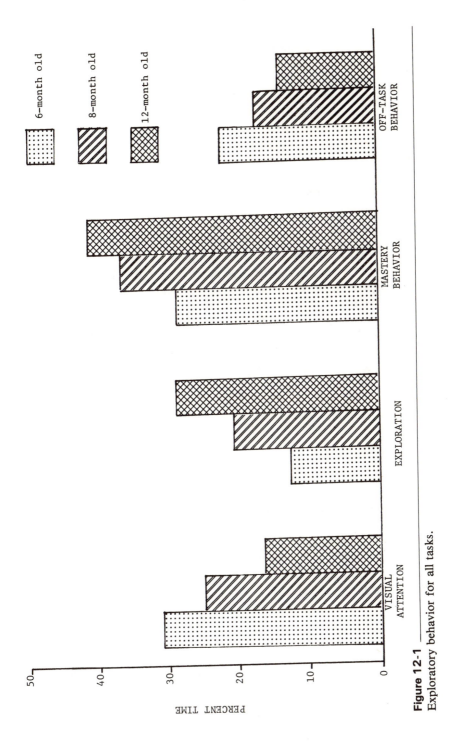

Figure 12-1 Exploratory behavior for all tasks.

there are two trends represented by the four measures depicted. Visual attention was the behavior showing the highest level at 6 months. It gradually declined from 6 to 12 months ($p < .005$), with only 16 percent of the time spent in looking alone by 1 year. Off-task behavior also declined, although the decline is not significant. The other two behaviors increased across the three age groups. Exploratory behavior went from 12.6 percent at 6 months to 28 percent at 12 months ($p < .001$), and mastery behavior increased from 28.5 percent to over 40 percent at 1 year ($p < .05$). Social behavior, not depicted here, showed a slight though nonsignificant increase across the three ages and represented only about 10 percent of the time.

Effect Production _____

The results for the Effect Production tasks are presented in Figure 12-2. As can be seen, visual attention decreased from 41 percent of the time at 6 months to 18 percent of the time at 12 months ($p < .005$). The overall decline from 6 to 12 months is significant ($p < .001$), as is that from 8 to 12 months ($p < .05$), with the difference between 6 and 8 months not being significant. At the same time, the change in exploratory behavior was not significant and represented less than 10 percent of the time. Mastery behavior increased from 30 percent to slightly over 50 percent ($p < .001$). The 6-month value was significantly lower than the 12-month value, but the intermediate differences were not significant. Off-task behavior did not change significantly, accounting for about 20 percent of the time.

Sensorimotor Skills _____

For the Sensorimotor Skills tasks (Fig. 12-3), visual attention decreased from 30 to 13 percent ($p < .001$) between the 6- and 12-month groups. This was accounted for by the change between 6 and 8 months ($p < .05$). There was also a significant increase in exploratory behavior, from 12 to 35 percent ($p < .001$), which was also accounted for by the increase between 6 and 8 months ($p < .005$). Mastery behavior increased also, but not significantly. Off-task behavior for this group of tasks decreased, although the change was not significant.

Problem Solving _____

For the Problem-Solving tasks (Fig. 12-4), visual attention also decreased across the three age groups, going from 27 percent at 6 months to 18 percent at 12 months ($p < .01$). This was accounted for by the difference between 8 and 12 months ($p < .005$) and the difference between 6 and 12 months ($p < .005$). Exploratory behavior doubled, from 20 percent at 6

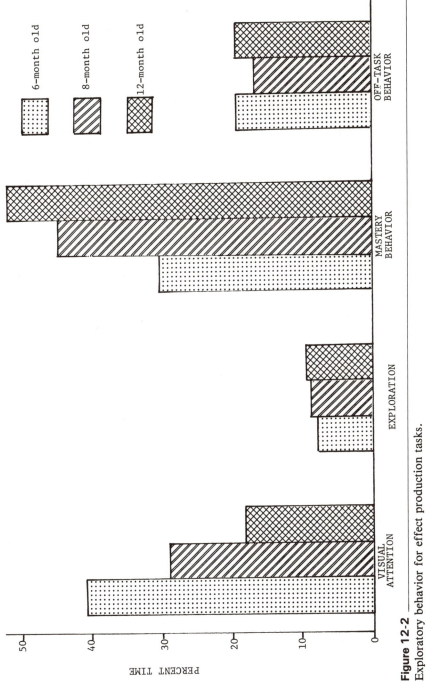

Figure 12-2

Exploratory behavior for effect production tasks.

261

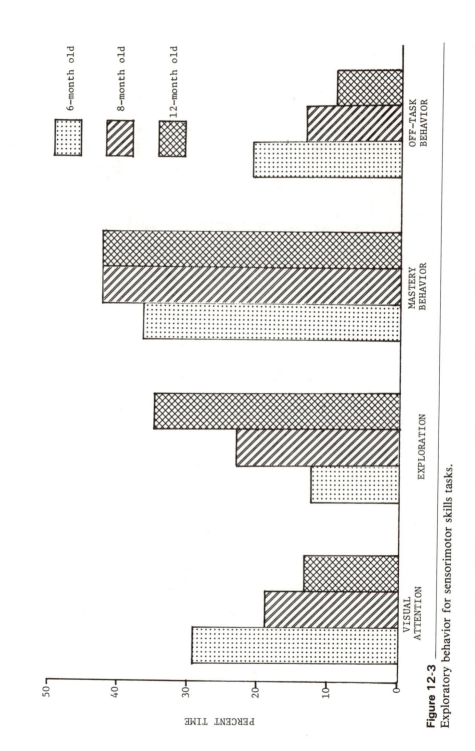

Figure 12-3

Exploratory behavior for sensorimotor skills tasks.

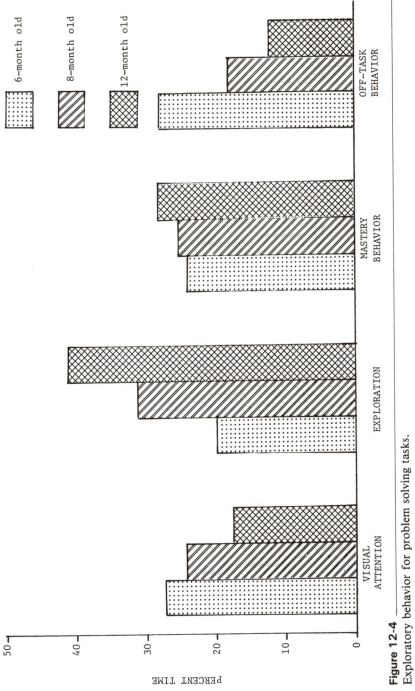

Figure 12-4
Exploratory behavior for problem solving tasks.

263

months to 40 percent ($p < .001$). This could be accounted for by the difference between the 6-month-olds and the 8- and 12-month-olds, respectively ($p < .05$ and $p < .005$). Mastery behavior showed a slight but nonsignificant increase between 6 and 12 months. Off-task behavior showed decreases, but none of the comparisons were significant.

Summary of Results

In general, results of these analyses indicated that the only consistent age difference across the three types of tasks was for looking. Looking at the materials was highest at 6 months and declined gradually through 8 months to the lowest level at 1 year. Exploratory behavior showed a general tendency to increase, though only for two of the three types of tasks, Sensorimotor Skills and Problem Solving. Mastery behavior also showed a tendency to increase across the three age groups for all the tasks, but the increase was only significant for the Effect Production tasks. Off-task behavior generally decreased as the infant groups increased in age, but this change was only significant for Problem Solving. The picture which emerges, then, is that as infants with Down's syndrome get older, they have increasing tendencies to explore and master objects which present some sort of problem, and decreasing tendencies merely to look at them. In the following section, these findings will be discussed in relation to a sample of nondelayed infants tested with the same tasks. In addition, implications for further research and for intervention will also be presented.

Correlations Between Bayley and Exploratory Behavior Measures

For the 6-month-old subjects, there were no significant correlations between either of the Bayley measures and any of the measures of exploratory behavior. The results for the 8-month-old infants yielded 4 significant correlation coefficients out of 32 correlations. This is below the chance level for a number of significant correlations. However, for the 1-year-old infants, more than 25 percent of the correlation coefficients were significant (see Table 12-4). These formed a consistent pattern, with significant positive relations between mastery behavior and the mental development raw score on the Bayley for two of the three types of tasks. Only the Sensorimotor Skills tasks did not yield a significant correlation. Furthermore, mastery behavior for the overall task measure was also significantly correlated with the mental development measure. All of the off-task measures were significantly negatively related to the mental development measure at this age. Finally, the exploration measures for the Effect Production and Problem-Solving tasks were significantly related to the motor development scale measure.

This pattern of results indicates that for the Down's syndrome infants

Table 12-4

Correlations Between Exploratory Behavior and Bayley Test Scores at 12 Months

	Bayley Mental Score	Bayley Motor Score
Effect Production		
Visual attention		
Exploration		.58
Mastery behavior	.87	
Off-task behavior	−.86	
Sensorimotor Skills		
Visual attention		
Exploration		
Mastery behavior		
Off-task behavior		
Problem Solving		
Visual attention		
Exploration		.63
Mastery behavior	.66	
Off-task behavior	−.75	
All Tasks		
Visual attention		
Exploration		
Mastery behavior	.80	
Off-task behavior	−.87	

at 12 months, measures of exploratory behavior which index mastery are correlated with a well-accepted measure of mental development. Visual attention was not related to mental development at any age. Furthermore, the fact that the time spent in non-task-related behavior is negatively correlated with mental development suggests that facilitating exploratory behavior, especially that which is challenging in some way, may facilitate mental development. The relations between exploration and motor development may be an indication that those infants whose fine motor development is more advanced may exhibit more exploratory behavior which is not directed to task solution.

DISCUSSION

The results of the present study indicate that at 6 months, infants with Down's syndrome spend an appreciable amount of time merely looking at toys and objects which are part of their culture and commonly available.

However, it is also clear that they are fully capable of exploring these materials and solving problems inherent in the materials. In order to put these results into perspective, a brief summary of a similar study with normal infants is in order. The previous study (Yarrow et al., 1983) had been conducted with 6-month-old normal infants utilizing the same materials as were used with the Down's syndrome infants. They spent about a tenth of the time looking at the materials without manually exploring them, while the 6-month-old Down's syndrome infants spent a third of the time merely looking. The normal infants also spent less time looking at the materials than the 12-month-old Down's syndrome infants. They spent more than twice as much time for the exploratory behavior measure compared with the 6-month-old Down's syndrome infants, and the same amount of time as the 12-month-old Down's syndrome infants. Finally, they spent more time engaged in mastery behavior than the Down's syndrome infants at any age. What might account for these differences? It is possible that the Down's syndrome infants did not have as much experience with toys or objects such as the ones we used in the assessment. We queried the mothers of the infants in the present study regarding the presence of toys in their homes such as the ones we were using. Most of them did have one or more of these toys. However, in the course of these discussions, it became evident that the infants had shown little interest in handling toys or objects. Some of the mothers indicated that since their children showed little interest in toys, they rarely gave the toys to them. One mother indicated that our assessment was the first time she had witnessed her baby playing with a toy. It is possible that the Down's syndrome infants, with their characteristic hypotonia, take longer to make contact with an object placed before them. Our results indicate that to be the case. Analyses of latency to contact the toys manually, still in progress, may provide firmer evidence for this. However, it may be possible that the care givers of these infants do not wait long enough for the infants to make contact and so the infants have limited experience with handling objects. It is also possible that it takes more effort for the Down's syndrome infants to contact and explore the objects.

It is clear that infants with Down's syndrome do explore objects and toys appropriately and are able to solve problems with them. The major difference between their performance and that of normal infants is in the level of behavior—the amount of time they spend in more instrumental behaviors such as manual exploration, or what we have called mastery behavior.

The present results cannot easily be compared with those of Miranda, Fantz, and Fagan (Miranda & Fantz, 1973, 1974; Fagan, 1971.) However, they too reported decreasing levels of visual attention with increasing age for Down's syndrome infants. Our results indicate, however, that such decreases in visual attention are accompanied by increasing manual exploration. These results suggest the importance of providing response modalities other than visual attention in studying infants with impaired capacity if we are to fully understand the range of abilities.

The results indicating that the mental development scales are related to the exploratory behavior measures at 12 months suggest that by this age cognitive functioning may be reciprocal with exploratory behavior. However, only mastery behavior is related to mental development. Since these are contemporaneous correlations, we can only speculate about the direction of effect. Nevertheless, it seems more plausible that the process measures for mastery behavior and mental development influence one another. Only more sophisticated analyses, precluded by the present sample size, could actually establish the causal direction of these relations. The present results are clear, however, in showing no strong relations between visual attention and mental or motor development measures. These findings conflict with the implications of Miranda's (1976) results. Our results strongly support the notion that manual exploration holds promise in further understanding the development of cognition in Down's syndrome children.

Finally, the present results suggest that the full range of exploratory behaviors must be considered in understanding the significance of exploration for the development of children with Down's syndrome. The observational system used in this study assumes an organization of the response repertoire of infants. The behavioral style of the infants can be studied, since the behaviors observed are mutually exclusive. Sroufe (1979) has outlined various aspects of the organization of development. Our data suggest that there is a progression in this organization for children with Down's syndrome with regard to exploration of the environment. This progression seems to begin with heavy reliance on visual attention to stimuli and becomes reorganized by the time the children are 1 year old so that they utilize manual exploration in the service of mastery. Future research which studies Down's syndrome infants longitudinally is necessary in order to understand this transformation more fully. It would also be important to study such groups of children well beyond their first year in order to observe the progression beyond the simple exploration which we have been studying.

To summarize, we have studied infants with Down's syndrome at 6, 8, and 12 months of age, using procedures designed to understand exploratory behavior in challenging situations. We have seen that the youngest children show extensive visual exploration which seems to change to manual exploration in order to master the problems presented to them. We have stressed the importance of examining different varieties of exploration. Finally, we have discovered that the exploration of toys and objects is related at 12 months to both mental and motor development. These results have implications for intervention aimed at facilitating the development of exploration, which in turn might affect developmental status in children with Down's syndrome.

REFERENCES _____

Carr, J. *Young children with Down's syndrome*, London: Butterworths, 1975.
Dicks-Mireaux, M. J. Mental development of infants with Down's syndrome. *American Journal of Mental Deficiency*, 1972, *77*, 26–32.
Fagan, J. F. Infants' recognition memory for a series of visual stimuli. *Journal of Experimental Child Psychology*, 1971, *11*, 244–250.
Hunt, J. M. Intrinsic motivation and its role in psychological development. In D. Levine (Ed.), *Nebraska Symposium on Motivation* (Vol. 13). Lincoln, Neb.: University of Nebraska Press, 1965.
McCall, R. B., Applebaum, M., & Hogarty, P. S. Developmental changes in mental performance. *Monographs of the Society for Research in Child Development*, 1973, *38*, 1–83.
McCall, R. B., Eichorn, D. H., & Hogarty, P. S. Transitions in early mental development. *Monographs of the Society for Research in Child Development*, 1977, *42*, 1–108.
Miranda, S. B. Response to novel visual stimuli by Down's syndrome and normal infants. *Proceedings of the 78th Annual Convention of the American Psychological Association*, 1970, 5, 46–47.
Miranda, S. B. Visual attention in defective and high risk infants. *Merrill-Palmer Quarterly of Development and Behavior*, 1976, *22*, 201–228.
Miranda, S. B., & Fantz, R. L. Visual preferences of Down's syndrome and normal infants. *Child Development*, 1973, *44*, 555–561.
Miranda, S. B., & Fantz, R. L. Recognition memory in Down's syndrome and normal infants. *Child Development*, 1974, *45*, 651–660.
Piaget, J. *The origins of intelligence in children*. New York: International Universities Press, 1952.
Sroufe, A. Socioemotional development. In J. Osofsky (Ed.), *Handbook of Infant Development*. New York: John Wiley & Sons, 1979.
White, R. W. Motivation reconsidered: The concept of competence. *Psychological Review*, 1959, *21*, 243–266.
Yarrow, L. J., McQuiston, S., MacTurk, R. H., McCarthy, M. E., Klein, R. P., & Vietze, P. M. The assessment of mastery motivation during the first year of life. *Developmental Psychology*, 1983, *19*, 159–171.
Yarrow, L. J., Morgan, G. A., Jennings, K. D., Harmon, R. J., & Gaiter, J. L. Infants' persistence at tasks: Relationships to cognitive functioning and early experience. *Infant Behavior and Development*, 1982, *5*, 131–141.
Vietze, P. M., Pasnak, C. F., Tremblay, A., McCarthy, M., Klein, R. P., & Yarrow, L. J. *A manual for assessing mastery motivation in 6 and 12 month-old infants*. Unpublished manuscript, 1981.

III Follow-up Assessments
During Childhood

13

Individual Differences in Infant Attention: Relations to Birth Status and Intelligence at Five Years

Marian D. Sigman

Newborn infants differ in their attentiveness to visual stimulation. Anyone who has spent any time in a newborn nursery has observed this variation. Some infants are quick to look at new faces or scenes; others remain for long periods staring attentively at unchanging vistas.

Parents, pediatricians, and researchers note these differences and wonder what they mean about the child. Is the child who examines the visual environment for long periods of time a child who is born curious, with an innate potential for careful analysis, or, on the contrary, is this child perhaps slower to take in visual input or less able to regulate his own attention processes? Are these differences in the infant's initial approach to the visual world responded to by the care takers? Does the kind of visual world provided in the first few days or weeks shape the infant's style of attention? The major questions in this chapter concern the origins and sequelae of these individual differences.

The research reported in this paper has been carried out for more than 12 years, has been supported by NICHD and the Grant Foundation, and has benefitted from the collaborative efforts of many individuals. Arthur H. Parmelee, M.D., has provided the conceptual and practical framework for the research investigation. Claire Kopp, Ph.D., and Wendell Jeffrey, Ph.D., made significant contributions to the development of many of the early assessment measures and, particularly, the term visual attention measure. Leila Beckwith, Ph.D., Sarale Cohen, Ph.D., Arthur H. Parmelee, M.D., and I have continued to document the developmental progress of this group of children. More recently, Peter Mundy, Ph.D., and Tracy Sherman, Ph.D., have shared their considerable breadth of knowledge and good judgment about early perceptual–cognitive development.

271

These questions prompted this research study aimed at understanding the significance of such obvious, early individual variations in behavior. I became interested in individual differences in neonates in 1964, when I had the opportunity to know a number of newborn infants and after a pediatrician described a neonate of my acquaintance as having "good cerebral connections." Although he appeared to be correct, the basis for this judgment was unclear to me. Shortly afterward, I collaborated in a short-term longitudinal study concerning the development of attention to faces administered by Genevieve Carpenter in collaboration with Gerald Stechler. We selected neonates as subjects with a 1-min test of attention to a single stimulus administered in the Newborn Nursery at Boston City Hospital. Those infants who showed adequate levels of attention were judged to be "attentive" and their mothers were invited to participate in the longitudinal study, which lasted from 2 to 8 weeks of age. The validity of this screening device was never tested, and I wondered whether the measure reflected a stable characteristic of infants. The original impetus in my studies of attention in neonates was to understand whether duration of attention represented a behavioral style with implications for neurological functions.

There are a number of ways in which one might conceptualize attentiveness and measure individual variability. One way to study individual differences might be to time-sample each infant's looking behavior repeatedly over extended periods of time in the hospital nursery or at home (Thoman, Acebo, Dreyer, Becker, & Freese, 1977). This would provide a measure of the percentage of time that the infant was in the awake, alert state and attentive to some stimulus in the environment. There is, however, great variability in the stimuli provided for infants from one environment to another and over time. Furthermore, the determination of what the infant is fixating can be very difficult unless the situation is structured. For these reasons, I decided to measure duration of infant attention over a brief period of time to a fairly simple stimulus, chosen because of its demonstrated attractiveness to newborns in many studies (Brennan, Ames, & Moore, 1966; Hershenson, 1964). This measure reflects a very different form of attentiveness than an assessment of the frequency of awake, alert behavior. Instead of assessing the predominance of a particular state, the attention duration measure would seem to reflect the infant's capacity to regulate responses to external and internal stimuli for a brief period of time, as well as the speed of information processing.

Several other considerations guided the research design. First, I wanted to study infants who were in an optimal state of alertness. While attentiveness in the neonate may relate partly to the infant's ability to regulate states of arousal, environments vary widely in their impact on infant states. Because behavior was sampled only at one time point, the environmental variables which might have an immediate effect on state of arousal needed to be controlled. For this reason, an attempt was made to provide those conditions which help infants to be most alert. Pilot work showed that measuring attention after a newborn's neurological examination provided many more neonates who were awake than simply testing the children without a previous arousing situation. On the other hand, most neonates reached the end of the neurological examination in a state of high arousal, so a brief feeding was included before the visual attention testing. This procedure seemed to be most effective in maximizing the number of infants who were alert when testing began.

Another major research consideration was the type of experimental paradigm to use in measuring attention. As compared to the presentation of single stimuli for fixed lengths of time, the visual habituation and dishabituation paradigm and preference for novelty paradigm have the advantage that changes in state of arousal are less confounded with maintenance of attention. The infant has to be aroused enough to demonstrate response recovery in one paradigm and a preference for novel stimuli in the other. While this is an important advantage in some regards, the infant's capacity to regulate state was of interest. Furthermore, both the habituation and novelty preference paradigms require that the infant remember whether he or she has previously seen a particular stimulus. A great deal of controversy exists as to whether the neonate possesses the necessary memory capacities to remember a stimulus that has been seen before (Olsen & Sherman, in press). Because of these reservations, the habituation or preference paradigms were not used, and the infant's attention to several presentations of stimuli presented singly was measured instead. This provided a measure of the infant's ability to marshal his or her attention to an inanimate stimulus, as well as the infant's proclivity to terminate visual scanning of the stimulus after a period of time.

In order to take advantage of the more sophisticated abilities and more advanced techniques suitable for older infants, the infants were also tested at a later age. At 4 months of age, preference for novelty using a paired comparison paradigm was assessed. Fantz, Fagan, and Miranda had demonstrated in a number of studies the sensitivity of this method for assessing group differences (Fantz & Nevis, 1967; Fantz, Fagan, & Miranda, 1976; Miranda & Fantz, 1974). While Les Cohen suggested at a somewhat later date that I use the infant control procedure and single-stimulus presentations, my early research had provided enough interesting leads to justify remaining with the paired comparison paradigm and fixed trial lengths. At 4 months preference for complexity and for regular versus scrambled facelike stimuli was also measured, since developmental trends in preferences had been demonstrated for these stimulus qualities (Brennan et al., 1966; Karmel, 1969; Haaf & Bell, 1964; McCall & Kagan, 1967).

STUDIES OF RISK FACTORS

Initial studies carried out in collaboration with Claire Kopp, Wendell Jeffrey, and Arthur Parmelee investigated the impact of several measures of risk status on the term infant's attentiveness to a single visual stimulus. We began with the hypothesis that neonates who are neurologically more intact should be better able to initiate and maintain their attention to visual stimuli. The testing procedure has been described in detail in a previous article (Sigman, Kopp, Parmelee, & Jeffrey, 1973). The neonate was shown a 2 × 2 checkerboard, 6 inches square, for a period of 1 min. Following this minute, the checkerboard was illuminated with flashing lights that alternated behind the white quadrants of the checkerboard. The third trial was a 1-min repetition of the first trial. Those infants who had shown little attention in the first three trials were removed from the infant seat and given tactile and vestibular stimulation and then retested for a further three trials. This intervention had so little effect that its use was discontinued after the first study.

The initial operational measures of attention were quite complex. The basic measure of visual fixation was the presence of the corneal reflection of the stimulus. However, differentiation between fixations with eyes opened wide and narrow as well as between fixations with and without eye movements was attempted. After the first study, the distinction between wide-eyed and narrow-eyed looking was eliminated because it seemed neither useful nor reliable. The second distinction was never used, because all infants, except one neonate who showed general paralysis, demonstrated at least some eye movements. Thus the dependent measure for the term visual attention measure became the length of the first fixation to each stimulus and the total duration of fixations on each of the three trials. In some analyses, the number and the average length of fixations were also examined.

The first study of a group of 25 full-term neonates, ranging in age from 24 to 48 hours, confirmed my original hypothesis that greater attentiveness was associated with better neurological integration (Sigman et al., 1973). Scores on a newborn neurological examination were significantly related to the length of the first fixation of each stimulus, as well as the total fixation time of the first stimulus. A reanalysis of these data in a later article showed that the relation was due to first fixation time rather than total fixation time (Sigman, Kopp, Littman, & Parmelee, 1977). Thus initial attentiveness to each new stimulus was related to neurological integration; full-term infants who fixated new stimuli for longer periods showed more normal reflex and organized behavior patterns.

In our second study, Claire Kopp, Wendell Jeffrey, Arthur Parmelee, and I aimed to replicate our observations with a sample of preterm infants tested at an equivalent conceptional age, the expected date of birth. Since preterm birth is often associated with obstetric and pediatric complications, the range of neurological functioning among preterm infants should be broader (Knobloch & Pasamanick, 1966) so that even stronger associations might be expected. The same procedure as in the first study was used, except that the preterm infants were brought back to a laboratory room in the department of pediatrics. To our surprise, we did not find any correlation between performance on the neurological assessment and visual attention (Kopp, Sigman, and Parmelee, & Jeffrey, 1975). Furthermore, the preterm infants appeared to show longer durations of fixation than the full-term infants and this was independent of the socioeconomic status and sex of the infant (Sigman et al., 1977). These differences seemed to involve both initial looking as well as the maintenance of attention.

One possible explanation for these group differences might have been that the behavioral responsiveness of the full-term infants was temporarily diminished by the effects of birth. The full-term neonates were tested within 2–3 days after birth. The preterm infants, however, were tested at 40 weeks conceptional age. Since all these preterm infants necessarily were born at gestational ages of 37 weeks or less, all were at least 3 weeks past birth. Thus the preterm infants might have been able to recover from the disruptive effects of birth, while the full-term infants were still disorganized by the birth experience.

In order to examine this hypothesis, a group of 15 full-term infants were tested twice, once within the first few days of life and again after 2 weeks. There was no significant increase in first fixation or total fixation time over this period. Therefore the explanation that the differences between preterm and full-term infants in their attention time could be attributed to transient birth effects was unsupported by the findings of our small longitudinal follow-up.

VISUAL PREFERENCES IN PRETERM AND FULL-TERM INFANTS

These preliminary studies of visual attention therefore revealed that preterm infants as a group showed longer fixation durations than full-term infants tested at the same conceptional age or after 2 weeks. Given these results, I was interested in whether group differences would also appear on the 4-month measure, particularly in terms of habituation and preference for novelty.

A new sample of 20 full-term and 20 preterm infants was recruited. Testing was carried out at matched conceptional ages, which was 4 months postnatal age for the full-term infants. Infants were tested at matched conceptional ages, since previous studies had shown that visual preferences varied with time from conception rather than time from birth (Fagan, Fantz, & Miranda, 1971; Fantz & Fagan, 1975). The stimuli, two-dimensional black and white figures, were presented as slides with a paired comparison technique. Each pair was shown for 20 sec.

Three different preferences were assessed. During the first eight slides, the infant was shown a series of checkerboards varying in the number of checks, including 2 × 2, 6 × 6, 12 × 12, and 24 × 24 checkerboards. The left–right positions of the complex and simple stimuli was varied over trials. The next four slides showed photographs and drawings of faces in regular or scrambled arrangements. The last series consisted of repeating the 24 × 24 checkerboards with four novel stimuli. These novel stimuli were chosen to be as attractive as the 24 × 24 checkerboard based on pilot data from a sample of 4-month-olds.

The results showed that both the preterm and full-term infants fixated the complex stimuli more than the simple stimuli (Sigman & Parmelee, 1974). There were no group differences in the degree of preference for the complex stimuli. When attention times to the four checkerboards were compared, both the full-term and preterm infants looked less at the simplest checkerboard compared to the other three checkerboards.

While preference for complex stimuli was similar for preterm and full-term infants, only the full-term infants showed a significant preference for the novel stimulus. The preterm infants looked for about equal amounts of time at the novel and familiar stimuli. There were no group differences in the amount of looking at the repeated trials of the 24 × 24 checkerboard; both groups showed evidence of a response decrement in the four familiarization trials. The major group difference in response to the face-like stimuli was that the full-term infants looked at these stimuli for longer periods of time.

To summarize the results at 4 months, the preterm and full-term infants no longer showed much difference in their total attention times to a variety of stimuli. While they looked at the stimuli for about equal lengths of time, the full-term infants showed a novelty preference that was not demonstrated by the preterm infants. These results suggest that preterm infants as a group may not process visual input at the same rate as full-term infants. If this hypothesis is true, then the differences noted at term also may relate to the infant's ability to encode information. The preterm infants tested at term may have looked for longer periods of time at the 2 × 2 checkerboards than did the full-term infants because some of them were slower to take in the visual information. The delay in visual information processing may be reflected in long attention times at term and in lesser degrees of preference for novel stimuli when fixed familiarization periods are used at later ages.

Other investigators have noted deficits in immediate recognition memory among preterm infants relative to the performance of full-term infants. Rose, Gottfried, and Bridger (1979) reported poorer performances on visual recognition of objects at 6 and 12 months after expected date of birth for preterm infants than for full-term infants. In addition, Rose (1980) found inferior performances on tests of visual recognition at 28 weeks corrected age by preterm infants who experienced ordinary hospital care. Interestingly, a group of preterm infants in an early intervention program were as responsive to novelty as the full-term infants. Caron and Caron (1981) found that full-term infants, tested at 52, 53, 61, and 64 weeks of age, recognized the invariant feature of the previously exposed stimuli, whereas preterm infants tested at equivalent conceptional ages did not.

While all these studies suggest that preterm infants are slower at encoding information, there is evidence that the deficiency can be ameliorated if the infants are allowed longer stimulus exposures. A study of exploratory behavior at 8 months corrected age compared the visual and tactile exploration of novel and familiar objects by 32 full-term and 32 preterm infants (Sigman, 1976). All infants were observed at 34–35 weeks of postnatal age for the full-term and at 34–35 weeks corrected age for the preterm. The term *corrected age* refers to the sum of the postnatal age and the estimated length of time before 40 weeks gestational age that the child was born. Each child was given a single object for 6 min. This object was then presented for 10 1-min trials with a set of 10 novel objects. All the novel objects were different, except that the first and tenth were both balloons. Although both groups played with the single object for equal amounts of time during the familiarization period, the preterm infants continued to play with the familiar toy for longer periods of time than the full-term infants, and the preterm infants showed a greater preference for the novel stimulus on the first trial. After the first 2 min, the group differences were no longer evident. The duration of exploration of the familiar stimulus declined among the preterm infants and they showed similar preference for the novel toys. Thus the preterm infants seem to have required additional experience with the object for familiarization to occur. When they had played with the familiar toy for two additional trials, they showed the same degree of preference for the novel objects as the full-term infants.

Similar results were reported by Rose (1980) in an investigation of visual preferences among 6-month-old infants. In the first study, preterm infants failed to differentiate between novel and familiar test stimuli following brief amounts of familiarization, whereas full-term infants showed significant novelty preferences on two of the three problems. In a second study, the familiarization periods provided for the preterm infants were lengthened so that the infants had an additional 5–10 sec of study time for each problem. With these lengthened study times, the preterm infants showed a subsequent preference for the novel stimulus on three of the four problems. A control group of preterm infants, with shorter study times, failed to differentiate between the patterns, replicating the original results. Group comparisons revealed that the major difference in attention during the test trials was in response to the familiar stimulus. The infants with the longer study times showed significantly less interest in the familiarization stimulus, but no difference was observed in the amount of time they spent looking at the novel stimulus. Thus both the results of my earlier study and those from the investigation carried out by Rose suggest that preterm infants are capable of storing the initial information and retrieving it from storage but register or process the information more slowly than full-term infants.

ATTENTION AND VISUAL PREFERENCES AS MEASURES OF INDIVIDUAL DIFFERENCES

The studies reported to this point, then, had a number of implications for my original questions and raised some new questions. First, initial levels of interest in a new stimulus, but not the tendency to sustain fixations, seemed to reflect better neurological integration in full-term infants; however, neither initial or sustained attention times had any association with neurological functioning in preterm infants. Preterm infants, as a group, demonstrated longer durations of attention to familiar stimuli and less preference for novelty than full-term infants when a fixed familiarization period was employed. The attention and visual preference measures seemed to be sensitive to birth group differences which might reflect the "risk" status of many preterm infants. These initial findings were consistent enough to suggest that visual attention and preference measures might reflect perceptual–cognitive abilities that were deficient in some medically at-risk infants. While the studies reported previously had uncovered group differences, it was clear that many preterm infants performed like the full-term infants. The clinically important issue was whether the preterm infants who showed very different patterns of behavior were also more affected by the correlates and sequelae of preterm birth and whether these behavior patterns would have any relation to their future development.

The opportunity to address these questions was presented with the initiation of the Infant Studies Project, a research investigation aimed at early assessment of factors placing the infant at risk for cognitive problems. The objective was to design an assessment battery that would identify infants with cognitive difficulties more effectively than standard developmental tests (Parmelee, Kopp, & Sigman, 1976). The infant attention and preference measures were included as early assessments of arousal control, interest in the environment, and information processing.

The design of the Infant Studies Project required that a risk score be constructed for each assessment. This was necessary since a portion of the sample was to participate in an intervention project beginning at 10 months of age. In order to select infants at this age, the formulators of the Infant Studies Project, directed by Arthur Parmelee, decided to use a mean score on our own assessment battery to determine which infants were in need of early intervention.

For the purpose of designing risk scores, each measure was administered to a sample of subjects, 85 percent of whom consisted of full-term infants and 15 percent of whom consisted of preterm and sick infants. A range of performance was observed and raw scores were converted to standardized scores based on these observations. For the term visual attention measure, the risk score consisted of a set of points that the child was assigned based on levels of fixation on each trial (see Fig. 13-1). For the 4-month visual preference measure, the following variables were included in the risk score: preference for the complex stimuli, preference for the novel stimuli, preference for the regular drawing of a face, preference for the photographed faces rather than geometric forms, and total attention time (see Fig. 13-1). Analyses of the data from the Infant Studies Project have often been carried out initially with the risk scores in order to limit the number of variables included in analyses.

The assessment battery administered to each infant included 16 measures of obstetric and medical complications, environmental observation, and developmental scales, such as the Gesell and Bayley Scales. Each infant was followed to 2 years of age, and a large number were tested with the Stanford-Binet IQ test at 5 years. Because a fairly large number of infants were assessed on all these parameters, the data from the Infant Studies Project are useful for addressing some of the questions regarding individual differences in attention duration and preferences, as well as the new questions regarding attention measures as clinical tools.

Before considering these data, the sample should be described. The major sample followed to 2 years included 126 preterm infants (Sigman & Parmelee, 1979). Prematurity was defined by a gestational age at birth of 37 weeks or less and a birth weight of 2500 grams or less. Subjects were from diverse ethnic backgrounds. Seventy-five children were from English-speaking families, 37 children were from Spanish-speaking families, and 14 children came from other language backgrounds. Socioeconomic status was determined using a weighting system which combined the years of maternal education with a rating of paternal occupation. Based on this scale, 54 children were from families considered to be of high socioeconomic status, while 72 children were from low socioeconomic status families. There were 76 males and 50 females in the sample. Three children maintained in the study had moderate cerebral palsy at age 2 years. A sample of 29 full-term

Newborn (Term) Visual Attention Measure

Add Points If	Trial 1	Trial 2	Trial 3	Points
Duration of first fixation is	≥ 2.0 sec	≥ 2.0 sec	≥1.0 sec	2
Duration of total fixation is	≥11.5 sec	≥12.5 sec	≥8.0 sec	2
Number of fixations is	>2 + <20	>2.2 + <10	≥2 + <9.9	1

Total points possible: 15

Four-Month Visual Attention Measure

Add Points (Maximum = 13 points) If

Total fixation time to complex stimuli > total fixation time to the simple stimuli (4 points)

Total fixation time to the novel stimuli > total fixation to the familiar stimuli (3 points)

Fixation time to novel stimuli on trials 1 and 2 > fixation time to familiar stimuli (1 point)

Fixation time to scrambled drawing > fixation time to regular drawing (1 point)

Fixation time to the photographed faces > fixation time to the geometric forms (1 point)

First fixation duration to the complex > first fixation duration to the simple (1 point)

First fixation duration to the novel > first fixation duration to the familiar (1 point)

Total fixation time > 130 sec (1 point)

Figure 13-1
Scoring for the risk scores.

280

neonates was also followed to 2 years of age; only 16 of these children were assessed with the term visual attention measures.

ATTENTION DURATION IN RELATION TO
GESTATIONAL AGE AND EARLY ILLNESS _____

One of the first risk measures to be investigated was gestational age and degree of illness (Sigman & Beckwith, 1980). There was a wide variation in the degree of prematurity among this sample. Furthermore, some preterm infants were born with few medical and neurological problems and were released after a short time in the hospital, whereas others were severely ill for an extended period of time. Of course, gestational age and medical complications were highly associated, so that very young, small preterm infants were sicker and had longer hospitalizations.

In order to investigate whether gestational age, the number of medical complications, or the length of hospitalization had any relation to attention durations, the group was subdivided according to the total fixation time on all three trials. Using a median split, half the male infants and half the female infants were placed in the brief-fixation group, while the other infants were placed in the long-fixation group. The data were analyzed with 2 × 2 analyses of variance (sex × fixation group), because sex differences have been reported in previous studies of infant attention.

My hypothesis was that the healthier infants would show briefer fixations, like the full-term infants. All the data to this point had suggested that long fixation durations were associated with risk status, so it seemed likely that infants who had been sick would fixate the stimuli for long periods of time. In fact, the group difference was contrary to the one hypothesized. Infants in the long-fixation group had been born after longer gestations, suffered less illness, and were hospitalized more briefly. Infants in the brief-fixation group had been born after shorter gestations, had suffered more illness, and were hospitalized for longer periods of time. These results were completely contrary to those expected based on what had been learned in the previous studies.

There are several possible explanations for these results. First, perhaps my hypotheses based on the comparisons between full-term and preterm infants were fallacious. Rather than the differences in mean duration between the preterm and full-term infants being attributed to the extended fixations of some very "high risk" preterm infants, they may be attributed to other factors, such as distinctive life experiences. It is possible that longer fixation durations do reflect better physiological integration within the preterm sample, just as longer initial looking relates to better neurological responses within the full-term sample. While the data on predictive outcome tend to negate this hypothesis, the explanation cannot be ruled out completely.

A second explanation is in terms of postnatal age. The brief-fixation and long-fixation groups differed not only in terms of gestational age, but also in terms of postnatal age. The infants who looked for long durations were about 1½ weeks younger than the preterm infants who looked briefly. Although I did not find differences in fixation durations over a 2-week period in full-term infants, many studies have reported a decline in attention among full-term infants over longer periods of time (Brennan et al., 1966; Fantz, 1965; Lewis, Goldberg, & Campbell, 1969; Wetherford & Cohen, 1973). While this explanation is not particularly convincing, perhaps the difference in postnatal age was sufficient among the preterm infants to account for the decline in attention times.

A third explanation stems from the fact that the preterm sample consisted of two subgroups. The infants from Spanish-speaking families were born after longer gestational periods, were heavier at birth, suffered fewer complications, and were hospitalized more briefly than infants from English-speaking families. Furthermore, the former group of infants showed longer fixation durations than the latter group. The infants from Spanish-speaking families had longer fixation durations on the first trial ($t = 2.56$, $df = 107$, $p = .01$) and somewhat longer fixations on all three trials ($t = 1.82$, $df = 107$, $p = .07$). Thus the associations between fixation durations and birth complications may have been attributable to the presence of two subgroups within the sample who varied both in terms of birth complications and visual responses.

ATTENTION DURATION IN RELATION TO CARE GIVER–INFANT INTERACTION AMONG PRETERM INFANTS

This line of evidence raised the issue of the relation between environmental factors and infant behaviors. Since most of the preterm infants had been home by 36 weeks gestational age, almost all were tested several weeks after discharge. Thus attention patterns may have been influenced by early experiences in the home. I wished to measure actual care-giving practices rather than relying on gross environmental measures of social class background. For these purposes, I was able to make use of Beckwith and Cohen's (in press) observations of care giver–infant interaction carried out in the home when the infants were 1 month corrected age.

The home observation has been described in several previous reports (Beckwith & Cohen, 1978; Beckwith, Cohen, Kopp, Parmelee, & Marcy, 1976). The naturalistic observations were made in the subject's home as the family proceeded with usual activities. The behaviors of the infant and primary care giver were time-sampled every consecutive 15 sec, using a checklist. The observed behaviors and the derived factors and their loadings, obtained by a principal-component factor analysis with varimax rotation to orthogonal structure, have been described in detail in a previous report (Beckwith et al., 1976). The five factors were named as follows: factor 1, social (defined by high loadings of the variables of affectionate touches, social play, contingent response to vocalization, and mutual gazing); factor 2, responsive holding (defined by attentiveness, long holds, soothing touches, and contingent response to distress); factor 3, verbal stimulation (defined by total talk comments, commands, and criticism); factor 4, mutual gazing (defined by three categories of mutual gazing); and factor 5, stressful holding (defined by stress musculature, interfering touches, and short holds). For the present report, factor scores were generated for the total sample derived from the weightings obtained in the original factor analysis. In addition, three infant behaviors, nondistress vocalization, fuss–cry, and duration of awake time, were also analyzed.

The factor scores of the infants in the brief and long-fixation groups were compared with 2 × 2 (sex × fixation group) analyses of variance (Sigman & Beckwith, 1980). To summarize the results, females who showed brief fixations were held more by the care givers, were talked to more, and were involved in somewhat more mutual gazing than female infants who showed long fixation durations. Males who showed brief fixations received more responsive holding and were stressed less motorically. Thus both the males and females who showed brief fixations received more optimal care taking. Whether it was the child's style of behavior that affected the parent or the quality of environmental stimulation that shaped the infant's behavior is impossible to ascertain with this data. The care giver may have responded to the child's behavioral style as manifested in attention, just as she did to factors associated with illness (Beckwith & Cohen, 1978). On the other hand, the infant's style of attention may have been shaped by the care giver's ministrations, affected to some degree by whether the infant had been ill or healthy. The association between previous illness and attention patterns may be attributable to the correlations of both factors with care giving.

There is one other line of evidence which supports this notion. As mentioned previously, the children from families who spoke Spanish tended to be healthier and of longer gestation and to have shorter hospitalizations. Furthermore, the longest fixation durations were shown by some of the healthiest preterm infants of Spanish-speaking families, and the infants from Spanish-speaking families had significantly longer fixation times. Care givers in these families, who were all of low socioeconomic background and frequently recent immigrants living in poor conditions, tended to furnish less optimal care for their children. These infants, then, deprived of much meaningful early stimulation, may have been slow to process visual information. The infants from more advantaged homes who received higher levels of care may have been better able to process the same visual input, despite their prior experience of more severe physical illnesses.

ATTENTION DURATION IN RELATION TO CARE GIVER–INFANT INTERACTION AMONG FULL-TERM INFANTS

The relation between total fixation time and care giver–infant interaction observed 1 month later was also examined for the full-term infants (Sigman & Beckwith, 1980). We expected to find that more attentive infants would receive more optimal care taking based on results from previous studies (Osofsky, 1976; Osofsky & Danzger, 1974). These expectations were confirmed in that full-term infants who looked for longer periods of time at the laboratory stimuli also cried less at home and were talked to more by their care givers. In the case of the full-term infants, the nature of the relationship can be attributed more clearly to the influence of the infant on the care giver. The visual attention assessment was carried out in the hospital before the home environment could have any impact. In summary, among the full-term infants, attentive infants were less irritable 1 month later and elicited more optimal interactions with their care givers. It must be kept in mind that total fixation times were much shorter for this full-term sample than for the preterm group.

VISUAL PREFERENCES IN RELATION TO CARE GIVER–INFANT INTERACTION IN PRETERM INFANTS

Since the preterm infants' attention patterns measured at the expected date of birth were related to environmental factors, the association between visual preferences at 4 months and previous care-giver–infant interaction was examined (Sigman, Cohen, & Forsythe, 1981). We hypothesized that infants who received more optimal care giving at 1 month corrected age would show greater preference for novel stimuli and more interest in social stimuli at 4 months. This hypothesis was supported for the 50 female preterm infants, but not for the male infants. Degree of preference for novelty was correlated with the total amount of social and verbal interaction between care givers and female infants. Furthermore, girls who had spent more time engaged in mutual gazing with their care givers at 1 month showed greater interest in social representations at 4 months. In summary, the infant's visual behaviors in the laboratory were associated with social interactions at home for the females, but not for the males. As noted previously, Rose (1980) has also reported effects of the early environment on novelty preferences measured 6 months later in a sample of preterm infants.

ATTENTION DURATION AND VISUAL PREFERENCES
AS PREDICTORS OF DEVELOPMENTAL OUTCOME _____

By way of introduction to the study of individual differences in preterm infants, I identified two important issues stemming from my earlier research comparing preterm and full-term groups in attention patterns and visual preferences. The first issue was whether the preterm infants who showed attention patterns differing from those of most full-term infants were more affected by the medical and environmental consequences of preterm birth. The results reviewed in the previous pages give somewhat conflicting answers to this question, particularly in regard to medical complications. What seems clearest is that the infant's visual fixation patterns are associated with the care-giving environment, though in different ways for full-term and preterm infants.

The second critical issue was whether attention duration and visual preferences would relate to subsequent development. If early attention patterns reflect stable individual differences either in the infant's self-regulating capacity or in his or her speed of information processing, then such stable qualities might well affect the infant's ability to learn from the environment. Alternatively, infant patterns of attention might shape the care-giving environment so that the child's learning experiences are enhanced or diminished. In either case, individual differences in style of attention might relate to subsequent learning and development. I tested the association between early attention and preferences and later development in the Infant Studies Project with developmental assessments in the second year of life and the Stanford-Binet Intelligence Test at 5 years.

RELATION OF THE TERM ATTENTION DURATION
MEASURE TO 2-YEAR OUTCOME _____

The preterm infants in this sample were administered a number of developmental measures in the second year of life. The Bayley Scale was administered at 18 and 25 months corrected age, while the Gesell Scale was administered at 24 months. In order to determine whether individual assessments of medical complications, behavioral development, or environmental factors were associated with developmental scores, two different approaches were used. First, Pearson product–moment correlations were calculated between the 16 risk scores and the outcome assessments. Second, multivariate regression analyses were used to identify those variables which most effectively predicted outcome.

The term visual attention risk score was significantly correlated with the 18-month Bayley mental scale, but not with the 24-month Gesell score or 25-month Bayley mental score (Sigman et al., 1981). While the visual attention risk score was included in the subset of measures predicting the

24-month Gesell score, it was the fifth measure to be included and added very little to the variance accounted for in the Gesell score (Sigman & Parmelee, 1979).

Although the risk score was not significantly associated with the 25-month Bayley mental score, total fixation time was significantly correlated with both Bayley mental scores. The correlations were very low, but significant ($r = -.23$, $df = 117$, $p < .05$ with the 18-month Bayley mental score and $r = -.20$, $df = 115$, $p < .05$ with the 25-month Bayley mental score). The fact that the correlations were negative indicates that infants who looked at the stimuli for longer periods of time had lower scores on the developmental measures. Thus those infants who showed brief fixations at term were likely to perform better on standard development assessments in the second year of life.

RELATION OF THE VISUAL PREFERENCE MEASURE TO 2-YEAR OUTCOME

In general, very little association was found between the measure of visual preferences administered at 4 months corrected age and developmental scores. The risk score was not correlated with any of the developmental scores and contributed even less to the best subset regression than the term visual attention risk score had contributed. Furthermore, analyses of the individual preference measures were not more productive. Almost all the preterm infants in the sample showed a preference for the complex stimuli and there was not sufficient variability to make this a useful measure. While there was variability among the preterm infants in terms of preference for novelty, the 67 infants who showed this preference did not have 2-year Gesell scores which were significantly different from those of the 23 infants who did not show preference for the novel stimuli. Thus the 4-month visual preference measure was not associated with outcome at 2 years.

RELATION OF THE TERM ATTENTION DURATION MEASURE TO INTELLIGENCE AT 5 YEARS

Of the group of 126 preterm infants followed intensively from birth to age 2 years, 100 returned for follow-up testing at age 5 years (Cohen & Parmelee, in press). At age 5, there were 62 children from English-speaking families, 28 from Spanish-speaking families, and 10 from other cultures.

The subjects lost did not differ significantly from the return group in terms of birth weight, gestational age, length of hospitalization, or socioeconomic factors. The mean birth weight was 1877 and the mean gestational age was 32.9 weeks. The 5-year outcome measure was the Stanford-Binet test. The approaches to data analyses were similar to those used for the 2-year measures; correlations of individual risk scores with IQ scores were calculated, as were multivariate stepwise regression analyses (Sigman, 1982).

The correlation between the term visual attention risk score and intelligence at 5 years was significant ($r = -.29$, $df = 98$, $p < .05$). The direction of the correlation corresponded to that noted at age 2 years. Those infants who looked at the stimuli for longer periods of time had lower intelligence quotients. The relation did not change with the deletion of the data on the three children with cerebral palsy. Furthermore, the relations were similar for both the English and Spanish subgroups, and significant for the English group alone ($r = -.25$, $df = 65$, $p < .05$).

The term visual attention measure was one of the major predictors from the early assessment measures to outcome at age 5 years. In a stepwise regression for the entire sample in which the demographic factors and the 16 risk scores were included, the term visual attention measure was the third variable selected (see Table 13-1). In fact, when the data collected on the three children with cerebral palsy were excluded, only socioeconomic status and the term visual attention measure were selected in the stepwise regression. The fact that this measure still contributed to the prediction of outcome after socioeconomic status had entered the regression indicates that the measure operated independently of the demographic factors. The term visual attention measure was also selected in similar fashion in stepwise regression analyses for the English-speaking sample alone (Cohen & Parmelee, in press).

Table 13-1

Stepwise Regression on Stanford-Binet Scores at Age 5 Years Using the Risk Scores and Demographic Factors as Predictors

Variable	Total Group ($n = 83$)	Without Outlyers	English Group Without Outlyers ($n = 47$)
Socioeconomic status	.16*	.22	.14
Gesell Scale—9 months	.24		.27§
Visual attention—term	.30	.26‡	.21
Manipulative schema—8 months	.33†		

*Numbers shown are the cumulative adjusted R² values given in stepwise fashion.

†$F_{(4,79)} = 11.77$, $p < .05$.

‡$F_{(2,77)} = 14.77$, $p < .05$.

§$F_{(3,45)} = 7.02$, $p < .05$.

RELATION OF THE VISUAL PREFERENCE MEASURE
TO INTELLIGENCE AT 5 YEARS

The visual preference risk score at 4 months did not correlate significantly with intelligence quotient at 5 years, nor was this risk score selected by the stepwise regression analysis. A comparison of the intelligence quotients of children who showed preference for novel stimuli with those who showed no novelty preference was not significant. Thus the novelty preference measure at 4 months showed no association with outcome at 2 or 5 years, a result somewhat at variance with other findings (Fagan & McGrath, 1981; Fagan & Singer, in press). In an extensive series of studies, Fagan and his colleagues have discovered strong relations between early measures of recognition memory and subsequent verbal abilities. Using the preference for novelty paradigm and vocabulary scores at 4 and 7 years of age, the associations between the novelty preference measures and later scores were significant with samples of normal full-term children. The failure in this study to uncover similar associations can be attributed to several methodological differences. First, Fagan used a number of novelty problems at each age and has presented evidence that prediction is more accurate with increasing numbers of test items. This study employed only one novelty preference problem, which may not have been sufficient to identify continuities in performance. Secondly, the novelty preference problem was made quite easy for the infants by the numerous presentations of the "familiar" 24×24 checkerboard first during the complexity series and then during the familiarization trials. Because of the repeated presentations of the familiar stimulus, three-fourths of the infants in this study's sample showed a preference for the novel stimulus. The ease of the novelty problem may have decreased its sensitivity as a measure of individual differences, which may account for the lack of predictive power.

In this light, recent preliminary analyses indicate that there was one component of the 4-month attention measure that did relate to outcome. As mentioned previously, the infant was shown the 24×24 checkerboard for four 20-sec trials as part of the complexity series. On each trial, one of the two simpler patterns was paired with the 24×24 checkerboard. Although all the infants tended to look far more at the 24×24 checkerboard than at the simpler ones, by the final trial some infants continued to show a long duration of fixation to the 24×24 checkerboard while other infants ignored both patterns. The length of fixation of the 24×24 checkerboard by the fourth exposure was negatively correlated with the Stanford-Binet Score at 5 years ($r = -.25$, $df = 89$, $p < .05$). Thus preterm infants who continued to look at this checkerboard after 1 min of exposure performed less well on the outcome measure.

In summary, significant negative relations were discovered between duration of fixation of a repeated pattern at term and at 4 months corrected age and intelligence at 5 years. In this regard, there is evidence that length of fixation to familiar stimuli is a sensitive measure of individual differences. Fagan and Singer (in press) reported no relations between rate of habituation and subsequent outcome. The only predictive study measuring habituation and response recovery to novel visual stimuli has somewhat ambiguous results. Lewis and Brooks-Gunn (1981) reported a significant relation between rate of response decrement and the Bayley score for one sample, but not for a second sample, while response recovery was associated with the Bayley score for both samples.

DISCUSSION

The first question raised in this chapter was whether the infant who examines stimuli for long periods of time is analyzing the world carefully or is slower to take in visual input or regulate his or her own attention processes. The research to date provides only a partial answer. For the preterm infants, and with moderately salient stimuli, long durations of attention are characteristic of children who will be less intellectually competent in the early years of school. However, I think that I have illuminated only a portion of the relation between attention duration and outcome (see Fig. 13-2).

The model that I would propose is a curvilinear model like the optimal

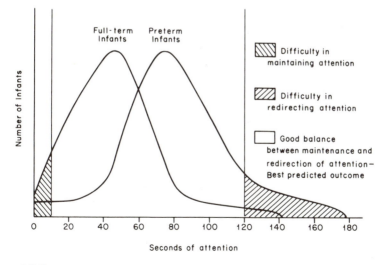

Figure 13-2
Hypothetical model for the relation between attention duration to moderately interesting stimuli and cognitive outcome in children born preterm and full-term.

arousal models of earlier times. Despite the lack of evidence from my studies, it does seem that infants need to spend a portion of time attending to visual stimuli in order to learn about their environment. Those infants who cannot maintain their attention to salient stimuli for even brief periods must be handicapped if this behavior is maintained. Perhaps the children with attention deficit disorders include some who are unable to sustain attention even briefly to important events from early on in life. This end of the spectrum may not have been uncovered in my research because of the stimuli employed. While checkerboards are moderately interesting to term infants, they are only moderately interesting. Some of the infants may have shown good judgment in not paying attention to them. However, there undoubtably are more complex, more arresting stimuli which should elicit a modicum of attention from all infants.

Within this model, two different curves may exist at term date. The curve for preterm infants may be somewhat removed from that for full-term infants. While these differences seem to exist early in life, the evidence is that they decline with age.

Another question left unanswered is the basis for these differences in attention duration. I have suggested that variations in attention durations may reflect the speed of encoding information and that this may be delayed in some preterm infants. However, another interpretation is that the duration of attention may reflect self-regulation of arousal mechanisms. Arthur Parmelee, Leila Beckwith, Sarale Cohen, & I are currently examining the association between measures of arousal in sleep–wake patterns and visual attention in order to clarify this issue.

The second set of questions raised in the beginning of the chapter concerned the relation between individual differences in infant attention patterns and environmental elicitors and responses. Again, the answers to these questions are incomplete. Full-term infants do seem to shape their caregiving environment either through their attention patterns or attendant arousal patterns. Attentive full-term infants in the hospital cry less at home and are talked to more by their mothers.

Associations between the fixation durations of the preterm infants and care giver behaviors have been identified, but the direction of effects is still unclear. Since the preterm infants in this study had been home for about 1 month before the laboratory assessment, their attention patterns may have already been shaped by the care-giving environment. On the other hand, their own characteristics may have influenced the nature of interactions. In order to delineate these relations more clearly, Peter Mundy and I, in collaboration with Leila Beckwith and Sarale Cohen, are beginning a study in which attention patterns will be examined before discharge from the hospital, as well as at 40 weeks conceptional age. Observations of care-giver–infant interaction will be made at 44 weeks conceptional age. These data may allow us to determine the direction of effects between child and care-giver behaviors.

The final issue concerns the nature of the continuity we have found between early infant behavior and subsequent child intelligence. Fagan and Singer (in press) suggested that the continuity they have discovered reveals a continuity in the process tapped by infant recognition memory tasks and vocabulary tests in childhood. Lewis and Brooks-Gunn (1981) have proposed that the continuity might be in rate of development through successive discontinuous states. In one of our previous chapters, we suggested that the continuity might stem from stabilities in the care-giving environment (Sigman & Parmelee, 1979). This conjecture was based in part on the very strong relations between the early care-giving environment and 2-year outcome revealed by our data analyses (Cohen & Beckwith, 1979; Sigman & Parmelee, 1979). However, the relationship between the early care-giving environment and intelligence at age 5 is not so strong (Beckwith & Cohen, in press; Cohen & Parmelee, (in press). Furthermore, the term visual attention measure seems to predict across different socioeconomic and cultural backgrounds. For these reasons, I am now more inclined to see the continuity as stability within the infant as much as within the care-giving environment. Whatever the nature of the origins, individual differences in infant attention seem to have significance for subsequent child development.

REFERENCES

Beckwith, L., & Cohen, S. E. Preterm birth: Hazardous obstetrical and postnatal events as related to caregiver–infant behavior. *Infant Behavior and Development*, 1978, *1*, 403–411.

Beckwith, L., & Cohen, S. E. Home environment and cognitive competence in preterm children in the first five years. In A. W. Gottfried (Ed.), *Home environment and early mental development*. New York: Academic, in press.

Beckwith, L., Cohen, S. E., Kopp, C. B., Parmelee, A. H., & Marcy, T. G. Caregiver–infant interaction and early cognitive development in preterm infants. *Child Development*, 1976, *47*, 579–587.

Brennan, W. N., Ames, E. W., & Moore, R. W. Age differences in infant's attention to patterns of different complexities. *Science*, 1966, *151*, 354–356.

Caron, A. J., & Caron, R. F. Processing of relational information as an index of infant risk. In S. L. Friedman & M. Sigman (Eds.), *Preterm birth and psychological development*. New York: Academic, 1981.

Cohen, S. E., & Beckwith, L. Preterm infant interaction with the caregiver in the first year of life and competence at age two. *Child Development*, 1979, *50*, 767–766.

Cohen, S. E., & Parmelee, A. H. Prediction of five year Stanford-Binet scores in preterm infants. *Child Development*, in press.

Fagan, J. F., Fantz, R. L., & Miranda, S. B. *Infants' attention to novel stimuli as a function of postnatal and conceptional age.* Paper presented at the meeting of the Society for Research in Child Development, Minneapolis, April 4, 1971.

Fagan, J. F., & McGrath, S. K. Infant recognition memory and later intelligence. *Intelligence*, 1981, *5*, 121–130.

Fagan, J. F., & Singer, L. T. Infant recognition memory as a measure of intelligence. In L. P. Lipsitt (Ed.), *Advances in infancy research* (Vol. 2). Hillsdale, N.J.: Ablex, in press.

Fantz, R. Visual experience in infants: Decreased attention to familiar patterns relative to novel ones. *Science*, 1965, *146*, 668–670.

Fantz, R. L., & Fagan, J. F. Visual attention to size and number of pattern details by term and preterm infants during the first six months. *Child Development*, 1975, *46*, 3–18.

Fantz, R. L., Fagan, J. F., & Miranda, S. B. Early visual selectivity as a function of pattern variables, previous exposure, age from birth and conception, and expected cognitive deficit. In L. B. Cohen & P. Salapatek (Eds.), *Infant perception: From sensation to cognition* (Vol. 1). New York: Academic, 1976.

Fantz, R. L., & Nevis, S. The predictive value of changes in visual preference in early infancy. In J. Hellmuth (Ed.), *The exceptional infant* (Vol. 1). Seattle: Special Child Publications, 1967.

Haaf, R. A., & Bell, R. O. A facial dimension in visual discrimination by human infants. *Child Development*, 1964, *38*, 893–899.

Hershenson, M. Visual discrimination in the human newborn. *Journal of Comparative and Physiological Psychology*, 1964, *58*, 270–276.

Karmel, B. The effect of age, complexity, and amount of contour on pattern preferences in human infants. *Journal of Experimental Child Psychology*, 1969, *7*, 339–354.

Knobloch, H., & Pasamanick, B. Prospective studies on the epidemiology of reproductive casualty: Methods, findings and some implications. *Merrill-Palmer Quarterly*, 1966, *12*, 27–43.

Kopp, C. B., Sigman, M., Parmelee, A. H., & Jeffrey, W. E. Neurological organization and visual fixation in infants at 40 weeks conceptional age. *Developmental Psychobiology*, 1975, *8*, 165–170.

Lewis, M., & Brooks-Gunn, J. Visual attention at three months as a predictor of cognitive functioning at two years of age. *Intelligence*, 1981, *5*, 131–140.

Lewis, M., Goldberg, S., & Campbell, H. A. A developmental study of information processing within the first three years of life: Response decrement to a redundant signal. *Monographs of the Society for Research in Child Development*, 1969, *34*.

McCall, R. B., & Kagan, J. Parameters of attention in the infant. *Child Development*, 1967, *38*, 938–952.

Miranda, S. B., & Fantz, R. L. Recognition memory in Down's syndrome and normal infants. *Child Development*, 1974, *45*, 651–660.

Olsen, G. M., & Sherman, T. Attention, learning, and memory in infants. In M. Haith & J. Campos (Eds.), *Manual of child psychology* (Vol. 2). New York: Wiley, in press.

Osofsky, J. B. Neonatal characteristics and mother–infant interaction in two observational situations. *Child Development*, 1967, *47*, 1138–1147.

Osofsky, J. B., & Danziger, B. Relationships between neonatal characteristics and mother–infant interaction. *Developmental Psychology*, 1974, *10*, 124–130.

Parmelee, A. H., Kopp, C. B., & Sigman, M. Selection of developmental assessment techniques for infants at risk. *Merrill-Palmer Quarterly*, 1976, *22*, 177–199.

Rose, S. A. Enhancing visual recognition memory in preterm infants. *Developmental Psychology*, 1980, *16*, 85–92.

Rose, S. A., Gottfried, A. W., & Bridger, W. H. Effects of haptic cues on visual recognition memory in full-term and preterm infants. *Infant Behavior and Development*, 1979, *2*, 55–67.

Sigman, M. Early development of preterm and full-term infants: Exploratory behavior in eight-month-olds. *Child Development*, 1976, *47*, 606–612.

Sigman, M. *The contribution of infant behavioral responses to prediction of intelligence at age five years*. Paper presented at the Third International Conference on Infant Studies, Austin, Texas, March 1982.

Sigman, M., & Beckwith, L. Infant visual attentiveness in relation to caregiver-infant interaction and developmental outcome. *Infant Behavior and Development*, 1980, *3*, 141–154.

Sigman, M., Cohen, S. E., & Forsythe, A. B. The relation of early infant measures to later development. In S. L. Friedman & M. Sigman (Eds.), *Preterm birth and psychological development*. New York: Academic, 1981.

Sigman, M., Kopp, C. B., Littman, B., & Parmelee, A. H. Infant visual attentiveness in relation to birth condition. *Developmental Psychology*, 1977, *13*, 431–437.

Sigman, M., Kopp, C. B., Parmelee, A. H., & Jeffrey, W. E. Visual attention and neurological organization in neonates. *Child Development*, 1973, *44*, 461–466.

Sigman, M., & Parmelee, A. H. Visual preferences of four-month-old premature and full-term infants. *Child Development*, 1974, *45*, 959–965.

Sigman, M., & Parmelee, A. H. Longitudinal evaluation of the preterm infant. In T. M. Field, A. M. Sostek, S. Goldberg, & H. H. Shuman (Eds.), *Infants born at risk*. New York: Spectrum, 1979.

Thoman, E. B., Acebo, C., Dreyer, C. A., Becker, P. T., & Freese, M. P. Individuality in the interactive process. In E. B. Thoman (Ed.), *Origins of the infant's social responsiveness*. Hillsdale, N.J.: Lawrence Erlbaum, 1977.

Wetherford, M. J., & Cohen, L. B. Developmental changes in infant visual preferences for novelty and familiarity. *Child Development*, 1973, *74*, 418–424.

14

The Prediction of Possible Learning Disabilities in Preterm and Full-Term Children

Linda S. Siegel

One of the primary areas of importance in the field of learning disabilities is the early detection of children who manifest learning problems. Because preterm children may be at risk for developmental problems, including learning disabilities, the present study is a report on an attempt to detect the presence of possible learning disabilities in preterm and full-term children. While there are a number of studies describing subsequent developmental problems in very low birthweight children (see Hunt, 1981, for a summary of the relevant studies), the incidence of specific learning disabilities, independent of general deficits, has typically not been examined. However, there are some suggestive data. Hunt (1981) has noted a higher incidence of visual–motor problems independent of IQ scores in preterm children at 4–8 years. Similar findings have been noted by Taub, Goldstein, and Caputo (1977) for 7- to 9-year-old children with birth weights below 2500 g. As

The author wishes to thank Kathy Deyo, Lorraine Hoult, Sheila McTavish, and Priyanthy Weerasekera for assistance with the data collection and analyses, and Richard A. Morton for assistance with the computer programming. This research was partially supported by Ontario Mental Health Foundation Grants Nos. 558, 732/77-79, and 800/80-82, and was aided by Social and Behavioural Sciences Grant No. 12-59 from the March of Dimes Birth Defects Foundation. Tiffany Field made many helpful suggestions on this chapter. The author wishes to thank the Special Enquiries and Grievance Committee of the McMaster University Faculty Association without whose assistance it would have been impossible to complete this project.

preterm children may be at significant risk for learning disabilities, it would seem important to predict these disabilities as early as possible so that remedial measures can be instituted.

However, attempts at the prediction of learning disabilities have typically been concentrated at the point at which the children enter school or in the early grades. These studies have been reviewed by Mercer (1979). The general finding is that it has not been possible to predict the outcome for an individual child. One notable exception and a reasonably successful system is that of Satz and his associates, in which children who subsequently will develop serious reading disabilities can be detected at age 5 with a reasonable degree of success (Fletcher & Satz, 1980; Satz & Friel, 1973, pp. 79–98, 1974; Satz, Friel, & Goebel, 1975).

As part of a longitudinal study of the development of preterm and full-term infants, the Satz battery of tests was administered when the children were 5 years old. The child's performance on the Satz battery was used as the measure of possible learning disabilities. On the basis of previous findings (Siegel, 1979, 1981, 1982a, b; Siegel, Saigal, Rosenbaum, Morton, Young, Berenbaum, & Stoskopf, 1982) of the value of both infant tests and a risk index for predicting language and cognitive development and detecting children whose development would be subsequently delayed, it was expected that the infant tests and risk index would show some relation with performance on the Satz battery. The present study is an attempt to examine that hypothesis.

METHOD

The subjects were part of a longitudinal study of the development of preterm and full-term infants. A total of 42 full-term and 44 preterm infants were administered the Satz battery at 5 years. The characteristics of the groups were as follows: males, 59 percent full-term, 50 percent preterm; firstborn, 36 percent full-term, 40 percent preterm; Hollingshead social classes 1–2, 33 percent full-term, 20 percent preterm; birth weight, full-term $\overline{X}$ = 3394 g, preterm $\overline{X}$ = 1236 g; gestational age, full-term $\overline{X}$ = 40 weeks, preterm $\overline{X}$ = 30.3 weeks. The Satz abbreviated battery (described in detail in Satz & Friel, 1973, 1974) included the following tests: the Peabody Picture Vocabulary Test, the Beery Developmental Test of Visual–Motor Integration, recognition discrimination, finger localization, and alphabet recitation. Prior to that time the infants were administered the following tests: Bayley Scales of Infant Development at 4, 8, 12, 18, and 24 months; Uzgiris–Hunt scales at 4, 8, 12, and 18 months; the Reynell Scales of Language Development (1969) at 2, 3, and 4 years; and the Stanford-Binet Intelligence Scale (1973) at 3 years.

Infant Tests

Bayley Scales

The Bayley Scales consist of two parts, a mental development index (MDI), which measures cognitive, language, and perceptual–motor functions, and a psychomotor development index (PDI), which measures gross and fine motor skills.

Kohen–Raz Scoring of the Bayley Scales

The Kohen-Raz (1967) scoring of the Bayley was used. This system separates the Bayley MDI score into a set of subscales: eye–hand coordination (e.g., reaches for dangling ring, puts three or more cubes in cup), manipulation (e.g., simple play with rattle, fingers holes in peg board), conceptual relations (e.g., uncovers toy, exploitive paper play), imitation and comprehension (e.g., responds to verbal request, imitates crayon strokes), vocalization-social (e.g., repeats performance, says "da-da" or equivalent).

The Uzgiris–Hunt Scale

This consists of tests of cognitive capacities of infants based on Piagetian theory and is described in Uzgiris and Hunt (1975). The following scales were used: (1) schemes, a test of the type of variety of activities that a child exhibits with familiar objects (e.g., car or doll); (2) visual pursuit and object permanence, a test of the child's ability to visually and/or manually search for hidden objects; (3) means–end thinking, the extent to which a child tries to influence the environment and to solve problems by, for example, using tools such as a stick to reach an object beyond immediate reach; (4) concepts of space, the child's capacity to understand containers and recognize obstacles; (5) gestural imitation, the child's ability to imitate familiar (e.g., stirring a spoon in a cup) and unfamiliar (e.g., scratching a surface) gestures; (6) vocal imitation, the child's ability to imitate familiar and unfamiliar words; and (7) causality, the child's ability to understand and try to activate some environmental event (e.g., pulling a string to make a music box work).

The Satz Battery

The Peabody Picture Vocabulary Test (PPVT). This is a vocabulary test in which the child must identify which of four pictures depicts a given word. Results are typically reported in terms of IQ scores.

The Beery Developmental Test of Visual-Motor Integration (VMI). For this test (Beery, 1967) the child has to copy an increasingly difficult series of geometric forms. Performance is compared with age norms and an IQ equivalent can be calculated based on the child's chronological age.

Recognition discrimination.   For this test the child has to select which of four alternatives matches the target stimulus. Performance is not timed and scores are the number of correct matches.

Alphabet recitation.   The child is asked to recite the alphabet. A hint can be given, for example, "say *a, b, c,* and what comes next." Performance scores are the number of letters named correctly.

Finger localization.   In this study's version of the task, rather than having the child blindfolded, as Satz and co-workers did, the child's hand was hidden through holes in a box and the fingers were lightly tapped with a paper clip in random order. The child had to point to the finger that was touched. There are 20 trials. The first 10 trials involve touching fingers on the right and left hands individually. The next 10 trials involve touching two fingers at the same time, one on each hand. The two fingers that are touched are always at different positions, for example, left ring finger and right middle finger. Performance scores are the number of correct identifications. This procedure was equivalent to task 1 of the finger localization task of the Satz battery.

Correction for Prematurity

As the children were administered the various tests at a particular chronological age, test scores, uncorrected for prematurity, were always used. In addition, corrected scores could be calculated for many of the tests.

Risk Index Variables

A risk index composed of reproductive, perinatal, and demographic variables was used for each child. Each variable was considered individually. A cumulative or weighted score was not used. The reproductive variables were birth order (gravidity), the number of cigarettes the mother smoked during pregnancy (none, less than 10, 10–20, over 20 cigarettes per day), and the number of previous spontaneous abortions. The perinatal variables included birth weight, 1- and 5-min Apgar scores, and, for the preterm infants, gestational age, severity of respiratory distress (RDS), birth asphyxia, and apnea. The following definitions for RDS were used: (1) severe, assisted ventilation, X-ray evidence of RDS, and/or O_2 levels above 80 percent; (2) moderate, assisted ventilation, continuous positive airway pressure (CPAP), and/or O_2 levels between 40 and 80 percent, and (3) mild, O_2 levels below 40 percent. For birth asphyxia, a 1-min Apgar score of less than 5 was defined as asphyxia. For apnea, a measure of the number of days in which apneic spells occurred was used, with periods of apnea greater than

20 sec. Socioeconomic status (Hollingshead), sex, and maternal and paternal educational levels were also included in the analyses.

RESULTS _____

Preterm and Full-Term Test Scores at 5 Years _____

The mean scores of the preterm and full-term children on the tests of the Satz battery at 5 years are shown in Table 14-1. All statistical comparisons are based on t tests. As it was possible to correct the PPVT and Beery VMI scores for the degree of prematurity because age norms are available for those tests, the corrected scores are included also. As can be seen from Table 14-1, preterm and full-term infants did not differ on the PPVT, a measure of vocabulary or single-word comprehension. They did, however, differ significantly on the Beery VMI, recognition discrimination,

Table 14-1 _____

Means and Standard Deviations for the Preterm and Full-Term Groups on the Tests of the Satz Battery at 5 Years

	Full-Term	Preterm
Uncorrected PPVT IQ		
X̄	111.8	107.1
SD	14.3	13.9
Corrected PPVT IQ		
X̄	111.8	107.3
SD	14.3	14.1
Uncorrected Beery VMI IQ		
X̄	102.0	89.6‡
SD	12.7	17.7
Corrected Beery VMI IQ		
X̄	102.0	93.7†
SD	12.7	12.4
Recognition discrimination		
X̄	12.9	3.4‡
SD	10.2	2.7
Alphabet recitation		
X̄	23.7	20.9*
SD	5.1	7.9
Finger localization		
X̄	18.4	17.7
SD	2.0	3.0

*$p < .05$.
†$p < .01$.
‡$p < .001$.

and the alphabet recitation task. The Beery VMI and recognition discrimination tasks involve perceptual–motor processes and attention. The lack of differences in finger localization probably represents a ceiling effect for this task.

A cutoff score was used which separated the lowest 10 percent (approximately) of the full-term group from the remaining full-term group. The percentages of full-term and preterm children with scores below this cutoff point are shown in Table 14-2. Statistical comparisons are based on chi-square tests. These results parallel those in Table 14-1 and provide further evidence for the differences between the preterm and full-term groups in perceptual–motor functioning. Even though the preterm and full-term groups were equivalent on a task involving language comprehension (PPVT), significantly more preterm children were delayed on the Beery VMI and the alphabet recitation task, and the difference between the groups on the recognition discrimination task did not reach conventional levels of statistical significance. These data support the idea that the differences between preterm and full-term children are more likely to be found in the perceptual–motor than in the language comprehension areas.

Correlations of Infant Test Scores with the Satz Battery

The correlations of the infant tests with the Satz battery are shown in Tables 14-3–14-7. For the purposes of simplicity, the correlations reported are for the preterm and full-term children together. There were few significant differences between the correlations for the preterm and full-term groups, so the combined correlations were used. Also, the correlations represent the relation between the scores not corrected for degree of prematurity. The correlations with the corrected scores were typically lower, although not significantly so. The infant tests were significantly correlated with the tests of the Satz battery, particularly the PPVT, the Beery VMI, and recognition discrimination.

As can be seen from Tables 14-3–14-7, scores on the infant tests are moderately correlated with the outcome measures. Many of the correlations with the Beery VMI were significant. The Beery test is a reasonably accurate measure of the perceptual–motor skills, which are probably related to maturation of the nervous system. It may be that the infant tests are also probably a measure of the maturation of the nervous system, at least in the first year of life. Therefore the relation between the infant tests and the Beery VMI may be a reflection of continuities in the development of the nervous system. In support of this position, Murphy and Liden (1982) have found strong relations between measures of neurological maturation and means–end thinking and the object concept in infants. The infant tests, though on the surface apparently very different, may also be measuring the

Table 14-2

Percentage of Children in Each Group with Scores in the Delayed Range

	Full-Term	Preterm
PPVT IQ < 90 ‡	9.3	9.5
VMI IQ < 90 §	9.3	47.7†
Alphabet recitation < 20	9.8	28.6*
Recognition discrimination < 9	11.6	25.0″
Finger localization < 16	9.5	10.5

*$p < .05$.
†$p < .001$.
‡The percentages were the same for both the corrected and uncorrected scores.
§If the corrected score was used, 31.8 percent of the preterm children were delayed. The difference between preterm and full-term children was significant ($p < .01$).
″$.05 < p < .10$.

Table 14-3

Correlations of Infant Tests with the Beery Visual–Motor Integration IQ at 5 Years

	Time of Administration (Months)				
	4	8	12	18	24
Bayley					
MDI	.43‡	.30†	.44‡	.36†	.36†
PDI	.43‡	.43‡	.34†	NS§	.42‡
Kohen–Raz					
Eye–hand coordination	.28†	.27†	.34†	.24*	NS
Manipulation	.40‡	.29†	NS	NS	CC″
Conceptual abilities	NS	.40‡	.40‡	NS	CC
Imitation–comprehension	CC	NS	.39‡	.33†	.37‡
Vocalization–social	CC	.25*	.22*	NS	.32†
Uzgiris–Hunt					
Schemes	.42‡	NS	NS	NS	
Object relations	.26*	.26*	.24*	NS	
Means–end thinking	.38‡	.46‡	NS	NS	
Space	.49‡	.44‡	.33†	.29†	
Gestural imitation	NS	NS	.24*	NS	
Vocal imitation	.33†	.34†	NS	NS	
Total	.44‡	.41‡	.33†	NS	

*$p < .05$.
†$p < .01$.
‡$p < .001$.
§NS, not significant.
″CC, cannot calculate.

Table 14-4

Correlations of the Infant Tests with the Peabody Picture Vocabulary IQ at 5 Years

	Time of Administration (Months)		
	12	18	24
Bayley			
MDI	.25*	.27*	.43‡
PDI	.25*	.24*	NS§
Kohen-Raz			
Eye–hand coordination	.28†	NS	NS
Manipulation	.23*	NS	CC″
Conceptual abilities	.24*	NS	CC
Imitation–comprehension	NS	.30†	.39‡
Vocalization-social	NS	NS	.40‡
Uzgiris–Hunt			
Schemes	.25*	NS	
Object relations	.41‡	.30†	
Vocal imitation	.27*	NS	
Total	.31†	.25*	

*$p < .05$.
†$p < .01$.
‡$p < .001$.
§NS, not significant.
″CC, cannot calculate.

developmental level of the same type of skills. The correlations with recognition discrimination, a measure of attention and perceptual skills, were also significant, indicating possible continuities in the development of the nervous system.

The infant tests at 4 and 8 months were not significantly correlated with the PPVT IQ score. At 12, 18, and 24 months some of the correlations were significant, particularly at 24 months. The Bayley MDI score at 24 months has a .43 correlation ($p < .001$) with the PPVT IQ at 5 years. While the magnitude of the correlations was lower, a similar pattern was found with the alphabet recitation task. These are both measures of verbal abilities and obviously infant tests are not detecting significant differences in verbal abilities in the first year of life. While there were very few significant correlations with the finger localization task, it is worth noting that most of the children had reached ceiling on this task.

The correlations followed the pattern noted previously (Siegel, 1979, 1981, 1982a). There appears to be a sequence in which the infant tests and subtests become significantly correlated with the outcome variables. The perceptual items of the Bayley Scale (eye–hand coordination, manipulation)

Table 14-5

Correlations of Infant Tests with Recognition Discrimination at 5 Years

	Time of Administration (Months)				
	4	8	12	18	24
Bayley					
MDI	NS§	.34†	.33†	.32†	.34†
PDI	.32†	.33†	.38‡	NS	NS
Kohen–Raz					
Eye–hand coordination	.30†	.27*	.37‡	NS	NS
Manipulation	.33†	.30†	.25*	NS	CC″
Conceptual abilities	NS	.28†	.40‡	NS	CC
Imitation–comprehension	CC	NS	.26†	NS	.28†
Vocalization–social	CC	.30†	NS	NS	.27*
Uzgiris–Hunt					
Schemes	.43‡	.22*	.26*	NS	
Object relations	.40‡	NS	NS	.24*	
Means–end thinking	.32†	.29†	NS	NS	
Space	.48‡	.30†	.39‡	NS	
Gestural imitation	NS	.36‡	NS	NS	
Vocal imitation	.37‡	.45‡	NS	NS	
Total	.47‡	.29†	.29*	NS	

*p < .05.
†p < .01.
‡p < .001.
§NS, not significant.
″CC, cannot calculate.

Table 14-6

Correlations of Infant Tests with Alphabet Recitation at 5 Years

	Time of Administration (Months)				
	4	8	12	18	24
Bayley					
MDI	NS‡	NS	NS	NS	29†
PDI	NS	.25*	.27*	NS	NS
Kohen–Raz					
Eye–hand coordination	.24*	NS	NS	NS	.27*
Manipulation	.28†	NS	NS	NS	CC§
Conceptual abilities	NS‡	NS	.23*	NS	CC
Imitation–comprehension	CC	NS	NS	.31†	.31†
Vocalization–social	CC	NS	NS	.30†	.26*
Uzgiris–Hunt					
Object relations	NS	NS	NS	.27*	
Means–end thinking	.25*	NS	NS	NS	
Space Concepts	.25*	NS	NS	NS	
Gestural imitation	NS	.23*	NS	.27*	
Total	.25*	NS	NS	.32†	

*p < .05.
†p < .01.
‡NS, not significant.
§CC, cannot calculate.

Table 14-7

Correlations of Infant Tests with Finger Localization at 5 Years

	Time of Administration (Months)			
	4	8	12	24
Bayley				
MDI	NS‡	NS	NS	.28*
Kohen–Raz				
Conceptual abilities	NS	.27*	NS	NS
Imitation–comprehension	CC§	NS	.29†	.27*
Uzgiris–Hunt				
Space concepts	.26*	.27*	NS	

*$p < .05$.
†$p < .01$.
‡NS, not significant.
§CC, cannot calculate.

were likely to be correlated early in development, somewhat later cognitive items (conceptual abilities) become correlated, and finally the language items (imitation–comprehension and vocalization-social) at the end of the first year and throughout the second year are significantly correlated with the Satz battery.

Correlations of the 3-Year Tests with the Satz Battery

The correlations of the Reynell and Stanford-Binet with the tests of Satz battery are shown in Table 14-8. The Reynell and the Stanford-Binet were significantly correlated with the Beery VMI and PPVT scores; the correlations with the other parts of the Satz were only significant in some cases. Several relations are worth noting: (1) the correlations between language comprehension measures (PPVT and Reynell) are high; (2) the 3-year Stanford-Binet, which includes some perceptual–motor items, is highly correlated with the Beery VMI; and (3) recognition discrimination and finger localization are correlated with language measures, although they are perceptual tasks.

Comparison of the Delayed and Nondelayed Children

While the correlations between the infant tests and the Satz battery tests were moderately high and statistically significant, they do not say much about the development of an individual child. A more important question is whether it was possible to predict the outcome for an individual. Several approaches to this question were used.

First of all, we used the cutoff scores indicated in Table 14-2 and con-

Table 14-8

Correlations of the Reynell Scales and the Stanford-Binet with the Satz Battery Tests at 5 Years

	PPVT	Beery VMI	Recognition Discrimination	Finger Localization	Alphabet Recitation
			2 Years		
Reynell					
Comprehension	.42‡	.35†	.34†	.38†	NS§
Expression	.48‡	.43‡	.31†	NS	.25*
			3 Years		
Comprehension	.49‡	.39‡	NS	.33†	NS
Expression	.41‡	.36†	NS	NS	NS
			4 Years		
Comprehension	.65‡	.37†	.24*	NS	.43‡
Expression	.46‡	.40‡	.32†	NS	.30†
			3 Years		
Stanford-Binet	.39†	.46‡	.31†	.32†	NS

*$p < .05$.
†$p < .01$.
‡$p < .001$.
§NS, not significant.

sidered children who fell below these cutoff scores as delayed. Obviously, only continued follow-up of these children into the early elementary grades will determine if these scores are meaningful in terms of learning disabilities. But on the basis of the data from the studies of Satz et al., it seems reasonably likely that these tests are predictive of subsequent learning disabilities. The scores on the infant tests (to 3 years inclusive) of the children who were delayed on each measure were compared to the children who were not delayed.

The infant test scores of the children who were delayed on the PPVT and those who were not are shown in Table 14-9. None of the 4-, 8-, or 18-month measures differentiated these groups. The 4- and 8-month tests do not have significant language components. The 2- and 3-year language measures did discriminate between the delayed and nondelayed children on the PPVT.

The infant test scores of the delayed and nondelayed children on the Beery VMI at 5 years are shown in Tables 14-10 and 14-11. As can be seen, many tests differentiated these groups. As noted previously, the common denominator may be that both measure maturation of the nervous system, and to the extent that the rate of nervous system development is predictable for an individual child, scores at one point in time may be predictable from an earlier point.

Table 14-9

Comparison of the Infant Test Scores of the Delayed and Nondelayed
Children on the PPVT at 5 Years

	Delayed	Nondelayed
12 Months		
Uzgiris–Hunt		
Schemes	7.4	9.3†
Object concept	1.6	5.4*
Kohen-Raz		
Manipulation	7.6	8.4*
2 Years		
Kohen-Raz		
Imitation-comprehension	11.8	13.7*
Reynell		
Expression	−1.5	−0.3*
3 Years		
Reynell		
Comprehension	−0.8	0.6*
Expression	−1.3	−0.3†

*$p < .05$.
†$p < .01$.

The tests which discriminated the delayed and nondelayed groups on the other tests of the Satz battery are shown in Tables 14-12 and 14-13. None of the tests discriminated those delayed on finger localization, probably because of ceiling effects on this task. The space concepts subtest on the Uzgiris–Hunt consistently differentiated those who were to become delayed on the recognition discrimination, and the language measures distinguished those who were to become delayed on the alphabet recitation. The early tests appear to be related to the significant components of either language (alphabet recitation) or perceptual functioning (recognition discrimination).

Prediction of Delayed Development Using a Risk Index

We also examined the extent to which a risk index (Siegel, 1982b; Siegel et al. 1982) would be related to the outcome variables. Some of these results are shown in Table 14-14. With some exceptions, the environmental-demographic variables are related to the language measure, while the perinatal and reproduction variables are related to the perceptual–motor measures.

The results of linear multiple discriminant function analyses for discriminating the delayed from the nondelayed children (see Table 14-2)

Table 14-10

Comparison of the Infant Test Scores of Delayed and Nondelayed 5-Year-Olds on the Beery Visual–Motor Integration Test

| | Time of Administration of Infant Tests | | | | | |
| | 4 Months | | 8 Months | | 12 Months | |
	Delayed	Nondelayed	Delayed	Nondelayed	Delayed	Nondelayed
Bayley						
MDI	73.5	92.9†	80.9	105.5†	76.6	96.2‡
PDI	81.4	99.5‡	68.6	92.9‡	73.9	86.6*
Kohen–Raz						
Eye–hand coordination	1.0	2.6†	7.2	8.9‡	10.7	12.0†
Manipulation	0.8	2.6‡	5.9	7.0†	7.9	8.5*
Conceptual abilities			3.7	5.4‡	6.6	8.2‡
Imitation–comprehension			0.4	1.3†	3.3	5.0‡
Vocalization–social			0.9	1.8†		
Uzgiris–Hunt						
Schemes	1.9	3.6‡				
Object concept	1.4	2.9‡	6.0	10.3*		
Means–end relations	1.7	3.2†	3.8	6.7‡		
Space concept	2.0	4.5‡	1.7	4.1‡	1.0	1.6*
Vocal imitation	1.9	2.7†	3.2	4.8‡		
Gestural imitation			1.3	2.3*	2.6	4.1‡
Total			22.9	35.8‡	23.1	27.4*

*$p < .05$.
†$p < .01$.
‡$p < .001$.

Table 14-11

Comparison of the Infant Test Scores of Delayed and Nondelayed
5-Year-Olds on the Beery Visual–Motor Integration Test

	Delayed	Nondelayed
18 Months		
Bayley		
MDI	82.6	94.1†
2 Years		
Kohen–Raz		
Eye-hand coordination	18.8	19.3†
Imitation–comprehension	12.7	13.8*
Vocalization	10.6	11.5*
3 Years		
Uzgiris–Hunt		
Space concepts	5.6	6.5†
Reynell		
Comprehension	0.0	0.7*
Expression	−0.8	−0.1*
Stanford-Binet	87.4	96.8†

*$p < .05$.
†$p < .01$.

Table 14-12

Comparison of the Infant Test Scores of the Delayed and Nondelayed
Children on Recognition Discrimination at 5 Years

	Delayed	Nondelayed
4 Months		
Uzgiris–Hunt		
Object concept	0.9	2.7*
Vocal imitation	1.1	2.7‡
Total	8.4	15.9*
8 Months		
Bayley		
MDI	80.2	98.7*
Uzgiris–Hunt		
Space concepts	1.7	3.6*
Vocal imitation	2.6	4.5†
12 Months		
Space concepts	0.5	1.6*
18 Months		
Space concepts	5.3	6.4*
3 Years		
Reynell		
Comprehension	10.8	11.7†

*$p < .05$.
†$p < .01$.
‡$p < .001$.

Table 14-13

Comparison of the Infant Test Scores of Delayed and Nondelayed
Children on Alphabet Recitation at 5 Years

	Delayed	Nondelayed
4 Months		
Uzgiris–Hunt		
Means–end relations	1.4	3.0*
Total	9.9	15.9*
Kohen–Raz		
Eye–hand coordination	0.9	2.3*
Manipulation	0.9	2.3*
8 Months		
Bayley		
PDI	76.5	89.5*
Uzgiris–Hunt		
Object concept	5.6	10.2*
Gestural imitation	1.1	2.2*
Total	25.6	34.2*
12 Months		
Bayley		
PDI	73.6	86.3*
18 Months		
Uzgiris–Hunt		
Object concept	10.1	14.3†
Total	45.5	53.6*
Kohen–Raz		
Imitation–comprehension	7.7	9.0*
Vocalization–social	5.7	7.5*
2 Years		
Bayley		
MDI	86.9	98.1*
Kohen–Raz		
Imitation–comprehension	12.2	13.9*
Vocalization–social	10.5	11.5*
3 Years		
Reynell		
Expression	−0.8	−0.2*

*$p < .05$.
†$p < .01$.

are shown in Tables 14-15 and 14-16. As can be seen, the risk index was
reasonably successful at discriminating the delayed from the nondelayed
children.

Regression analyses and discriminant function analyses were con-

Table 14-14

Multiple Regression Results of the Risk Index Variables and the 5-Year Scores*

PPVT IQ

Full-Term		Preterm	
Socioeconomic status	.49	Socioeconomic status	
		Sex	
		Maternal education	.63

Beery VMI IQ

Maternal smoking	.27	Maternal smoking	
		Sex	.51

Finger Localization

Maternal smoking		Maternal smoking	
Sex		Sex	.64
Apgar—5 min	.53		
Maternal education			

Alphabet Recitation

Birth order		Gestational age	
Maternal smoking		Socioeconomic status	
Maternal education	.67	Severity of RDS	.61
Sex		Birth order	

Recognition Discrimination

Socioeconomic status		Gestational Age	.37
Previous spontaneous abortions	.53		
Birth order			

*Only variables which entered significantly into the regression are noted.

ducted with a combination of various infant test scores and the risk index variables. While the infant test scores were themselves significantly correlated with the outcome variables, they typically did not contribute much to the regression or discriminant function analysis variance. For example, the multiple regression for the full-term group using the Uzgiris–Hunt object relations at 12 months and socioeconomic status yielded a multiple correlation of .62. Similarly, the risk index variables and the object relations score at 12 months resulted in 87.9 and 84.4 percent correct predictions for the full-term and preterm groups, respectively.

DISCUSSION

On the bases of these data analyses it appears that preterm children are at subsequent risk for learning disabilities, and the infant test scores and a risk index can be used as predictors of these disabilities.

Table 14-15

Results of the Discriminant Function Analyses of the Risk Index and the Tests of the Satz Battery

	True Positive	False Positive	True Negative	False Negative	Overall Percentage of Prediction (%)
PPVT IQ					
Preterm					
Birth order	4	4	30	0	89.5
Socioeconomic status					
Sex					
Apgar—1 min					
Apnea					
Full-term					
Socioeconomic status	3	5	30	0	86.4
Maternal smoking					
Previous spontaneous abortions					
Birth order					
Beery VMI					
Preterm					
Birth asphyxia	15	4	19	6	77.3
Maternal smoking					
Birth weight					
CPAP					
Apnea					
Full-term					
Socioeconomic status	3	11	23	1	68.4
Maternal smoking					

Table 14-16

Discriminant Function Analyses of the Risk Index Variables and the Variables of the Satz Battery

	True Positive	False Positive	True Negative	False Negative	Overall Percentage of Prediction (%)
Finger Localization					
Preterm	2	3	24	1	86.7
Maternal smoking					
Sex					
Gestational age					
Maternal education					
Birth weight					
Full-term	3	6	28	0	83.8
Sex					
Maternal smoking					
Previous spontaneous abortions					
Socioeconomic status					
Apgar—5 min					
Alphabet Recitation					
Preterm	8	11	15	4	60.5
RDS					
Gestational age					
Sex					
Birth weight					
Apgar—5 min					
Full-term	3	3	33	1	90.0
Birth order					
Sex					
Maternal smoking					
Maternal education					
Recognition Discrimination					
Preterm	7	9	18	3	67.57
Socioeconomic status					
Apgar—1 min					
Full-term	3	2	32	0	95.6
Socioeconomic status					
Sex					
Birth order					
Apgar—5 min					

These results indicate significant continuities in development between infancy and early childhood. The underlying factor that may explain these continuities is that infant tests may be sensitive to the maturation of the nervous system at a particular point in time. A child who is delayed at one point in time is likely to be delayed at another point in time. For example, early in development, perceptual and motor functions such as the eye-hand coordination or manipulation items of the Bayley MDI or PDI are the best predictors of subsequent outcome, whether it is language (PPVT, alphabet recitation) or perceptual motor (recognition discrimination or Beery VMI score). The more cognitive items of the Bayley become predictive at 8 months, but it is not until 12 months that the language items become predictive.

Tests of early cognitive functioning as measured by the Uzgiris–Hunt test appear to be useful predictors of subsequent scores. These relations may be a result of the fact that score scales such as means–end thinking, space concepts, and object concepts are a reflection of the level of neurological maturation. In support of this supposition, the correlations between the infant tests and the Beery VMI, a measure of maturation of perceptual–motor functions, were the strongest. To the extent that the rate of development is relatively constant for an individual child, this would be reflected in the strong relations between infant and later behaviors.

While these correlations may be statistically significant, they do not account for a major proportion of the variance. However, when one considers the differences in the early test scores between the children who subsequently become delayed and those who do not, there are clear differences between the groups. Discriminant function analyses using a risk index are also able to detect many of the children who will subsequently become delayed, although the rate of false positives is frequently high. It should be noted that the environmental and demographic variables contributed more to the prediction of language functioning and delay, while the perinatal and reproductive variables contributed more to the prediction of perceptual–motor functions.

SUMMARY _____

Very low birth weight (under 1500 g) preterm children were found to perform significantly differently from a demographically matched group of full-term children on perceptual–motor tests at 5 years. The variables associated with prematurity appear to be associated with specific impairments of perceptual–motor functioning in childhood. There were no significant differences between the groups on language comprehension.

15

Five-Year Follow-up of Preterm Respiratory Distress Syndrome and Post-Term Postmaturity Syndrome Infants

Tiffany Field
Jean Dempsey, H. H. Shuman

Shortened or prolonged gestations per se are not necessarily risk factors if the maternal, fetal, and placental systems have been functioning optimally and if the neonate does not experience perinatal or postnatal complications (DiVitto & Goldberg, 1979; Sostek, Quinn, & Davitt, 1979). Unfortunately, a nonterm delivery is often symptomatic of dysfunction in these systems, and the infant is thus vulnerable to complications, particularly respiratory complications.

A preterm infant who develops respiratory distress is considered medically at risk, even though recent technological advances have drastically reduced the mortality and morbidity rates. The developmental progress reported for these infants has varied according to a number of factors, including gestational age, birth weight, severity of the respiratory distress syndrome (RDS), the type of treatment, and the time of the study. Earlier studies suggest that the higher birth weight survivors of *less severe* RDS experienced early developmental delays but had normal IQ scores at age 4 (Ambrus, Weintraub, Niswander, Fischer, Fleishman, Bross, & Ambrus,

We would like to thank the mothers and infants who participated in this study. For assistance with data collection, additional thanks go to Catherine Benson, Cyrus Dabiri, Norma Hallock, Judith Hatch, Sally Leeds, Catherine Larned, and George Ting. This study was supported in part by grants from the Public Health Department of Massachusetts and the March of Dimes National Foundation. An earlier version of this paper was presented at the American Psychological Association Meeting, Los Angeles, California, August 1981.

1970; Fisch, Bilek, Miller, & Engel, 1975). Recent survivors of *more severe* RDS requiring mechanical ventilation have been reported to experience a higher incidence of neurological and developmental problems (Harrod, L'Heureaux, Wangensteen, & Hunt, 1974; Johnson, Malachowski, Grobstein, Daily, & Sunshine, 1974; Outerbridge & Stern, 1972; Stahlman, Hedwall, Dolanski, Foxelius, Burko, & Kirk, 1973).

Infants born after a prolonged pregnancy have often experienced nutritional deficiency and fetal distress due to placental insufficiency. Although infants with symptoms of Clifford's (1954) stage 1 postmaturity syndrome are not considered medically at risk, they may experience developmental delays associated with this subtle perinatal insult. Developmental outcomes reported for the post-term postmaturity syndrome infant range from no problems to delayed social development (Lovell, 1973), severe illness, and sleep disturbances (Zwerdling, 1967), reading disabilities (Butler & Alberman, 1969), neurological handicaps (Wagner & Arndt, 1968), and cerebral palsy (Drillien, 1968).

The variability of outcomes reported for both of these nonterm groups suggests the importance of examining closely their developmental course. The purpose of the present study was to review the first 5 years of the development of these two groups of nonterm infants and a group of healthy term infants. In addition to comparing the developmental course of these infants, multivariate regression analyses were conducted to determine whether any of our measures were predictive of developmental delays. Because the first 2 years of data for this longitudinal study have been described elsewhere (Field, Dempsey, & Shuman, 1979; Field, Dempsey, & Shuman, 1981; Field, Hallock, Ting, Dempsey, Dabiri, & Shuman, 1978), they will be briefly summarized here, and greater consideration will be given to the 3 to 5-year outcome data.

METHODS AND RESULTS

The subjects were 194 infants born during the period of February 1975 to April 1977. The preterm RDS group, which consisted of 56 infants (27 females, 29 males), averaged 1600 g in birth weight and 32 weeks gestation, and experienced 3 days mechanical ventilation (minimum of 12 hours) and 32 days of intensive care. The 57 post-term postmaturity syndrome infants (32 females, 25 males), averaged 3600 g in birth weight, 42 weeks gestation, and had a mean of two postmaturity symptoms (for example, meconium staining, long fingernails, parchmentlike skin, a long thin body, and a wizened look). The healthy term group was comprised of 81 infants (42 females, 39 males), who averaged 3300 g in birth weight and 40 weeks gestation. The infants were born to white, middle-income, high-school-educated mothers who averaged 25 years of age. Most of the infants were later born.

Several assessments were made at 4-month intervals during the first year of life and at 1-year intervals thereafter through the age of 5 years. A variety of different measures were selected in an attempt to describe the early behavioral, social, mental, and motor development of these infants. All assessment dates were calculated from the mother's expected date of delivery rather than the infant's real birthdate as an adjustment for differences between groups on gestational age. Multivariate and univariate analyses of variance were performed, the multivariate analyses to determine whether the group of variables measured at each assessment period yielded significant differences and the univariate analyses to examine individual variables. In order that the error rate per comparison might conform to an experiment-wise error rate of .05, a fairly conservative level of significance was adopted. Findings are reported only if the probability that they resulted by chance is less than .001.

Perinatal Assessments _____

In addition to the traditional measures of gestational age, birth measurements, and Apgar scores, we included Littman and Parmelee's Obstetric and Postnatal Complications Scales (OCS) (Littman & Parmelee, 1978) and the Brazelton Neonatal Behavior Assessment Scale (Brazelton, 1973). All infants were tested with the Brazelton just prior to discharge from the hospital (average age of term and post-term infants was 2 days and the preterm RDS infants averaged 5 weeks of age). Although this age range itself might account for differences between the groups, we did not want to assess the preterm RDS infants until they were medically stable, and we felt it was important to assess the infants as they might present themselves to their parents upon discharge.

Table 15-1 summarizes the significant group differences on the perinatal assessments. As evidenced by their lower, less optimal scores on the OCS, both nonterm groups experienced obstetric complications. Pregnancy problems common to both groups included hypertension, toxemia, and bleeding. As expected, the birth measurements and Apgar scores were lower for the preterm RDS group.

Both nonterm groups received inferior Brazelton interactive and motoric process scores, but for different reasons. The RDS babies were typically floppy, hypotonic, difficult to arouse and alert, and had weak reflexes and flat affect. Conversely, the postmature newborns tended to be very active, hyperirritable, extremely labile, hypertonic, and difficult to console. Similarly, on the Mother's Assessment of the Behavior of Her Infant (Field, Dempsey, Hallock, & Shuman, 1978), an adaptation of the Brazelton for mothers' administration, the nonterm infants were assigned lower scores than term infants on both the interactive and motoric process dimensions. The mothers' scores were comparable to the testers', except on

Table 15-1

Means for Perinatal Assessments Which Yielded Significant Group
Differences at $p < .001$

Variables	Preterm RDS	Normal Term	Post-Term Postmature
Obstetric complications scale	78	117	102
Birth measurements			
Weight (grams)	1597	3338	3581
Length (cm)	41	54	58
Head circumferences (cm)	28	34	
5-min Apgar	7	9	
Brazelton interactive process†	2.30	1.70	2.21
Brazelton motoric process†	2.63	1.88	2.25
Postnatal complications scale	71	152	

*Scores are not given when comparisons are not significant.
†Lower scores are optimal.

the interactive process dimension, where the mothers tended to assign less optimal scores. Although the Brazelton testers may have been more successful than the mothers in maintaining alertness and responsiveness to stimulation, it is interesting to note that the mothers' ratings were accurate and objective, even when the infants were considered "difficult" and fragile and when contact with their infants during hospitalization had been limited.

Postnatal complications of the RDS group, particularly hyperbilirubinemia and respiratory and metabolic disturbances, were relatively severe, resulting in significantly less optimal scores on the Postnatal Complications Scale. Although the postmatures may have experienced some perinatal anoxia related to placental deterioration, their postnatal complication scale scores did not significantly differ from those of the term group.

Four-Month Assessments

When the infants were 4 months corrected age, they were seen at the hospital for a pediatric examination, the Denver Developmental Screening Test (Frankenburg & Dodds, 1967), and an assessment of mother–infant interaction during feeding and playing (Field, 1980). The mothers were also asked to describe their infant's temperament on the Carey Temperament Questionnaire (Carey, 1970), which includes ratings of activity, regularity of feeding and sleeping, adaptability, intensity, threshold, distractability, persistence, and mood.

As can be seen in Table 15-2, the 4-month weight measures were significantly lower for the RDS and higher for the post-term infants. Both

Table 15-2
Means for 4-Month Assessments Which Yielded Significant Group
Differences at $p < .001$

Variable	Preterm RDS	Normal Term	Post-Term Postmature
Weight (grams)	5872	6428	6603
Denver developmental*	1.83	1.14	1.52
Carey temperament*	2.89	1.83	2.66
Interaction ratings*			
Face to face	2.20	1.71	2.28
Feeding	2.38	1.45	

*Lower scores are optimal.

nonterm groups received inferior ratings on the Denver (the postmatures scoring lower on personal–social items, while the RDS infants scored lower on personal–social as well as fine and gross motor items). This pattern of scores is consistent with their newborn performance on the Brazelton Scale, the postmatures having been particularly weak on the Brazelton interactive process items and the RDS infants weak on both the Brazelton interactive and motor items. The Carey scores indicate that both groups of nonterm infants were viewed by their mothers as having "difficult" temperaments and being particularly difficult to console. Further evidence for the difficult temperaments of the nonterm infants was suggested by their excessive fussiness, restlessness, and gaze aversion during filmed face-to-face interactions with their mothers. The mothers of RDS and post-term infants were more active than mothers of term infants in their attempts to elicit attention and responses from their infants. They were also less imitative and less attentive to their infant's interaction signals. Difficult interactions also occurred during feedings, yielding less optimal ratings on the feeding interactions for the preterm infants and their mothers. Whereas mothers of preterm infants tended to stimulate their infants only when they were not sucking, mothers of preterm infants engaged in almost continuous "coaxing to feed" behaviors.

Eight-Month Assessments

The 8-month assessments, which were conducted in the infants' homes, included the Bayley Scales of Infant Development (Bayley, 1969), the Carey Questionnaire, and the Caldwell Home Stimulation Inventory (Caldwell, Heider, & Kaplan, 1966). As a measure of test taking behaviors, the Bayley Infant Behavior Record was also analyzed using Matheny's (Matheny, Dolan, & Wilson, 1974) clusters of intercorrelated items: The Primary Cognition Composite Score, which is the sum of ratings on object orientation, goal directedness, attention span, reactivity, and gross and fine motor coordination; and the Extraversion Composite Score, which includes the ratings on social orientation to the examiner, cooperation, and emotional tone.

Table 15-3 summarizes the significant differences at 8 months. The continuing motor deficit of the RDS infants was evident not only in their delayed motor scores, but also in the lower mental scores. The RDS infants appeared to have the requisite cognitive abilities (e.g., object permanence), but not the coordination and fine motor skills needed to pass many of the mental items.

The postmatures also scored lower than the term infants on the Bayley mental subscale. Short attention span and restlessness, which were noted as problems on their behavior records, may have contributed to these low scores. Although the groups did not differ on the Extraversion Composite Score (social orientation, cooperation, emotional tone), the preterm infants did score significantly lower on the Primary Cognition Composite Score (object orientation, goal directedness, attention span, reactivity, and gross motor and fine motor coordination). The Carey scores indicate that the mothers again rated their nonterm infants as having difficult temperaments, suggesting some stability of infant temperament and/or stability of the mothers' assessment of temperament during early infancy (Field, Dempsey, Hallock, & Shuman, 1978; Sostek & Anders, 1977). Despite the consistent mental, motor, and behavioral differences between term and nonterm infants, their home environments (as assessed by the Caldwell Scale) did not differ. Although this may indicate that the parents were not treating their nonterm infants differently and were sensitive to the importance of developmentally appropriate toys and experiences, the inventory of home stimulation may simply be less sensitive to the differences within a homogeneous socioeconomic group. That is, it may be a better discriminator of environments across rather than within socioeconomic groups.

Table 15-3

Means for 8-Month Assessments Which Yielded Significant Group Differences at $p < .001$

Variable	Preterm RDS	Normal Term	Post-term Postmature
Bayley mental	88	104	82
Bayley motor	77	106	
Bayley behavior record			
Primary cognition composite score	25.40	28.88	
Carey temperament*	2.72	1.57	2.48

*Lower scores are optimal.

One-Year Assessments

At 1 year of age the infants were seen at the hospital for developmental and physical examinations. Littman and Parmelee's (1978) Pediatric Complications Scale, which notes the presence of medical problems such as abnormal rates of growth, occurrences of illness, injury or hospitalization, and physical and neurological problems, was used to quantify our pediatrician's findings. In addition, the Ainsworth Strange Situation Procedure was conducted (Ainsworth & Witting, 1969).

As can be seen in Table 15-4, the preterm RDS infants averaged lower weights and lengths and the postmatures greater head circumference measurements than the term infants at 1 year. The scores on the Pediatric Complications Scale indicate that the preterm RDS infants had the greatest number of complications in their first year of life, while the term infants had the fewest. No differences were noted between groups on the Ainsworth Strange Situation Procedure. The 1-year Bayley scores for the nonterm groups are similar to the 8-month findings; that is, the postmatures tended to score lower on the mental scale, whereas the preterm RDS infants received significantly lower mental, motor, and Primary Cognition Composite Scores.

Two-Year Assessments

In addition to the measures used at 1 year, the 2-year assessments included Quay and Peterson's (1975) Behavior Problem Checklist, the Vineland Social Maturity Scale (Doll, 1965), and an analysis of mother-infant verbal interaction during a 10-min free play situation (Field, Dempsey, & Shuman, 1981).

Table 15-4

Means for 1-Year Assessments Which Yielded Significant Group Differences at $p < .001$

Variable	Preterm RDS	Normal Term	Post-Term Postmature
Weight (grams)	9,280	10,208	
Length (cm)	73	77	
Head circumference (cm)		46	47
Pediatric complications scale	91	118	
Bayley mental	90	110	86
Bayley motor	80	105	
Bayley behavioral			
Primary cognition composite score	28.69	32.00	

Table 15-5

Means for 2-Year Assessments Which Yielded Significant Group
Differences at $p < .001$

Variable	Preterm RDS	Normal Term	Post-Term Postmature
Weight (grams)	11,413	12,231	12,987
Length (cm)		86	89
Head circumference (cm)		48	51
Pediatric complications scale	99	123	
Bayley mental	95	118	104
Bayley motor	92	115	102
Bayley behavior record			
Primary cognition composite score	30.07	35.51	
Vineland Social Maturity Scale	110	123	
Behavior problem checklist*	31	26	
Language ratings			
Mother's Imperatives	20	17	
Questions	55	48	
Statements	25	32	
Infant's Verbosity	82	155	
Working vocabulary	30	54	
MLU	1.3	1.8	

*Lower scores are optimal.

The significant group differences at age 2 are summarized in Table
15-5. The RDS infants continued to weigh less than the term infants. The
postmatures weighed more, were longer, and had larger head circumference
measurements than the term infants. Pediatric complications in the second
year of life were again greater for the preterm group. Both nonterm groups
received lower Bayley mental and motor scores and the preterm RDS infants continued to score lower on the Primary Cognition Composite Score.
The RDS infants received lower social quotients on the Vineland than the
term infants, though their scores were within normal limits for that scale.
On the Behavior Problem Checklist, mothers in the preterm RDS group
rated their infants as having significantly more problems (especially
restlessness, irritability, and short attention span). The language recordings
of free play between mothers and infants revealed the following differences:
the mothers of the preterm infants used fewer statements and more imperatives and questions in their conversations. The preterm infants were less
verbose, had a smaller working vocabulary, and a shorter mean length of
utterance. An inverse relation was noted for mother's imperatives and the
infant's mean length of utterance (MLU) and vocabulary score.

Three- to Five-Year Assessments _____

For the 3-, 4-, and 5-year follow-up assessments, we continued to use the Quay and Peterson Behavior Problem Checklist, the Vineland Social Maturity Scale, and an analysis of mother–child verbal interaction during a 10-min free play situation. These scales had differentiated the groups at 2 years, and we wondered if those differences would persist. In addition, we administered the McCarthy Scales at these periods. These were used instead of the more popular Stanford-Binet Scale, because in previous samples the Stanford-Binet had failed to differentiate children who had experienced RDS, suggesting either no differences by age 4 or an insensitive instrument. In addition, the McCarthy Scales have more interesting items for children, cover a broader range of skills, and yield subscale scores for verbal, perceptual, quantitative, memory, and motor skills. They are also considered more continuous than other preschool scales with the Bayley Scales of Infant Development (Kaufman & Kaufman, 1977).

At 3 years the RDS children were of lower weight than the term children, and of lower mental age (although the mental ages of both groups are greater than the chronological age of 36 months). In addition, the RDS children exhibited more behavior problems according to the questionnaires completed by their mothers (Table 15-6). On the McCarthy Scales the children of both the RDS and postmature groups received less optimal verbal, quantitative, and general cognitive scores (which is a summary of the verbal and quantitative scale scores). The RDS group also received inferior McCarthy motor scores (Table 15-6). All of these scores are percentile scores. As can be seen in Table 15-6, the language records of the free play sessions revealed a greater number of imperatives used by the mothers of RDS and postmature children. The RDS children had a shorter mean length of utterance and a smaller vocabulary and were less verbose.

At 4 years the data look very much the same, with a weight and a height difference for the RDS group and inferior mental age, Vineland social, and behavior problem scores (Table 15-6). Again, it is noteworthy that the mental ages of all infants are slightly above their chronological age. The particular scales on which the RDS and normal groups differ are, again, the verbal, quantitative, general cognitive, and motor scales. The postmature group differed from the normal only on the verbal and general cognitive scales (Table 15-6). Again, at 4 years the RDS children had inferior language production measures, as did the postmature children, although the mean length of utterance of the postmature group did not differ from that of the normal term group (Table 15-6). The mothers of the RDS children emitted more imperatives and more questions.

At 5 years the results are consistent with those at 4 years. The RDS group are of lower weight and lower mental age than the normal group

Table 15-6
3-, 4-, and 5-Year Assessments

Variable	Group Means		
	Preterm RDS	Term Normal	Post-Term Postmature
3 Year			
Height	95	95	96
Weight	13,257*	14,057	14,102
Head circumference	49	49	50
Mental age	37*	42	40
Behavior problem score	60*	18	28
Number of behavior problems	9	6	8
McCarthy Scale %			
Verbal	62*	75	62*
Perceptual-performance	63	68	65
Quantitative	40*	78	58*
General cognitive	59*	76	64*
Memory	66	73	70
Motor	50*	68	66
Language records			
Mother Statements	35	34	40
Questions	51	45	51
Imperatives	21*	9	14*
Child Statements	80	83	84
Questions	13	11	10
Imperatives	7	7	6
Mean length utterance	2.2*	2.8	2.4
Verbosity	271*	349	289*
Working vocabulary	121*	141	130
4 Year			
Height	96*	102	103
Weight	15,516*	15,942	16,662*
Head circumference	51	51	51
Mental age	50*	56	54
Vineland SQ	116*	133	125*
Behavior problem score	33*	17	27*
Number of behavior problems	16*	6	11*
McCarthy Scale %			
Verbal	68*	82	70*
Perceptual-performance	67	72	68
Quantitative	63*	76	71
General cognitive	76*	88	76*

Variable		Preterm RDS	Term Normal	Post-Term Postmature
		4 Year (continued)		
Memory		69	75	70
Motor		56*	70	68
Language records				
Mother	Statements	37	41	44
	Questions	60*	42	49
	Imperatives	31*	12	18
Child	Statements	58	59	64
	Questions	13	15	14
	Imperatives	11	9	13
	Mean length utterance	2.4*	3.1	2.7
	Verbosity	289*	357	301*
	Working vocabulary	130*	163	144*
		5 Year		
Height		109	110	114
Weight		17,358*	18,217	18,730
Head circumference		51	51	51
Mental age		66*	71	69
McCarthy Scale %				
Verbal		74*	84	83
Perceptual		66*	85	68*
Quantitative		63*	75	70
General cognitive		70*	85	77*
Memory		75	80	76
Motor		53*	73	65
Behavior Problem Scale		24*	9	10
Vineland Social Scale		63	68	67
Sociability		20	23	18
Emotionality		13	10	20
Activity		19*	13	20*
Attention span		17*	24	19
Reaction to food		13	11	13
Soothability		18*	10	20*

*Group differences significant at $p < .001$.

(Table 15-6). However, note that their mental age is 66 months, or 5½ years. Despite their falling within the normal range, they continue to lag behind the normal group by 5 months, and although their mean McCarthy scores are above the 50th percentile, they are significantly lower than the normal group on all subscales but memory (Table 15-6). As can seen in

Table 15-6, they still have more behavioral problems according to their mothers. Also, at this stage we asked mothers to assess their infants' temperament on the Colorado Childhood Temperament Inventory. The mothers of the children in the RDS and postmature groups rated their children as more active, but more soothable. The children of the RDS group were also considered by their mothers to have a shorter attention span.

Finally, we conducted a series of stepwise regression analyses to answer two questions: (1) which variables were significant predictors of mental and motor development measured yearly during the 5-year period, and (2) how much of the variance in performance on the developmental scales could be explained by performance on earlier measures. The stepwise regression analyses were performed in a cumulative fashion; first-year measures were entered in the analyses on 1-year Bayley mental and motor scores, first- and second-year measures on the 2-year Bayley scores, and first-, second-, and third-year measures on the McCarthy Cognitive Index and Motor Scale scores. The 5-year analysis included a composite of all measures. These analyses were not conducted separately for each of the three groups because of insufficient sample sizes relative to the number of variables entered.

As can be seen in Table 15-7, the 8-month Bayley motor scale score explained 42 percent of the variance on the 1-year Bayley mental scale with the 8-month Bayley mental scale score and the 4-month Denver Developmental scale score, adding a minimal but significant amount for a total of 49 percent of the outcome variance. While it is surprising that the 8-month Bayley motor score contributed to a significantly greater proportion of the variance on the 1-year Bayley mental scale than did the 8-month Bayley mental scale performance, many of the 1-year Bayley mental scale items require motor skills for their successful completion. For example, several of the motorically delayed RDS infants appeared to have mastered the object permanence task judging from visual search behavior, but were unable to complete the task because of limited motor control. The 8-month Bayley motor scale score also contributed to most of the variance (61%) on the 1-year Bayley motor scale, with gestational age and 4-month Denver scores contributing an additional 4 percent.

As can be seen in Table 15-7, similar amounts of the Bayley mental scale variance at 1 and 2 years were accounted for by our measures (49 and 41 percent, respectively). However, a much lower proportion of the 2-year than the 1-year Bayley motor scale variance was accounted for by our measures (28 percent versus 65 percent). The order in which the measures entered the analysis on 2-year Bayley mental scale scores was 8-month Bayley motor scale, sex, 1-year Bayley motor scale, 4-month mother interaction rating, and the Obstetric Complications Scale score. Thus, for the 2-year Bayley mental score, as for the 1-year Bayley mental score, the 8-month Bayley motor scale score continued to be the most efficient predictor. The first appearance at 2 years of the Obstetric Complications Scale

Table 15-7

One- and Two-Year Bayley Mental and Motor

Variable	R	R^2
1 Year		
Bayley Mental		
Bayley motor		
8 months	.64	.42
Bayley mental		
8 months	.69	.48
Denver developmental		
4 months	.70	.49
Bayley Motor		
Bayley motor		
8 months	.78	.61
Gestational age	.79	.63
Denver developmental		
4 months	.81	.65
2 Year		
Bayley Mental		
Bayley motor		
8 months	.55	.30
Sex	.58	.34
Bayley motor		
1 year	.60	.36
Mother interaction rating		
4 months	.62	.39
Obstetric complication scale	.64	.41
Bayley Motor		
Bayley motor		
1 year	.42	.17
Diagnostic group	.47	.22
Weight		
4 months	.51	.26
Gestational age	.53	.28

score and the 4-month mother interaction rating is difficult to interpret except as having "sleeper" or transactional effects, suggesting the need for a more complex form of regression analysis such as path analysis or structural equations analysis. On the 2-year Bayley motor scale regression the 1-year Bayley motor scale contributed to the largest proportion of the variance, with significant increments contributed by the diagnostic category of the infants, 4-month weight, and gestational age variables.

Table 15-8 suggests that at 3 years similar amounts of the variance were accounted for, as had been accounted for at 2 years by our earlier measures.

Table 15-8

Three-, Four-, and Five-Year McCarthy Cognitive Index and Motor Score

Variable	R	R^2
3 Year		
McCarthy Cognitive Index		
Bayley Mental		
2 years	.63	.40
McCarthy Motor Score		
Bayley Mental: 2 years	.49	.24
Weight: 4 months	.54	.29
Infant interaction rating: 4 months	.58	.33
4 Year		
McCarthy Cognitive Index		
Bayley Mental 2 years	.53	.28
MLU 2 years	.75	.56
Bayley motor 8 months	.79	.63
Maternal education	.82	.67
MLU 3 years	.85	.72
McCarthy Motor Score		
Bayley mental 2 years	.37	.13
Mother interaction rating—1 year	.60	.36
Maternal education (number of years)	.68	.46
MLU 3 years	.75	.56
5 Year		
McCarthy Cognitive Index		
McCarthy cognitive index	.69	.48
MLU 3 years	.72	.52
Brazelton interactive process rating	.75	.56
McCarthy Motor Score		
McCarthy motor score 4 years	.69	.48
Bayley motor score 8 months	.73	.53
Birthweight	.77	.59
Postnatal complications scale	.79	.62
Infant interaction rating—4 months	.81	.66
Maternal education	.83	.69

The 2-year Bayley mental scale score explained most of the variance on both the 3-year McCarthy Cognitive Index and the 3-year McCarthy motor scale score. On the motor scale, the 2-year Bayley mental scale, 4-month weight, and 4-month infant interaction ratings also accounted for significant proportions of the variance.

While 8-month Bayley motor scale scores appeared to be the most efficient predictor of both 1- and 2-year mental and motor scale performance on the Bayley, it appears that the 2-year Bayley mental scale performance is the most efficient predictor of both 3- and 4-year mental and motor scale performance on the McCarthy Scales. Item analyses of the Bayley 8-month motor composite and 2-year mental composite might reveal the more specific skills which contribute to the predictive validity of their more global scores. If the 8-month Bayley motor scale and the 2-year Bayley mental scale appear to have similar predictive validity values in other samples, those two measures may be the most cost-effective assessments during the first 4 years of development, and their component skills might be the most cost-effective intervention exercises.

Surprisingly, at 4 years the 2-year Bayley mental scale again was the first variable to enter both the McCarthy cognitive and motor scale regression analyses (see Table 15-8). The 3-year McCarthy Scale scores would be expected to explain more of the variance by virtue of their being the same scale as the outcome measures and being administered closer in time to the outcome measure (1 year instead of 2 years prior to the 4-year outcome measure). It is also surprising that the variance explained by our measures increases considerably from the 3-year to the 4-year McCarthy Scale scores, that is, 72 percent at 4 years versus 40 percent at 3 in the case of the McCarthy Cognitive Scale and 56 versus 33 percent years in the case of the McCarthy Motor Scale. Unlike the previous regression analyses results, a relatively small proportion of the variance was explained by the first variables to enter the equations, with each of the subsequent variables entered adding a considerable amount to the total variance. For example, the 2-year Bayley mental scale score contributed 28 percent of the variance in 4-year McCarthy cognitive scores and the step 2 variable, 2-year mean length of utterance, added another 28 percent to the variance. This was followed by the 8-month Bayley motor scale entering at step 3, maternal education at step 4, and 3-year mean length of utterance at step 5. Similar variables, mother interaction ratings at 1 year, maternal education, and 3-year mean length of utterance, also entered the analysis on the McCarthy Motor Scale. Thus maternal education variables and child language variables first emerge as significant predictors of performance measures at 4 years, a finding that is consistent with other longitudinal data (Broman, Nichols, & Kennedy, 1975) and which suggests again the transactional nature of these measures (Sameroff & Chandler, 1975).

Finally, at 5 years (see Table 15-8) more than half of the variance was accounted for by our earlier measures (56% of the variance on the McCarthy cognitive index and 69% on the McCarthy Motor Scale). For this period, the 4-year McCarthy cognitive index contributed to the most variance on the 5-year McCarthy cognitive index and the 4-year McCarthy Motor Scale contributed to most of the variance on the 5-year McCarthy Motor Scale. Other measures which significantly contributed to the variance on the 5-year McCarthy cognitive index were the 3-year mean length of utterance and the Brazelton interactive process rating. On the 5-year McCarthy Motor Scale, additional variance was explained by the 8-month Bayley Motor Scale, birth weight, the Postnatal Complications Scale Score, 4-month infant interaction ratings, and maternal education, again suggesting the "sleeper" effects of some of our earlier measures.

DISCUSSION

Those variables which most frequently entered the stepwise regression analyses were the 8-month Bayley motor scale score, the 2-year Bayley mental scale score, the 4-month mother-infant interaction ratings, and years of maternal education. That the 8-month Bayley motor and 2-year Bayley mental scale scores were predictive of 4-year cognitive performance is inconsistent with several longitudinal studies which failed to show a relation between infant developmental assessments and later IQ scores. This inconsistency might be explained by the greater correspondence between Bayley and McCarthy scale items than between Bayley and the traditionally used Stanford Binet Scale items. The predictive validity of the early mother–infant interaction ratings is consistent with other longitudinal data (Sigman & Parmelee, 1981) as is the predictive validity of maternal education (Broman et al., 1975; Sameroff & Chandler, 1975). Thus to predict school entry performance in samples varying in risk status, these early measures might be the most efficient. Path analysis or structural equations may reveal the specific paths by which these early measures relate to later performance.

Using various assessment scales throughout the first 5 years of life, we were thus able to identify consistent differences between term and nonterm infants in the areas of physical, mental, motor, social, language, and behavioral development. The most critical intervention needs identified by our follow-up include the motor delays of the preterm infants and the social interaction problems experienced by both nonterm groups.

The mild but persistent developmental delays shown by our preterm infants are difficult to interpret. RDS may exacerbate the effects of prematurity or gestational age adjustments may not compensate for differences between preterm and term groups. Because we did not include a preterm-without-RDS control group, it is not possible to determine the degree to which RDS contributed to these effects.

Although the nonterm infants continued to score lower than the term group on the McCarthy Scales, it is important to note that their scores improved from year to year and were within the normal range on these scales by 2 years. These "normal" scores of the RDS survivors make a positive prediction for their cognitive development. However, their language production delays and problems with hyperactivity, distractability, and short attention span indicate that they remain at risk for learning disabilities. Our findings suggest that assessments of children with a history of prematurity and RDS should include traditional developmental and IQ tests, as well as specialized assessments which are more sensitive to these minimal deficits.

Just as the neonatal problems of the postmature are more subtle than those of the preterm RDS group, an interpretation of their developmental delays is more complex. It is not clear whether prenatal stress, large birth size, some form of anoxia, or other factors contributed to these delays. Nonetheless, their delayed mental and social skills suggest that despite the absence of postnatal complications, the effects of the postterm postmaturity syndrome are not confined to the perinatal period and the development of these infants should be closely monitored. Being born not at term is not necessarily a risk factor, but when compounded by syndromes such as respiratory distress or postmaturity, the risk for developmental delays appears to be more pronounced.

REFERENCES

Ainsworth, M., & Wittig, B. Attachment and exploratory behavior of one-year-olds in a strange situation. In B. M. Foss (Ed.), *Determinants of infant behavior.* London: Methuen, 1969.

Ambrus, C., Weintraub, D., Niswander, K., Fischer, L., Fleishman, J., Bross, L., & Ambrus, J. Evaluation of survivors of the respiratory distress syndrome. *Journal of Pediatrics*, 1970, *120*, 296–302.

Bayley, N. *Manual for the Bayley Scales of Infant Development.* New York: Psychological Corporation, 1969.

Brazelton, T. B. *Neonatal Behavioral Assessment Scale.* London: Spastics International, 1973.

Broman, S. H., Nichols, P.L. & Kennedy, W. A. *Preschool IQ: Prenatal and early developmental correlates.* Hillsdale, N.J.: Lawrence Erlbaum Associates, 1975.

Butler, N. R., & Alberman, E. D. *Perinatal problems: The second report of 1958 British perinatal mortality survey.* London: Livingston, 1969.

Caldwell, B. M., Heider, J., & Kaplan, B. *The inventory of home stimulation.* Paper presented at the meeting of the American Psychological Association, New

York, September 1966. (Available from Center for Early Development and Education, 814 Sherman, Little Rock, Arkansas 72202)

Carey, W. B. A simplified method of measuring infant temperament. *Journal of Pediatrics*, 1970, *77*, 188–194.

Clifford, S. H. Postmaturity with placental dysfunction: Clinical syndrome and pathological findings. *Journal of Pediatrics*, 1954, *44*, 1–13.

DiVitto, B., & Goldberg, S. The effects of newborn medical status on early parent-infant interaction. In T. Field, A. Sostek, S. Goldberg, & H. H. Shuman. (Eds.), *Infants born at risk.* New York: Spectrum, 1979.

Doll, E. A. *Vineland Social Maturity Scale.* Minnesota: American Guidance Service, 1965.

Drillien, C. M. Studies in mental handicap, II: Some obstetric factors of possible actiological significance. *Archives of Disease in Childhood*, 1968, *43*, 283–288.

Field, T. Interactions of preterm and term infants with their lower- and middle-class teenage and adult mothers. In T. Field, S. Goldberg, D. Stern, & A. Sostek (Eds.), *High-risk infants and children: Adult and peer interactions.* New York: Academic, 1980.

Field, T., Dempsey, J., Hallock, N., & Shuman, H. H. The mother's assessment of the behavior of her infant. *Infant Behavior and Development*, 1978, *1*, 156–167.

Field, T., Dempsey, J., & Shuman, H. H. Developmental assessments of infants surviving the respiratory distress syndrome. In T. Field, A. Sostek, S. Goldberg, & H. H. Shuman (Eds.), *Infants born at risk.* New York: Spectrum, 1979.

Field, T., Dempsey, J., & Shuman, H. H. Developmental follow-up of pre- and post-term infants. In S. Friedman & M. Sigman (Eds.), *Preterm birth and psychological development.* New York: Academic, 1981.

Field, T., Hallock, N., Ting, G., Dempsey, J., Dabiri, C., & Shuman, H. H. A first year follow-up of high-risk infants: Formulating a cumulative risk index. *Child Development*, 1978, *49*, 119–131.

Fisch, R., Bilek, M., Miller, L., & Engel, R. Physical and mental status at 4 years of age of survivors of the respiratory distress syndrome. *Journal of Pediatrics*, 1975, *86*, 497–503.

Frankenburg, W. K., & Dodds, J. B. The Denver Developmental Screening Test, *Journal of Pediatrics*, 1967, *71*, 181–191.

Harrod, J. R., L'Heureaux, P., Wangensteen, D. O., & Hunt, C. D. Long-term follow-up of severe respiratory distress syndrome treated with IPPV. *Journal of Pediatrics*, 1974, *84*, 277.

Johnson, J. D., Malachowski, N. C., Grobstein, R., Daily, W. J. R., & Sunshine, P. Prognosis of children surviving with the aid of mechanical ventilation in the newborn period. *Journal of Pediatrics*, 1974, *84*, 272.

Kaufman, A., & Kaufman, N. *Clinical evaluation of young children with the McCarthy scales.* New York: Grune & Stratton, 1977.

Littman, D., & Parmelee, A. Medical correlates of infant development. *Pediatrics*, 1978, *61*, 470–474.

Lovell, K. E. The effect of postmaturity on the developing child. *Medical Journal of Australia*, 1973, *1*, 13–17.

Matheny, A. P., Dolan, A. B., & Wilson, R. S. Bayley's Infant Behavior Record:

Relations between behaviors and mental test scores. *Developmental Psychology*, 1974, *10*, 697–702.

Outerbridge, E. W., & Stern, L. Developmental follow-up of artifically ventilated infants with neonatal respiratory failure. *Pediatric Research*, 1972, *6*, 412.

Quay, H., & Peterson, D. W. *Manual for the behavior problem checklist.* Unpublished manuscript, 1975.

Sameroff, A. J., & Chandler, M. J. Reproductive risk and the continuum of caretaking casualty. In F. D. Horowitz, E. Mavis Hetherington, S. Scarr-Salatpatek,   G. M. Siegel (Eds.), *Review of child development research*. Chicago: University of Chicago Press, 1975.

Sostek, A. M., & Anders, T. F. Relationships among the Brazelton Neonatal Scale, Bayley Infant Scales, and early temperament. *Child Development*, 1977, *48*, 320–323.

Sostek, A., Quinn, P., & Davitt, M. K. Behavior, development and neurologic status of premature and full-term infants with varying medical complications. In T. Field, S. Sostek, S. Goldberg, & H. H. Shuman (Eds.), *Infants born at risk*. New York: Spectrum, 1979.

Stahlman, M., Hedwall, G., Dolanski, E., Foxelius, G., Burko, H., & Kirk, V. A six-year follow-up of clinical hyaline membrane disease. *Pediatric Clinics of North America*, 1973, *20*, 433.

Wagner, M. G., & Arndt, R. Postmaturity as an aetiological factor in 124 cases of of neurologically handicapped children. In *Studies in infancy*. London: Heinemann, 1968.

Zwerdling, M. A. Factors pertaining to prolonged pregnancy and its outcome. *Pediatrics*, 1967, *40*, 202–212.

Index

a
b
3 c
4 d
5 e
6 f
7 g
8 h
9 i
8 0 j